"*Eliminating Race-Based Mental Health Disparities* does an excellent job of addressing the impacts of racism on the mental health of people-of-color communities. The editors did an excellent job of speaking to the need for self-reflection, cultural humility, and interrogating one's privilege in the context of mental health care. I would highly recommend this book as a primer for all clinicians, researchers, and trainees in the social sciences."

—**Sand Chang, PhD**, (they/them), Chinese American nonbinary psychologist, educator, and advocate based in Oakland, CA; and coauthor of *A Clinician's Guide to Gender-Affirming Care*

"*Eliminating Race-Based Mental Health Disparities* provides an extensive, much-needed exploration of intrapersonal, interpersonal, institutional, and structural sources of race-based inequity and harm in clinical and education settings, as well as evidence-based practices for promoting equity and culturally responsive care. Every clinician, educator, researcher, and person in training should read this book. Readers will learn realities that all mental health professionals and educators (and citizens) need to face, and be guided through a host of thoughtful, expansive, anti-racist approaches that range from essential intrapersonal work to structural interventions. I will share this with all my colleagues and trainees."

—**Lizabeth Roemer, PhD**, professor in the department of psychology at the University of Massachusetts Boston, and coauthor of *Worry Less, Live More*

"*Eliminating Race-Based Mental Health Disparities* not only meets the editors' goal of being both 'timely and timeless,' but also seamlessly weaves the theoretical with the practical, and the empirical with the clinical. Breadth and depth are demonstrated by documenting epidemiological and structural inequities alongside specific advice about how to restore social justice in clinical settings and other institutions. I spend a good deal of my professional time consulting with mental health agencies about how to meet the needs of their diversifying client base. This is a book that will put me out of business!"

—**Nnamdi Pole, PhD**, professor in the department of psychology and social work at Smith College in Northampton, MA

"This is the most comprehensive book addressing race-based mental health disparities and promoting culturally responsive care that I have had the privilege to read. The editors, ranging from senior experts to graduate students with new perspectives, cite compelling evidence on the underestimated impact of racism in multiple contexts. Grounded in science and cultural humility, they provide multidimensional models, best practices, and personal road maps so we can work collectively to achieve mental health equity across settings. This volume belongs in the library of anyone who yearns to make a difference personally or professionally."

—**Mavis Tsai, PhD**, coauthor of *A Guide to Functional Analytic Psychotherapy*, and research scientist and clinical faculty at the University of Washington

"This book is needed more than ever in today's current sociopolitical landscape, and will remain essential reading so long as we live in a diverse and multicultural society. Its thoughtful examination of the current state of disparities faced by people of color lays the groundwork for evidence-based strategies to guide individual practitioners and training programs. This book has taken the most complex and difficult social issues of our time, and provided a critical framework to understand and approach the work. Woven beautifully throughout, empirically sound strategies—fundamental to any practitioner new to the field, or experienced veteran—provide the tools for culturally responsive care."

—**Christy Matta, MA**, is a health manager at Stanford's Health Improvement Program, an instructor for Stanford's BeWell Program, and author of *The Stress Response*

"This edited book is a primer on not only what race-based mental health disparities 'look like' in the real world, but also (and more importantly) how clinicians can address these disparities in our everyday mental health practice, research, education, training, and advocacy. In an era where anti-Blackness, anti-Latinx, anti-immigrant sentiments, and more are escalating these disparities, this book is a practical guide for next steps for countering these negative messages and developing a more racially just world."

—**Anneliese Singh, PhD, LPC**, professor and associate dean of diversity, equity, and inclusion at the University of Georgia, and author of *The Racial Healing Handbook* and *The Queer and Transgender Resilience Workbook*

"A timely, pragmatic, and exquisite resource for students, teachers, researchers, and practitioners who are seeking an empirically sound, current book that captures the layered complexity and urgency to address mental health disparities for people of color. This book is a scholarly masterpiece; a courageous deep dive into the morass of historical and contemporary sociopolitical issues that create and sustain barriers to mental health for marginalized populations, and particularly for clients of color. Williams, Rosen, and Kanter set a high bar for those who are committed to understanding and meeting the challenges of learning, teaching, and practicing with cultural humility, deep empathy, and equity for all."

> —**Olivia Moorehead-Slaughter, PhD**, Center for Multicultural Training in Psychology (CMTP) Boston University School of Medicine and Boston Medical Center

"Race-based trauma has defined our collective history, and remains a daunting challenge to contemporary sociopolitical relationships and individual well-being. *Eliminating Race-Based Mental Health Disparities* addresses this reality head-on by expanding and deepening our understanding of the psychological impacts of racism, the debilitating role of bias, barriers to access, and implications across multiple treatment settings. This is an invaluable resource for all mental health professionals in the twenty-first century who righteously aspire toward culturally responsive and affirming best practices."

> —**Anatasia S. Kim, PhD**, associate professor at The Wright Institute, and coauthor of *It's Time to Talk (and Listen)*

Eliminating Race-Based Mental Health Disparities

Promoting Equity and Culturally Responsive Care Across Settings

Edited by

Monnica T. Williams, PhD
Daniel C. Rosen, PhD
Jonathan W. Kanter, PhD

CONTEXT PRESS
An Imprint of New Harbinger Publications, Inc.

Publisher's Note

Printed in the United States of America

Distributed in Canada by Raincoast Books

Copyright © 2019 by Monnica T. Williams, Daniel C. Rosen, and Jonathan W. Kanter
      Context Press
      An imprint of New Harbinger Publications, Inc.
      5674 Shattuck Avenue
      Oakland, CA 94609
      www.newharbinger.com

Cover design by Sara Christian

Acquired by Tesilya Hanauer

Edited by Jennifer Eastman

Indexed by James Minkin

All Rights Reserved

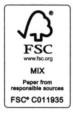
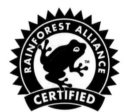

Library of Congress Cataloging-in-Publication Data on file

21   20   19

10 9 8 7 6 5 4 3 2 1   First Printing

To our families, who support us; the many individuals who have shaped and influenced us to be better at what we try to do; and the health and well-being of all communities.

—MTW, DCR, and JWK

Contents

Foreword: Evidence-Based Practices and Recommendations for
Clinicians and Educators ix

    Patricia Arredondo, *Arredondo Advisory Group*

Acknowledgments xiii

Introduction 1

    Monnica T. Williams, *University of Connecticut;*
    Daniel C. Rosen, *Bastyr University;*
    Jonathan W. Kanter, *University of Washington*

PART 1   Creating Context: Understanding Disparities

1   Understanding Mental Health Disparities 9

    Amanda NeMoyer, *Massachusetts General Hospital;*
    Kiara Alvarez, *Harvard Medical School and Massachusetts General Hospital;*
    Margarita Alegría, *Harvard Medical School and Massachusetts General Hospital*

2   Barriers to Mental Health Treatment for African Americans:
    Applying a Model of Treatment Initiation to Reduce Disparities 27

    Erlanger A. Turner, *University of Houston–Downtown;*
    Celeste M. Malone, *Howard University;*
    Courtland Douglas, *Texas Southern University*

3   The Science of Clinician Biases and (Mis)Behavior 43

    John F. Dovidio, *Yale University;*
    Ava T. Casados, *Yale University*

4   Strategies for Promoting Patient Activation, Self-Efficacy, and Engagement
    in Treatment for Ethnic and Racial Minority Clients 61

    Margarita Alegría, *Harvard Medical School and Massachusetts General Hospital;*
    Naomi Ali, *Massachusetts General Hospital;*
    Larimar Fuentes, *Massachusetts General Hospital*

5   The Impact of Racism on the Mental Health of People of Color 79

    Shawn C. T. Jones, *University of Pennsylvania;*
    Enrique W. Neblett Jr., *University of North Carolina at Chapel Hill*

6   Using Contextual Behavioral Science to Understand Racism and Bias 99

    Jonathan W. Kanter, *University of Washington;*
    Daniel C. Rosen, *Bastyr University;*
    Katherine E. Manbeck, *University of Washington;*
    Adam M. Kuczynski, *University of Washington;*
    Mariah D. Corey, *University of Washington;*
    Heather M. L. Branstetter, *Bastyr University*

PART 2   Best Practices in Training and Psychotherapy

7   Cultural Competence 101: Teaching About Race and Racism   129
      Monnica T. Williams, *University of Connecticut*

8   Becoming an Antiracist White Clinician   147
         Daniel C. Rosen, *Bastyr University;*
         Jonathan W. Kanter, *University of Washington;*
         Matthieu Villatte, *Bastyr University;*
         Matthew D. Skinta, *Roosevelt University;*
         Mary Plummer Loudon, *The Seattle Clinic*

9   Culturally Responsive Assessment and Diagnosis for Clients of Color   169
         Jessica R. Graham-LoPresti, *Suffolk University;*
         Monnica T. Williams, *University of Connecticut;*
         Daniel C. Rosen, *Bastyr University*

10   Supervising Therapist Trainees of Color   187
         Linda A. Oshin, *University of Connecticut;*
         Terence H. W. Ching, *University of Connecticut;*
         Lindsey M. West, *The Medical College of Georgia and Augusta University*

11   White Parents Raising Black Kids   203
         Anne Blakely Steketee, *Chapman University*

PART 3   Structural Mental Health Disparities

12   Strategies for Increased Racial Diversity and Inclusion in Graduate
      Psychology Programs   227
         Erin N. Arney, *Bastyr University;*
         Sharon Y. Lee, *University of Connecticut;*
         Destiny M. B. Printz, *University of Connecticut;*
         Catherine E. Stewart, *University of Connecticut;*
         Sylvie P. Shuttleworth, *Bastyr University*

13   Promoting Diversity and Inclusion on College Campuses   243
         Monnica T. Williams, *University of Connecticut;*
         Jonathan W. Kanter, *University of Washington*

14   Barriers to Outpatient Psychotherapy Treatment   277
         Camelia Harb, *Georgetown University Medical Center;*
         Jessica Jackson, *VA Los Angeles Ambulatory Care Center;*
         Alfiee M. Breland-Noble, *Georgetown University Medical Center*

15   Racial Disparities in University Counseling Centers   291
      M. R. Natacha Foo Kune, *University of Washington;*
      Agnes Kwong, *Interconnections Healing Center;*
      Ellen B. Taylor, *Washington State University*

16   Mental Health Treatment Disparities in Racial and Ethnic Minority
      Military Service Members and Veterans   307
      Elizabeth M. Goetter, *Massachusetts General Hospital;*
      Allyson M. Blackburn, *Harvard Medical School*

17   Refugee Communities   327
      Victoria A. Schlaudt, *Nova Southeastern University and University of Michigan;*
      Alisa B. Miller, *Boston Children's Hospital and Harvard Medical School*

      Index   347

Evidence-Based Practices and Recommendations for Clinicians and Educators

Patricia Arredondo,
Arredondo Advisory Group

The cornerstones of the multicultural competency movement were laid in the late 1960s, fueled by the passage of the Civil Rights Act of 1964. Counseling and psychology educators and practitioners, persons of color and allies alike, recognized the historic disparities in access and treatment contributing to race-based mental health disparities and created proactive movements in academia to address inequities and to prepare more culturally responsive mental health professionals. In 1992 and 1996, many of us used aspirational and pragmatic language to inspire individuals' development of *awareness*, *knowledge*, and *skills*, the three domains of the multicultural counseling competency (MCC) model, also designed to address inequities and to promote social justice principles. Early MCC standards and guidelines articulated a rationale that serves as the foundation to this powerful book, *Eliminating Race-Based Mental Health Disparities: Promoting Equity and Culturally Responsive Care Across Settings*. The book goes beyond the aspirations of MCC documents and provides current research about disparities, new information on waves and targets of racism, and, of course, evidence-based practices to implement aspirations. The goal of the authors is to engage educators and practitioners in promoting and practicing equity and excellence across settings and communities.

Eliminating Race-Based Mental Health Disparities: Promoting Equity and Culturally Responsive Care Across Settings is critically relevant in the contemporary sociopolitical context, in which many elected leaders are perpetuating White nationalism and heteropatriarchy in the United States on a daily basis. Vitriolic discourse about immigrant children, women victims of sexual assault, Muslim people, school shootings, and ethnic minority men as a danger to society functions to oppress and engender anxiety and fear in many communities. Hate crimes have struck Jewish synagogues, Black men in their own homes, and immigrants seeking asylum. As is pointed out by various authors, such violence has an impact on mental health. All of us hear the same divisive statements through the media, but with different cognitive and emotional reactions. If you are the person of color being verbally assaulted by White men in macro-settings, such as televised political rallies, you may wish you were not a member of a visible ethnic minority group. Why? Because you know that this form of dog-whistle politics is not going to benefit you, your family, or your community. If you are a White person, however, these racist diatribes likely heighten latent perceptions that people of color are not trustworthy, are dangerous, and take advantage of government benefits.

In chapter 2, "Barriers to Mental Health Treatment for African Americans," the authors remind us that the predominant mental health providers are White men and women, generally well meaning, but underprepared to address health and mental health disparities in the delivery of care or to recognize "everyday racism" faced by persons of color or those from underrepresented religious, cultural, and gender identity groups. As the authors state, biases and prejudices will heighten interpersonal barriers with persons of color and affect the delivery of culturally responsive and authentic services, whether it is a college counseling setting, a graduate program classroom, or a clinic where family services are intended for low-income Black families. Context and culture are inextricably linked, and with each chapter of this book, this paradigm is given meaning.

The book is structured in such a way that parallels the multicultural counseling competency development model of awareness, knowledge, and skills, with social justice themes woven throughout. The first part, "Creating Context: Understanding Disparities," provides research-informed context about the increase in mental health disparities for persons of color, particularly those who are financially disenfranchised. The chapters throughout this section point to the perpetuation of issues of access, provider bias, mistrust of White providers by communities of color, and the effects of racism on mental health. This section is an extension of early data and themes reported for the 1992 multicultural counseling competencies rationale and in the report by the Surgeon General in 1999 on health disparities. In short, little has changed, except, perhaps, greater intentionality on the part of educators, clinicians, and researchers to eliminate mental health disparities, as discussed in the book.

In chapter 6, Kanter and colleagues provide a very compelling discussion about the use of contextual behavioral science (CBS) to understand the influences and effects of racism and bias on behavior. Discussions of race-based stress and trauma, as well as proposed interventions, provide further knowledge for educators, researchers, and practitioners. Yet, each time clients, students, or persons of color in general hear racist rants, they are retraumatized and perhaps even more fearful of seeking help, according to Jones and Neblett in chapter 5. For positive change to occur, that is beneficial for clients of color, agency leaders and supervisors need to recognize the harm of the macro-context on the mental health of persons of color and assume responsibility at their local level.

Part 2, "Best Practices in Training and Psychotherapy," addresses multiple contexts for promoting the elimination of race-based disparities. All of the chapters in this section have a culture-centered framework with practical applications. The starting point, as discussed by the authors, is to embed empirically informed practices into all forms of therapist preparation, from assessment and diagnosis of persons of color to supervision of clinicians of color and supervision of White clinicians working with clients of color. It is impossible to recognize structural, interpersonal, and cross-cultural biases if one has never examined these, as they succinctly point out.

Teaching about race, racism, and cultural competence is an art and a science, and various authors in this section address both teaching and competence development for those who are educators, clinicians, and supervisors. In chapter 7, "Cultural Competence 101: Teaching About Race and Racism," Williams outlines key points to address when teaching about race and racism. She emphasizes that instructors must have full awareness of their preparation to address others' biases, resistance, egocentrism, and other defense mechanisms that often emerge when teaching. Recognizing the barriers that may occur during teaching, she encourages the use of empathy, statements of caring, and self-disclosure. The latter can disarm a participant who is reluctant and a defensive learner.

Chapter 9, "Culturally Responsive Assessment and Diagnosis for Clients of Color" addresses inequities by pointing to misinterpretations of symptoms of distress for clients of color and how this leads to misdiagnosis. The authors remind us that the use of instruments with White, middle-class norms does not serve less-educated or immigrant clients. In fact, they can do more harm and are a form of unethical practice. The authors share empirically informed best practices for the assessment and diagnosis of clients of color.

Part 3, "Structural Mental Health Disparities," tightens the focus to specific settings and populations, such as veterans, refugee communities, and psychology training programs. Though there is variance among the settings discussed, the thread across the chapters is the identification of structural barriers and provider biases that impede access to inclusion and participation.

Chapter 14, "Barriers to Outpatient Psychotherapy Treatment," discusses research on provider bias and the responsibility of institutions, be they hospitals or college counseling centers, to prioritize culturally responsive training, supervision, and practice; they have an ethical obligation to do no harm. So often in MCC-based education and training, the focus is on the client, not clinicians and our inherent biases. The authors point out that at the provider level, psychotherapists in solo practice and practitioner groups have unique situations where biases may emerge. In delivering outpatient therapy, they make decisions about who they will or will not see. Their racial bias, perhaps masked, will be apparent if they see only White clients. If a solo practitioner chooses, he or she may not accept any individuals of color and offer justification as well. Individuals in public-agency settings do not have the privilege to refuse to see a client based on ethnicity, race, or language capability, yet if this barrier is gone, many more individuals will not be seen.

Eliminating race-based mental health disparities and promoting culturally responsive care is a life-long process, as articulated by the coeditors. In each chapter, there are key points that emerge and guidelines for best practices. There are personal roadmaps, cultural and clinical models, and excellent new research with different cultural groups.

The authors are steadfast in their chapter-by-chapter approach, leading readers to relevant practices to eliminate race-based mental health disparities. By emphasizing the consequences of race and racism in the multiple contexts in which clinicians and educators work, they are also recommending opportunities to work collectively to achieve mental health equity across settings and in different cultural groups, but especially on behalf of clients of color.

Acknowledgments

The authors would like to acknowledge the following undergraduate research assistants at the University of Connecticut, who assisted with developing the powerpoint presentations included with this volume: Michael Cruz, Hayley Rowe, Emma Turner, Jessica Barber, and Tiana Robinson. We would also like to acknowledge Jessica Gee at Bastyr University for help formatting and organizing the final manuscript for publication.

Introduction

Monnica T. Williams,
University of Connecticut

Daniel C. Rosen,
Bastyr University

Jonathan W. Kanter,
University of Washington

Race-based mental health disparities exist at a much larger scale than most mental health clinicians, teachers, and researchers realize. We know, for example, that most White people in the United States vastly underestimate the continued extent and impact of racism on people of color in this country. The first problem addressed by this book is simply delineating the scope of the problem as it exists today, across the multiple settings in which mental health practitioners work. The first problem, as is said, is admitting we have a problem.

The second problem concerns what to do. Learning what to do has not been easy, as we the editors—a Black woman and two White men—have learned from our collective experiences. While each of our learning curves and trajectories has been unique, we resonate strongly, collectively, as a group with these experiences. Some of our learning has been what not to do. The early efforts of the first editor, Monnica Williams, in trying to teach multicultural psychology are a good example. She applied the framework she had used successfully to teach abnormal psychology: work through the textbook, present interesting facts, and ask the students to write papers. It didn't work. The students became angry and disengaged. Several wrote abusive comments in their course evaluations. She wondered if she should stop teaching about race altogether and go back to the comfort and familiarity of abnormal psychology.

In addition to being able to relate well to Dr. Williams's experience, the second editor, Dan Rosen, found that his learning curve has not been linear. Having taught culture-focused courses since 2002, he has felt the ground shift under him, most recently and significantly with the 2016 presidential election and the resurgence of visible White nationalism. His teaching strategies felt less effective, his lessons less relevant, and neither sufficiently addressed the elephant that had grown in the room—emotion. How to educate and train clinicians to effectively care for their patients amid increased levels of anxiety, fear, shame, anger, and hopelessness emerged as central questions.

The third editor, Jonathan Kanter, first approached the problem of teaching this material committed to an active and fully experiential learning approach, based on effective training strategies developed within contextual behavioral science (CBS). He was not prepared for how quickly an active and experiential approach could spin out of control when the content was race and racism. He was not prepared for the intensity of emotion that was elicited in his trainees and in himself.

We know this material cannot be taught from the neck up, with just facts and figures. We have learned that what students need may change rapidly, rendering our previous learning obsolete. We have learned that emotional engagement is important to learning, but emotional dysregulation and its counterpoint, suppression, are toxic to the process.

This book is an effort to produce the resource we wish we had had earlier in our careers, as we aspired to become clinicians, educators, and researchers. It reflects how each of us has grappled with important questions around race that our field and our training have left us unprepared to answer. Published in 2019, this collection is situated in a clear moment in time when the work is harder than it has been in years. We are alarmed and appalled by the sharp increase in explicit acts of hatred that have occurred recently, demonstrating in blunt form how racism, xenophobia, and other forms of oppression are deeply rooted in our societies. That said, we recognize that oppression has existed for centuries, and many of the themes addressed here were important before this current moment and will remain important if and when the sociopolitical landscape changes.

Contextual behavioral science aims to consider the many layers of the human experience (context) and put this understanding into focused applications to alleviate human suffering and promote well-being. This book reflects our belief that CBS harbors an untapped potential for addressing many of the problems facing society, and at the same time, clarifies that there is much yet to do. CBS efforts are still in their infancy, and there are many settings and areas of problems that CBS simply has not touched. To date, only small and largely unfunded CBS efforts have occurred in this arena. While most contextual behavioral clinicians strongly endorse equity and denounce racism, this book shows that committed actions, across clinical practice, teaching, and research, are not being generated on a meaningful scale. We aim to bridge the gap in values and practice by providing information clinicians, educators, and researchers can use to promote equity in their own contexts.

Roadmap to Action

The book is comprised of three distinct parts. The first part, "Creating Context: Understanding Disparities," delves into the state of racial disparities in mental health care and the science that allows us to understand them. The first chapter, "Understanding Mental Health Disparities," provides context for the chapters that follow, explaining the problem of people of color being largely excluded from access to quality mental health treatment. Chapter 2, "Barriers to Mental Health Treatment for African Americans," explains how this came to be, based on the history of racism in psychology. Chapter 3, "The Science of Clinician Biases and (Mis)Behavior," cowritten by leading racism researcher Jack Dovidio, shows how these problems are maintained via intrapersonal variables (e.g., implicit bias) that influence clinical behavior and prevent the formation of effective therapeutic relationships and culturally responsive care. To address this, chapter 4, "Strategies for Promoting Patient Activation, Self-Efficacy, and Engagement in Treatment for Ethnic and Racial Minority Clients," describes the role of participatory action research and the empirical findings that inform best practices in engaging communities and people of color, within both public health and psychotherapy contexts.

Structural and individual racism, including microaggressions and racial discrimination, impact the mental health of people of color (POC) across their whole lives. Chapter 5, "The Impact of Racism on the Mental Health of People of Color," dives deep into the empirical literature to reveal the resulting major mental health outcomes: anxiety and stress, mood disorders, substance use disorders, race-based stress, and trauma. As mentioned above, we believe CBS offers unique insights and underutilized tools for surfacing and countering racialized bias in mental health care. Chapter 6, "Using Contextual Behavioral Science to Understand Racism and Bias," illuminates how the concept of race-based experiential avoidance helps us understand—and intervene on—core problems like implicit bias, colorblindness, White privilege, and microaggressions.

The second part of the book, "Best Practices in Training and Psychotherapy," provides hands-on practical approaches for educators and clinicians. Chapter 7, "Cultural Competence 101: Teaching About Race and Racism," describes cutting-edge approaches for developing courses, workshops, and seminars for reducing racism and engaging mental health clinicians in developing culturally responsive care practices, including step-by-step guidance on the delivery of challenging material to diverse trainees. It is infused with CBS principles, such as functional analytic psychotherapy, to make the material more palatable for learners. The slides that accompany this chapter were developed and used for the authors' anti-racism training and research interventions.

Chapter 8, "Becoming an Antiracist White Clinician," uses principles from CBS treatment approaches (e.g., acceptance and commitment therapy, functional analytic psychotherapy) explicated in chapter 6 to guide clinicians in overcoming bias in clinical encounters and building a strong working alliance across racial differences. This is followed by chapter 9, "Culturally Responsive Assessment and Diagnosis for Clients of Color," which describes empirically informed best practices for the assessment and diagnostic process with clients of color, including the intake process and culturally informed diagnostic considerations.

Chapter 10, "Supervising Therapist Trainees of Color," tackles a largely neglected area of clinical training, providing examples of the unique challenges faced by therapists who may experience racism from clients, peers, and supervisors alike. Likewise, chapter 11, "White Parents Raising Black Kids," addresses the common emotional and identity challenges faced by Black children who are raised without the benefit of the normal

African American racial-socialization process. The chapter's author, a White mother of three adopted children of color, shares how therapists can support parents in addressing racial issues throughout their child's development.

The third part of the book, "Structural Mental Health Disparities," takes a broader look at problems across multiple domains. Chapter 12, "Strategies for Increased Racial Diversity and Inclusion in Graduate Psychology Programs," explores issues central to recruiting and retaining students of color to diversify the mental health delivery workforce. Likewise, chapter 13, "Promoting Diversity and Inclusion on College Campuses," focuses on psychologists working on college campuses, tackling issues related to curriculum, faculty recruitment and retention, structural and leadership issues within the university system, and the psychological harms caused by a lack of diversity.

The remainder of the book is about disparities in specific mental health settings, with a focus on access to care, quality of care, and treatment outcomes. Chapter 14, "Barriers to Outpatient Psychotherapy Treatment," addresses outpatient therapy, with an emphasis on solo practice and practitioner groups. And the last three chapters examine these issues on college campuses, among service members and veterans, and among refugees: chapter 15, "Racial Disparities in University Counseling Centers"; chapter 16, "Mental Health Treatment Disparities in Racial and Ethnic Minority Military Service Members and Veterans"; and chapter 17, "Refugee Communities."

Overall, this book represents a tremendous effort of our authors, who range from the most senior and respected scholars in the field to new graduate students with fresh perspectives on diversity issues. We pushed ourselves and our authors into new ground to ensure the work is both timely and timeless, fearless in its representation of the problems we as a society face, creative in its proposed solutions, anchored in evidence and theory, and pragmatic for immediate, on-the-ground uptake and utility. We hope we have succeeded in creating the book we desired early in our careers, and we hope it inspires current graduate students, clinicians, and researchers to action in their classrooms, organizations, clinics, and communities. These topics are not easy ones—this book may result in strong emotions and even a desire to turn away from the challenges we face. Even so, we encourage our readers to also be curious, fearless, self-reflective, creative, responsive, and committed to cultural humility and continued learning, taking valued action in the service of equity and access for everyone whose lives we touch in the course of our work.

References

Carter, E. R., & Murphy, M. C. (2015). Group-based differences in perceptions of racism: What counts, to whom, and why? *Social and Personality Psychology Compass, 9*(6), 269–280.

Constantine, M. G. (2007). Racial microaggressions against African American clients in cross-racial counseling relationships. *Journal of Counseling Psychology, 54*(1), 1–16. https://doi.org/10.1037/0022-0167.54.1.1

Jones, R. P., Cox, D., & Navarro-Rivera, J. (2014, September 23). Economic insecurity, rising inequality, and doubts about the future. Findings from the 2014 American Values Survey. Public Religion Research Institute (PRRI). Washington, DC.

Kugelmass, H. (2016). "Sorry, I'm not accepting new patients": An audit study of access to mental health care. *Journal of Health and Social Behavior, 57*(2), 168–183. https://doi.org/10.1177/0022146516647098

Masuda, A. (Ed.) (2014). *Mindfulness and acceptance in multicultural competency: A contextual approach to sociocultural diversity in theory and practice.* Oakland, CA: New Harbinger.

Sue, D. W., & Sue, D. (2016). *Counseling the Culturally Diverse* (7th ed.). New York, NY: Wiley.

PART 1

Creating Context
Understanding Disparities

CHAPTER 1

Understanding Mental Health Disparities

Amanda NeMoyer,
Massachusetts General Hospital

Kiara Alvarez,
Harvard Medical School and Massachusetts General Hospital

Margarita Alegría,
Harvard Medical School and Massachusetts General Hospital

Introduction

In 2001, the Department of Health and Human Services identified a need to address "striking" disparities in mental health, noting that members of racial and ethnic minority groups consistently had less access to mental health care and received poorer-quality care than Whites. Nearly two decades later, racial and ethnic disparities remain in mental health disorder prevalence, access to care, service quality, and care outcomes. These disparities—which we define as racial and ethnic differences that do not arise from varying clinical needs or treatment appropriateness—contribute to an increased disability and disease burden among minority populations (LaVeist et al., 2011). Individuals who wish to reduce disparities—whether on an individual basis as providers or on a broader scale via policy reform—must first understand these disparities, the factors that promote and maintain them, and current, promising strategies for addressing them. We aim to provide that information in this chapter, as we briefly discuss mental health disparities observed among racial and ethnic groups, review contributing factors, and identify major approaches to addressing racial and ethnic disparities in mental health.

Disparity Statistics

To provide an overview of the research to date on racial and ethnic disparities in mental health, we first review statistics on mental health disorder prevalence, access to care, utilization of care, and quality of care.

Disorder Prevalence

Research has suggested that non-Latinx Whites demonstrate higher lifetime prevalence rates of most mental health disorders than members of many racial and ethnic minority groups, including Black, Latinx, and Asian individuals (Breslau et al., 2006; Harris et al., 2005). However, these data typically exclude certain vulnerable populations—such as individuals who are homeless, hospitalized, or incarcerated—where both racial and ethnic minorities and individuals with mental illness are overrepresented; therefore, findings from these data may underestimate prevalence among racial and ethnic minority groups (Primm et al., 2010). Additionally, despite lower lifetime *prevalence* rates, Black and Latinx individuals frequently demonstrate greater rates of *persistent* mental health disorders than Whites (Breslau et al., 2005; Grant et al., 2012) and can experience disproportionate disability and mortality from these disorders (LaVeist et al., 2011).

Unlike members of other racial and ethnic minority groups, American Indians and Alaska Natives (AI/ANs) frequently demonstrate *increased* prevalence of certain mental health disorders than Whites (Brave Heart et al., 2016; Harris et al., 2005). However, the term AI/AN itself masks substantial heterogeneity across nearly six hundred federally recognized tribes (Brave Heart et al., 2016). Similarly, although data for certain racial and ethnic minority groups (e.g., Native Hawaiians and Pacific Islanders, Asian Americans) are typically grouped together for the purposes of statistical presentation, this practice masks prevalence differences among ethnic subgroups (Ta et al., 2008; Wong, Hosotani, & Her, 2012).

Access to and Utilization of Services

Racial and ethnic disparities in mental health care access and utilization have been well documented: for example, AI/ANs living on tribal reservations are less likely than the general US population to seek mental health treatment (Primm et al., 2010) and Asians are less likely than Whites to seek or receive such care (Abe-Kim et al., 2007; Ta et al., 2008). Compared to Whites, Black and Latinx individuals make fewer mental health care visits (both to general and specialty mental health providers) and are less likely to fill initial prescriptions for psychiatric medication—these disparities persist even when controlling for socioeconomic and health status (Cook et al., 2010; Dobalian & Rivers, 2008; Olfson et al., 2016; Satre et al., 2010). Some evidence even suggests disparities have *worsened* over time, particularly for Black and Latinx individuals regarding mental health care and psychotropic medication use (Cook et al., 2017).

Similar disparities emerge when examining substance use disorder treatment: Black men and women are less likely than members of other racial groups to engage in chemical-dependency programs (Satre et al., 2010) and just 39 percent of surveyed AI/AN individuals with substance use disorders reported seeking help (Beals et al., 2006). Access and utilization statistics may also reflect the fact that members of racial and ethnic minority groups are more likely than Whites to lack a regular health care provider, who could assist in identifying mental health needs and facilitate treatment referrals (Burgess et al., 2008). Of note, because members of racial and ethnic minority groups are under-represented in outpatient mental health treatment, they tend to be *overrepresented* in inpatient or emergency treatment settings, at greater cost to patients, health systems, and taxpayers (Samnaliev, McGovern, & Clark, 2009; Snowden, Hastings, & Alvidrez, 2009).

Quality of Services

Once members of racial and ethnic minority groups enroll in mental health services, they often receive poorer-quality care, as Black and Latinx individuals are less likely to receive guideline-based care than Whites (Primm et al., 2010) and Black patients with psychotic disorders are less likely than Whites to receive novel treatments (Mallinger, Fisher, Brown, and Lamberti, 2006). Asian individuals may also receive lower than stan-dard care compared to Whites, though fewer studies examine this difference (Satre et al., 2010). Likely as a result, racial and ethnic minority patients typically demonstrate greater dropout rates than Whites, even when controlling for language and socioeconomic status (Gone & Trimble, 2012; Jimenez, Bartels, Cardenas, Daliwal, & Alegría, 2012; Satre et al., 2010).

Factors Contributing to Disparities

Given the complexity of the disparities described above, there is no single cause for these differences. Instead, several factors operate to maintain and further these disparities at the patient, provider, and systemic or institutional levels. Here, we examine these factors in more detail.

Patient-Level Factors

Individual patient characteristics such as socioeconomic status, insurance status, language proficiency, patient preferences, and stigma or mistrust can all contribute to existing racial and ethnic disparities in mental health. Additionally, it is important to note that these factors cannot be discussed in isolation, as they are often linked to each other and to race or ethnicity.

SOCIOECONOMIC STATUS

Researchers have frequently observed a significant relationship between socioeco-nomic status (SES)—often measured via education level and income—and mental health variables, including disorder prevalence (Everson, Maty, Lynch, & Kaplan, 2002) and access to and use of needed services (Wang et al., 2005). Longstanding structural racism—through mechanisms such as educational and workplace segregation leading to fewer opportunities for high-paying jobs and wealth accumulation—has contributed to observed links between racial and ethnic minority status and low SES (Gee & Ford, 2011; Gone & Trimble, 2012; Williams, Priest, & Anderson, 2016). As a result, SES has been thought to contribute to observed mental health disparities, especially for Latinx and Black adults (Cook et al., 2010; Williams, Yu, & Jackson, 1997). Individuals with low SES likely struggle to access typical mental health services because of inflexible work scheduling, limited sick time, childcare obligations, and lack of reliable transportation (Krupnick & Melnikoff, 2012). Further, residential segregation has contributed to provider shortages and limited access to quality health care in geographic areas with high proportions of Black and Latinx residents and residents with low SES—particularly in rural areas (White, Haas, & Williams, 2012).

INSURANCE STATUS

Given that health insurance can reduce out-of-pocket expenses for mental health treatment, a lack of sufficient coverage reduces access to needed care, especially for individuals with low income (Cook et al., 2010). Prior to implementation of the Affordable Care Act (ACA), Black, Latinx, and AI/AN men and women were less likely to have insurance coverage than Whites (Cook et al., 2010; Foutz, Squires, Garfield, & Damico, 2017), and foreign-born residents were nearly three times as likely as US-born residents to lack insurance coverage (Primm et al., 2010). Although uninsured rates have decreased across the race and ethnicity spectrum since the ACA took effect, people of color are still significantly more likely than Whites to be uninsured (Foutz et al., 2017). Further, although coverage inequities appear to contribute to observed racial and ethnic disparities, similar disparities have also been observed in countries with universal health insurance (Tiwari & Wang, 2008).

LANGUAGE PROFICIENCY

Members of racial and ethnic minority groups—especially those who identify as Latinx or Asian—are more likely than Whites to have limited English proficiency (Sentell & Braun, 2012). Language barriers further limit access to behavioral health services, such that in a survey of non-English speakers with mental health needs, just 8 percent of Latinx people and 11 percent of Asian and Pacific Islanders reported receiving services (Kim et al., 2011; Ohtani, Suzuki, Takeuchi, & Uchida, 2015; Sentell, Shumway, & Snowden, 2007). Even if individuals with limited English proficiency *do* access care, they often receive poorer-quality care, as language barriers increase the chances of misdiagnosis, reduce patients' understanding of their diagnoses, and decrease the likelihood patients will correctly adhere to discharge plans (Betancourt, Green, Carrillo, & Ananeh-Firempong, 2003).

PATIENT PREFERENCES

When deciding whether to seek mental health care, individuals consider their personal beliefs about the underlying causes of mental health disorders, typical mental health treatments, and treatment providers (e.g., Jimenez et al., 2012). Such beliefs arise from a combination of educational experiences, personal experience, family tradition, and cultural values (Barksdale & Molock, 2009) and can have a significant impact on whether individuals recognize a need for mental health care and initiate help-seeking behavior (Jorm, 2012). Racial and ethnic minorities may be more likely than Whites to believe that mental health treatment does not work or that they can address mental health symptoms without professional assistance, and they are more likely to seek assistance through nontraditional sources of support, such as a family member or spiritual leader (Cooper et al., 2003; Gone & Trimble, 2012; Jimenez et al., 2012). Professional treatment preferences can also vary by race and ethnicity; for example, Black and Latinx individuals seeking treatment often prefer incorporating psychotherapy into their care and may leave care that emphasizes psychotropic medications alone (Blanco et al., 2007; Cooper et al., 2003). Finally, many racial and ethnic minorities prefer clinicians from similar backgrounds (Cabral & Smith, 2011) and prefer treatment in their native language (Kim et al., 2011). However, national shortages of providers from minority racial and ethnic groups and with foreign language proficiency (Santiago & Miranda, 2014) limit access for these individuals and can reduce treatment satisfaction.

STIGMA OR MISTRUST

Although mental health stigma can prevent individuals across the racial and ethnic spectrum from seeking necessary treatment, members of racial and ethnic minority groups may be more likely than Whites to perceive such stigma (Cook et al., 2010). For example, Asian and Arabic minority groups may be more likely to identify mental health stigma as a barrier to help-seeking, and Black individuals may report concerns related to perceived personal weakness or family stigma more frequently than White individuals (Clement et al., 2015). Stigma impedes treatment seeking, thereby increasing the likelihood that mental health needs will escalate to crisis level and require emergency or inpatient care (Chow, Jaffee, & Snowden, 2003; Primm et al., 2010). Minority racial and ethnic group members also frequently report feeling less trusting of providers (Dobalian & Rivers, 2008), perhaps given local community perceptions of clinicians, their effectiveness, and their likelihood to unfairly judge or stereotype (Campbell & Long, 2014).

Provider-Level Factors

Beyond recognizing patient characteristics that contribute to racial and ethnic disparities in mental health, providers should acknowledge the ways in which they and their colleagues might further these differences. Below, we describe three provider-level examples that, if addressed, might help to reduce existing disparities.

LACK OF RACIAL AND ETHNIC MINORITY PROVIDERS

Many US regions suffer from a critical lack of mental health providers, especially in rural areas, communities with low income, and communities of color (Thomas, Ellis, Konrad, Holzer, & Morrissey, 2009). Additionally, despite representing nearly 40 percent of the US population, racial and ethnic minority group members represent just 21 percent of psychiatrists, 13 percent of social workers, and 8 percent of psychologists (Santiago & Miranda, 2014). Rates of AI/AN providers are particularly low, even within programs supported by the Indian Health Service (Gone & Trimble, 2012; SAMHSA, 2012). Addiction treatment and recovery service specialists have a more diverse workforce: racial and ethnic minority men and women comprise 36 percent of direct care providers in this field (Ryan, Murphy, & Krom, 2012); however, services from these providers are not always covered by insurance and are therefore less accessible. Multilingual clinicians are also in limited supply, despite thousands of US residents who require or prefer care in a language other than English (Blanco et al., 2007; Kim et al., 2011). Beyond discouraging individuals from seeking care, language discordance between individuals and their available providers can promote poor quality of care (Betancourt et al., 2003). Overall, racial and ethnic minority and multilingual providers are more likely than White providers to serve underserved populations and patients of color (Alegría, Alvarez, Ishikawa, DiMarzio, & McPeck, 2016); therefore, continued shortages foster ongoing racial and ethnic disparities in mental health treatment.

LACK OF APPROPRIATE TRAINING AND TOOLS

Although symptom presentation can vary across racial and ethnic groups, many providers have not received significant training in conducting culturally competent assessment and treatment. Further, few diagnostic tools have been developed or adapted for use with minority populations. Providers, therefore, are often less able to accurately identify mental health disorders for racial and ethnic minority patients than for White patients (Cook et al., 2010). These challenges can result in both over- and underdiagnosis of certain mental health disorders: for instance, understandable behaviors among members of a minority group may be interpreted as symptomatic by providers from the majority group (e.g., distrust of health care systems based on historical mistreatment could be perceived as paranoia) and result in unnecessary diagnosis and treatment. On the other hand, providers with little cross-cultural familiarity may feel uncomfortable asking questions that could help identify mental health symptoms for racial and ethnic minority patients (Alegría, Alvarez, Pescosolido, & Canino, 2017).

In addition to a lack of training and tools for culturally competent assessment, a dearth of evidence-based services designed or adapted for racial and ethnic minorities means that properly diagnosed individuals from these groups can still fail to receive appropriate treatment. Historically, clinical research has been conducted with predominantly White male populations, leading the National Institutes of Health (NIH) to issue a policy requiring researchers to recruit women and members of ethnic minority populations into NIH-funded studies (Miranda, 1996). Regardless, many clinical trials are conducted without sufficient racial and ethnic minority group representation and thus fail to determine whether treatments that are efficacious with a majority group will generalize to other groups. And, given the need for larger sample sizes to conduct between-group comparisons, few clinical trials specifically examine the impact of participant race or ethnicity on treatment outcomes (Santiago & Miranda, 2014).

A review of barriers and facilitators to health-research participation among Asian, Latinx, Black, and Pacific Islander individuals identified common barriers such as mistrust, competing demands, stigma, lack of information access, and limited insurance coverage (George, Duran, & Norris, 2014). Overall, studies point to the need for active and sustained work by researchers to engage diverse populations in research. This work might include active recruitment, budgeting for increased outreach costs, and maintaining strong relationships with diverse collaborators (Shavers-Hornaday, Lynch, Burmeister, & Torner, 1997). Further, because equitable access to research has been identified as a relevant barrier to research participation for racial and ethnic minority individuals—sometimes even more so than mistrust—it is important that future efforts focus on making health research more accessible, rather than focus solely on changing perceived individual attitudes toward research participation (Green, Verges, Jackson, Rivers, & McCallum, 2006; Wendler et al., 2006).

BIAS AND DISCRIMINATION

Whether conscious or unconscious, provider biases also contribute to racial and ethnic disparities in mental health, especially when providers rely on group stereotypes to make diagnostic and treatment decisions. For example, physicians have rated Black patients as less intelligent, less educated, more likely to abuse alcohol or drugs, and less likely to comply with medical advice than demographically and clinically similar White patients (van Ryn & Burke, 2000). Such perceptions can influence providers' diagnoses, recommendations, and referrals for future treatment. Within behavioral health clinics, provider biases can affect patient trajectories as early as the initial intake, as providers gather different types of diagnosis-relevant information or weigh similar information differently depending on patient race or ethnicity (Alegría et al., 2008). Differing procedures likely contribute to disparate rates of diagnosis for certain disorders across racial and ethnic groups: for example, Black and Latinx individuals are frequently overdiagnosed with psychotic disorders and underdiagnosed with mood disorders compared to Whites (Choi et al., 2012). Accurate and comprehensive diagnostic assessments are critical to determining appropriate treatment plans; providers who inconsistently gather information risk misdiagnosing patients, making inappropriate treatment recommendations, damaging therapeutic relationships, and further contributing to racial and ethnic disparities in mental health.

Biased perceptions among providers likely influence their behaviors during patient interactions, such that they indicate, even subtly, their negative expectations for patient outcomes, leading to patient discouragement and reduced motivation (Alegría et al.,

2017). When meeting with minority patients, White providers may appear more verbally dominant, less patient-centered, less informative, and less inclusive of patients during decision making (Dovidio et al., 2008). These behaviors are often apparent to patients, as individuals from racial and ethnic backgrounds report feeling disrespected or discriminated against during clinical encounters more frequently than Whites; these patients were then less likely to adhere to provider recommendations or return for future care (Shavers et al., 2012). Spanish-speaking individuals have also reported perceiving impatience and unhelpfulness from providers and other health care personnel when their limited language proficiency becomes apparent, leaving them less satisfied with their care and less likely to seek care (Nápoles-Springer, Santoyo, Houston, Perez-Stable, & Stewart, 2005).

Institutional and Systemic Factors

Finally, adequate understanding of existing mental health disparities must include awareness of the ways in which broader systems and structures contribute. To address these factors, clinicians should consider advocating for change within their associated institutions.

INSURANCE PLANS

Although differences in insurance status across racial and ethnic groups contribute to observed mental health disparities, even individuals with insurance—especially public insurance—can face prohibitive limits to coverage for behavioral health services. For example, plans might be strict in defining care that meets "medical necessity" criteria or in approving promising emerging treatments, leading insurers to deny behavioral health care more frequently than they deny medical health services (Alegría et al., 2016). Given that members of racial and ethnic minority groups are overrepresented in government-sponsored insurance programs (e.g., Medicaid), they are also increasingly vulnerable to federal and state policy changes designed to reduce public spending (Alegría et al., 2017). Chronic underfunding of the Indian Health Service has substantially limited AI/AN access to mental health programs, as less than 10 percent of the service's clinical funds are dedicated to mental health and substance abuse treatment (Gone & Trimble, 2012). Additionally, Medicaid programs vary by state in eligibility criteria, mental health treatment coverage, and reimbursement policies (Cook et al., 2010). These differences have a disproportionate impact on individuals with low SES, who are largely racial, ethnic, and linguistic minorities, and further impede access to care (Alegría et al., 2017). Further, federal policy prevents immigrants with lawful status from obtaining public coverage for five years, and some immigrants are permanently excluded from public coverage (Alegría et al., 2017).

HEALTH CARE SYSTEMS

Health care system policies and practices often play a role in furthering disparities. For example, systems may be less inclined to serve racial, ethnic, and linguistic minorities, who are often perceived as needing more intensive treatment and referrals to additional support services (Alegría et al., 2017). These concerns are supported by statistics suggesting that psychiatrists refuse to accept new Medicaid patients (a disproportionate number of whom are racial, ethnic, and linguistic minorities) more frequently than other physicians and that their acceptance rates for this population have declined over time (Bishop, Press, Keyhani, & Pincus, 2014). Such policies reduce the number of providers available to serve racial and ethnic minority patients with low income, further limiting access to needed care.

Despite the need to improve provider interactions with racial and ethnic minority patients, few health care systems support their providers in developing necessary cultural competence and overcoming bias, for example by encouraging them to utilize shared decision-making strategies, elicit more information about patient preferences, and develop mutual understanding (Alegría et al., 2016). Similarly, organizations that lack required care resources in a patient's preferred language reduce patient satisfaction and provide poorer-quality care (Betancourt et al., 2003). Underfunded systems predominantly serving low-income and racial and ethnic minority populations—faced with low reimbursement rates and productivity requirements—struggle to support the use of evidence-based practices, even those designed to address service barriers (Alegría et al., 2017).

Finally, like the pervasive dearth of racial and ethnic minority providers, health care leadership teams have historically been made up of predominantly non-Latinx White men and women (Betancourt et al., 2003). For example, members of racial and ethnic minority groups represent just 14 percent of hospital leadership and governance (American Hospital Association, 2012). Limited diversity in health care leadership suggests that system administrators are disconnected from minority patients, often failing to design practices and policies that adequately address their unique needs (Betancourt et al., 2003; Blanco et al., 2007).

Major Approaches to Addressing Racial and Ethnic Disparities in Mental Health

Over the last two decades, a wealth of information about successfully reducing disparities in access and service quality has emerged. Advancements point to three central ideas: (1) addressing social determinants of health; (2) payment model and policy reform; and (3) improving quality of care.

Addressing Social Determinants of Health

Given the frequent overlap between social and mental health needs for racial and ethnic minority groups, addressing social determinants of health has recently become an important method of tackling mental health disparities. For example, states and local jurisdictions that provide increased funding to social services and community health care tend to have better health and mental health outcomes (Bradley et al., 2016). Additionally, many national social-service initiatives have been modified to better address mental health disparities among different racial and ethnic groups. Supported housing programs, which combine housing and support services to assist individuals facing homelessness or health and behavioral health challenges, have demonstrated great promise as an integrated method of treating severe mental illness and as a potential way to reduce racial and ethnic disparities in health outcomes (Nelson, Aubry, & Lafrance, 2007). For example, Housing First programs, serving adults experiencing homelessness and mental illness, have implemented anti-racism and anti-oppression practices meant to improve housing stability and community functioning for racial and ethnic minorities (Stergiopoulos et al., 2016). Supported housing participants can experience enriched quality of relationships; increased access to resources such as food, clothing, and employment; fewer days in shelters; and reduced rates of psychiatric hospitalization (Culhane, Metraux, & Hadley, 2002; Nelson, Clarke, Febbraro, & Hatzipantelis, 2005).

Individuals with mental illness identify their diagnoses as a significant barrier to pursuing education (Fernando, King, & Loney, 2014); this challenge may be linked to elevated high school dropout rates for racial and ethnic minorities. Supported education programs are designed to help these individuals attain their educational goals and have demonstrated some success: participants in a hospital-based program offering inpatient and outpatient classes reported feeling improved self-confidence, leading to more ambitious educational and vocational goals (Fernando et al., 2014). Similarly, supported employment programs have demonstrated improved paid-work outcomes for racial and ethnic minority group members with mental illness (Mueser et al., 2014). Serving racial and ethnic minority groups through faith-based initiatives has also demonstrated effectiveness in facilitating access to mental health care, particularly for low-income families.

Payment Model and Policy Reform

By expanding public insurance programs, subsidizing private plans for low- and middle-income individuals, and identifying mental health and substance abuse treatment as essential benefits, the ACA targeted health care access disparities for low-income and racial and ethnic minority populations (Zuckerman & Holahan, 2012). Some evidence suggests that the ACA has improved insurance coverage rates and access to behavioral health treatment; however, these improvements have not been observed across all racial and ethnic groups (Schoen et al., 2010). Beyond increased insurance coverage, providers—especially providers who accept public insurance—must become more available in areas where racial and ethnic minority populations are overrepresented (Bishop et al., 2014; Cook, Doksum, Chen, & Alegría 2013).

Additionally, policies that increase health care efficiency may facilitate disparity reduction. For example, accountable care organizations (ACOs)—health care providers, clinics, and hospitals responsible for the outcomes of an identified group of individuals—are incentivized to efficiently use resources and promote positive outcomes. It remains to be seen whether ACOs will lessen disparities, but their novel payment models and flexible delivery methods could promote innovations that increase access to high-quality care for racial and ethnic minorities and individuals with low income.

Finally, through $181 million of annual funding to states, the Comprehensive Addiction and Recovery Act aims to decrease the abuse of methamphetamines, opioids, and heroin, and to promote treatment and recovery. Though funding can be used to improve substance use disorder identification and provide evidence-based treatment, studies have yet to examine whether this act has diminished previously observed racial and ethnic disparities related to substance use disorder prevalence and treatment access. Of note, 40 percent of US counties have no outpatient substance use treatment facilities that accept Medicaid—especially counties with a high percentage of Black, rural, and uninsured residents (Cummings, Wen, Ko, & Druss, 2014). Policies that monitor the availability of providers and facilities that offer, fund, or facilitate behavioral health care could be key in reducing both access and outcome disparities.

Improving Quality of Care

Although the use of evidence-based practices has improved treatment quality for some disadvantaged groups, these improvements have not always been observed within racial and ethnic minority populations (Aisenberg, 2008). Enhancements and better tailoring of evidence-based treatments for racial and ethnic minority populations could reduce the frequency of early termination of treatment for these groups, thereby decreasing treatment outcome disparities. Boosting the quality of mental health care for individuals with limited English proficiency requires addressing language barriers in care (Kim et al., 2011; Wafula & Snipes, 2013), for example, by ensuring availability and competency of interpreter services (Bauer & Alegría, 2010). Further, more attention should be centered on provider practices within safety net facilities, as few implement evidence-based treatments (Saxena, Thornicroft, Knapp, & Whiteford, 2007). Finally, increasing education and training to a diverse workforce should facilitate an adequate supply of culturally competent and linguistically appropriate mental health providers and paraprofessionals that can deliver effective care to racial and ethnic minority patients.

Conclusion

Despite recognition for the need to address racial and ethnic disparities in mental health, this challenge persists, contributing to disproportionate negative outcomes for people of color in the United States. Future reform efforts should be grounded in an adequate understanding of the complexity of these disparities and how they are maintained via patient-level, provider-level, and system- and institutional-level factors. The chapters that follow will further explore the challenges identified here and present meaningful, multidimensional, and promising strategies for addressing disparities.

KEY POINTS FOR CLINICIANS

- Racial and ethnic disparities in disorder prevalence, access to care, service quality, and care outcomes contribute to increased disability and disease burden among minority populations.

- On an individual or patient level, factors such as socioeconomic status, insurance status, language proficiency, personal preference, and stigma or mistrust can all contribute to existing mental health disparities, often in combination.

- Providers, whether knowingly or unknowingly, can also contribute to racial and ethnic disparities in mental health when they lack appropriate training or tools or rely on conscious and unconscious biases when making diagnostic and treatment decisions.

- At a broader systems level, insurance provider and health care system policies that increase out-of-pocket costs for behavioral treatment and do not adequately encourage the use of culturally competent, evidence-based practices work to further existing racial and ethnic disparities in mental health.

- Efforts to address identified disparities might focus on addressing social determinants of health, reforming models of payment for care, and improving quality of care for disadvantaged groups.

References

Abe-Kim, J., Takeuchi, D. T., Hong, S., Zane, N., Sue, S., Spencer, M. S., Alegría, M. (2007). Use of mental health–related services among immigrant and US-born Asian Americans: Results from the National Latino and Asian American study. *American Journal of Public Health*, 97(1), 91–98.

Aisenberg, E. (2008). Evidence-based practice in mental health care to ethnic minority communities: Has its practice fallen short of its evidence? *Social Work*, 53(4), 297–306.

Alegría, M., Alvarez, K., Ishikawa, R., DiMarzio, K., & McPeck, S. (2016). Removing obstacles to eliminate racial and ethnic disparities in behavioral health care. *Health Affairs*, 35(6), 991–999.

Alegría, M., Alvarez, K., Pescosolido, B. A., & Canino, G. (2017). A socio-cultural framework for mental health and substance abuse service disparities. In B. Sadock, V. Sadock, & P. Ruiz (Eds.), *Kaplan & Sadock's comprehensive textbook of psychiatry* (10th ed.) (pp. 4377–4386). Philadelphia, PA: Wolters Kluwer.

Alegría, M., Nakash, O., Lapatin, S., Oddo, V., Gao, S., Lin, J., & Normand, S. (2008). How missing information in diagnosis can lead to disparities in the clinical encounter. *Journal of Public Health and Managing Practice*, 14(Suppl.), S26–S35.

American Hospital Association. (2012). *Diversity and disparities: A benchmark study of US hospitals.* Chicago, IL: Author.

Barksdale, C. L., & Molock, S. D. (2009). Perceived norms and mental health help seeking among African American college students. *Journal of Behavioral Health Services & Research*, 36(3), 285–299.

Bauer, A., & Alegría, M. (2010). Impact of patient language proficiency and interpreter service use on the quality of psychiatric care: A systematic review. *Psychiatric Services*, 61(8), 765–773.

Beals, J., Novins, D. K., Spicer, P., Whitesell, N. R., Mitchell, C. M., Manson, S. M., & the AI-SUPER-PFP Team. (2006). Help seeking for substance use problems in two American Indian reservation populations. *Psychiatric Services*, 57(4), 512–520.

Betancourt, J. R., Green, A. R., Carrillo, J. E., & Ananeh-Firempong, O. (2003). Defining cultural competence: A practical framework for addressing racial/ethnic disparities in health and health care. *Public Health Reports*, 118(4), 293–302.

Bishop, T. F., Press, M. J., Keyhani, S., & Pincus, H. A. (2014). Acceptance of insurance by psychiatrists and the implications for access to mental health care. *JAMA Psychiatry*, 71(2), 176–181.

Blanco, C., Patel, S. R., Liu, L., Jiang, H., Lewis-Fernandez, R., Schmidt, A. B., … & Olfson, M. (2007). National trends in ethnic disparities in mental health care. *Medical Care*, 45(11), 1012–1019.

Bradley, E. H., Canavan, M., Rogan, E., Talbert-Slagle, K., Ndumele, C., Taylor, L., & Curry, L. A. (2016). Variation in health outcomes: The role of spending on social services, public health, and health care, 2000–09. *Health Affairs*, 35(5), 760–768.

Brave Heart, M. Y. H., Lewis-Fernández, R., Beals, J., Hasin, D. S., Sugaya, L., Wang, S., … & Blanco, C. (2016). Psychiatric disorders and mental health treatment in American Indians and Alaska Natives: Results of the National Epidemiologic Survey on Alcohol and Related Conditions. *Social Psychiatry and Psychiatric Epidemiology*, 51(7), 1033–1046.

Breslau, J., Aguilar-Gaxiola, S., Kendler, K. S., Su, M., Williams, D., Kessler, R. C. (2006). Specifying race-ethnic differences in risk for psychiatric disorder in a USA national sample. *Psychological Medicine*, 36(1), 57–68.

Breslau, J., Kendler, K. S., Su, M., Gaxiola-Aguilar, S., Kessler, R. C. (2005). Lifetime risk and persistence of psychiatric disorders across ethnic groups in the United States. *Psychological Medicine*, 35(3), 317–327.

Burgess, D. J., Ding, Y., Hargreaves, M., van Ryn, M., & Phelan, S. (2008). The association between perceived discrimination and underutilization of needed medical and mental health care in a multi-ethnic community sample. *Journal of Health Care for the Poor and Underserved, 19*(3), 894–911.

Cabral, R. R., & Smith, T. B. (2011). Racial/ethnic matching of clients and therapists in mental health services: A meta-analytic review of preferences, perceptions, and outcomes. *Journal of Counseling Psychology, 58*(4), 537–554.

Campbell, R. D., & Long, L. A. (2014). Culture as a social determinant of mental and behavioral health: A look at culturally shaped beliefs and their impact on help-seeking behaviors and service use patterns of Black Americans with depression. *Best Practices in Mental Health, 10*(2), 48–62.

Choi, M. R., Eun, H., Yoo, T. P., Yun, Y., Wood, C., Kase, M.,…& Yang, J. (2012). The effects of sociodemographic factors on psychiatric diagnosis. *Psychiatry Investigation, 9*(3), 199–208.

Chow, J. C., Jaffee, K., & Snowden, L. (2003). Racial/ethnic disparities in the use of mental health services in poverty areas. *American Journal of Public Health, 93*(5), 792–797.

Clement, S., Schauman, O., Graham, T., Maggioni, F., Evans-Lacko, S., Bezborodovs, N., … & Thornicroft, G. (2015). What is the impact of mental health-related stigma on help-seeking? A systematic review of quantitative and qualitative studies. *Psychological Medicine, 45*(1), 11–27.

Cook, B. L., Doksum, T., Chen, C., Carle, A., & Alegría, M. (2013). The role of provider supply and organization in reducing racial/ethnic disparities in mental health care in the US. *Social Science & Medicine, 84*, 102–109.

Cook, B. L., McGuire, T. G., Lock, K., & Zaslavsky, A. M. (2010). Comparing methods of racial and ethnic disparities measurement across different settings of mental health care. *Health Services Research, 45*(3), 825–847.

Cook, B. L., Trinh, N. H., Li, Z., Hou, S. S., & Progovac, A. M. (2017). Trends in racial-ethnic disparities in access to mental health care, 2004–2012. *Psychiatric Services, 68*(1), 9–16.

Cooper, L. A., Gonzales, J. J., Gallo, J. J., Rost, K. M., Meredith, L. S., Rubenstein, L. V., … & Ford, D. E. (2003). The acceptability of treatment for depression among African-American, Hispanic, and White primary care patients. *Medical Care, 41*(4), 479–489.

Culhane, D. P., Metraux, S., & Hadley, T. (2002). Public service reductions associated with placement of homeless persons with severe mental illness in supportive housing. *Housing Policy Debate, 13*(1), 107–163.

Cummings, J. R., Wen, H., Ko, M., & Druss, B. G. (2014). Race/ethnicity and geographic access to Medicaid substance use disorder treatment facilities in the United States. *JAMA Psychiatry, 71*(2), 190–196.

Dobalian, A., & Rivers, P. A. (2008). Racial and ethnic disparities in the use of mental health services. *Journal of Behavioral Health Services Research, 35*(2), 128–141.

Dovidio, J. F., Penner, L. A., Albrecht, T. L., Norton, W. E., Gaertner, S. L., & Shelton, J. N. (2008). Disparities and distrust: The implications of psychological processes for understanding racial disparities in health and health care. *Social Science & Medicine, 67*, 478–486.

Everson, S. A., Maty, S. C., Lynch, J. W., & Kaplan, G. A. (2002). Epidemiologic evidence for the relation between socioeconomic status and depression, obesity, and diabetes. *Journal of Psychosomatic Research, 53*(4), 891–895.

Fernando, S., King, A., & Loney, D. (2014). Helping them help themselves: Supported adult education for persons living with mental illness. *The Canadian Journal for the Study of Adult Education (Online), 27*(1), 15.

Foutz, J., Squires, E., Garfield, R., & Damico, A. (2017). *The uninsured: A primer. Key facts about health insurance and the uninsured under the Affordable Care Act.* Menlo Park, CA: The Henry J. Kaiser Family Foundation.

Gee, G. C., & Ford, C. L. (2011). Structural racism and health inequities: Old issues, new directions. *Du Bois Review, 8*(1), 115–132.

George, S., Duran, N., & Norris, K. (2014). A systematic review of barriers and facilitators to minority research participation among African Americans, Latinos, Asian Americans, and Pacific Islanders. *American Journal of Public Health, 104*(2), e31.

Gone, J. P., & Trimble, J. E. (2012). American Indian and Alaska Native mental health: Diverse perspectives on enduring disparities. *Annual Review of Clinical Psychology, 8,* 131–160.

Grant, J. D., Verges, A., Jackson, K. M., Trull, T. J., Sher, K. J., & Bucholz, K. K. (2012). Age and ethnic differences in the onset, persistence and recurrence of alcohol use disorder. *Addiction, 107*(4), 756–765.

Green, B. L., Arekere, D. M., Katz, R. V., Rivers, B. M., & McCallum, J. M. (2006). Awareness and knowledge of the US public health service syphilis study at Tuskegee: Implications for biomedical research. *Journal of Health Care for the Poor and Underserved, 17*(4), 716–733.

Harris, K. M., Edlund, M. J., & Larson, S. (2005). Racial and ethnic differences in mental health problems and use of mental health care. *Medical Care, 43*(8), 775–784.

Jimenez, D. E., Bartels, S. J., Cardenas, V., Daliwal, S. S., & Alegría, M. (2012). Cultural beliefs and mental health treatment preferences of ethnically diverse older adult consumers in primary care. *American Journal of Geriatric Psychiatry, 20*(6), 533–542.

Jorm, A. F. (2012). Mental health literacy: Empowering the community to take action for better mental health. *American Psychologist, 67*(3), 231–243.

Kim, G., Aguado Loi, C. X., Chiriboga, D. A., Jang, Y., Parmelee, P., & Allen, R. S. (2011). Limited English proficiency as a barrier to mental health service use: A study of Latino and Asian immigrants with psychiatric disorders. *Journal of Psychiatric Research, 45*(1), 104–110.

Krupnick, J. L., & Melnikoff, S. E. (2012). Psychotherapy with low-income patients: Lessons learned from treatment studies. *Journal of Contemporary Psychotherapy, 42*(1), 7–15.

LaVeist, T. A., Gaskin, D., & Richard, P. (2011). Estimating the economic burden of racial health inequalities in the United States. *International Journal of Health Services, 41*(2), 231–238.

Mallinger, J. B., Fisher, S. G., Brown, T., & Lamberti, J. S. (2006). Racial disparities in the use of second-generation antipsychotics for the treatment of schizophrenia. *Psychiatric Services, 57*(1), 133–136.

Miranda, J. (1996). Introduction to the special section on recruiting and retaining minorities in psychotherapy research. *Journal of Consulting and Clinical Psychology, 64*(5), 848–850.

Mueser, K. T., Bond, G. R., Essock, S. M., Clark, R. E., Carpenter-Song, E., Drake, R. E., & Wolfe, R. (2014). The effects of supported employment in Latino consumers with severe mental illness. *Psychiatric Rehabilitation Journal, 37*(2), 113.

Nápoles-Springer, A. M., Santoyo, J., Houston, K., Perez-Stable, E. J., & Stewart, A. L. (2005). Patients' perceptions of cultural factors affecting the quality of their medical encounters. *Health Expectations, 8*(1), 4–17.

Nelson, G., Aubry, T., & Lafrance, A. (2007). A review of the literature on the effectiveness of housing and support, assertive community treatment, and intensive case management interventions for persons with mental illness who have been homeless. *American Journal of Orthopsychiatry, 77*(3), 350–361.

Nelson, G., Clarke, J., Febbraro, A., & Hatzipantelis, M. (2005). A narrative approach to the evaluation of supportive housing: Stories of homeless people who have experienced serious mental illness. *Psychiatric Rehabilitation Journal, 29*(2), 98.

Ohtani, A., Suzuki, T., Takeuchi, H., & Uchida, H. (2015). Language barriers and access to psychiatric care: A systematic review. *Psychiatric Services, 66*(8), 798–805.

Olfson, M., Blanco, C., & Marcus, S. C. (2016). Treatment of adult depression in the United States. *JAMA Internal Medicine, 176*(10), 1482–1491.

Primm, A. B., Vasquez, M. J. T., Mays, R. A., Sammons-Posey, D., McKnight-Eily, L. R., Presley-Cantrell, L. R., … & Perry, G. S. (2010). The role of public health in addressing racial and ethnic disparities in mental health and mental illness. *Preventing Chronic Disease, 7*(1), A20.

Ryan, O., Murphy, D., & Krom, L. (2012). *Vital signs: Taking the pulse of the addiction treatment workforce, a national report*. Kansas City, MO: Addiction Technology Transfer Center.

Samnaliev, M., McGovern, M. P., Clark, R. E. (2009). Racial/ethnic disparities in mental health treatment in six Medicaid programs. *Journal of Health Care for the Poor and Underserved, 20*(1), 165–176.

Santiago, C. D., & Miranda, J. (2014). Progress in improving mental health services for racial-ethnic minority groups: A ten-year perspective. *Psychiatric Services, 65*(2), 180–185.

Satre, D. D., Campbell, C. I., Gordon, N. P., & Weisner, C. (2010). Ethnic disparities in accessing treatment for depression and substance use disorders in an integrated health plan. *International Journal of Psychiatry in Medicine, 40*(1), 57–76.

Saxena, S., Thornicroft, G., Knapp, M., & Whiteford, H. (2007). Resources for mental health: Scarcity, inequity, and inefficiency. *The Lancet, 370*(9590), 878–889.

Schoen, C., Osborn, R., Squires, D., Doty, M. M., Pierson, R., & Applebaum, S. (2010). How health insurance design affects access to care and costs, by income, in eleven countries. *Health Affairs, 29*(12), 2323–2334.

Sentell, T., & Braun, K. (2012). Low health literacy, limited English proficiency, and health status in Asians, Latinos, and other racial/ethnic groups in California. *Journal of Health Communication, 17*(Suppl 3), 82–99.

Sentell, T., Shumway, M., & Snowden, L. (2007). Access to mental health treatment by English language proficiency and race/ethnicity. *Journal of General Internal Medicine, 22*(Suppl 2), 289–293.

Shavers, V. L., Fagan, P., Jones, D., Klein, W. M. P., Boyington, J., Moten, C., & Rorie, E. (2012). The state of research on racial/ethnic discrimination in the receipt of health care. *American Journal of Public Health, 102*(5), 953–966.

Shavers-Hornaday, V. L., Lynch, C. F., Burmeister, L. F., & Torner, J. C. (1997). Why are African Americans under-represented in medical research studies? Impediments to participation. *Ethnicity & Health, 2*(1–2), 31–45.

Snowden, L. R., Hastings, J. F., & Alvidrez, J. (2009). Overrepresentation of Black Americans in psychiatric inpatient care. *Psychiatric Services, 60*(6). 779–785.

Stergiopoulos, V., Gozdzik, A., Misir, V., Skosireva, A., Sarang, A., Connelly, J., … & McKenzie, K. (2016). The effectiveness of a housing first adaptation for ethnic minority groups: Findings of a pragmatic randomized controlled trial. *BMC Public Health, 16*(1), 1110.

Substance Abuse and Mental Health Services Administration. (2012). *Mental Health, United States, 2010*. HHS Publication No. (SMA) 12-4681. Rockville, MD: Author.

Ta, V. M., Juon, H, Gielen, A. C., Steinwachs, D., & Duggan, A. (2008). Disparities in the use of mental health and substance abuse services by Asian and Native Hawaiian/other Pacific Islander women. *Journal of Behavioral Health Services Research, 35*(1), 20–36.

Thomas, K. C., Ellis, A. R., Konrad, T. R., Holzer, C. E., & Morrissey, J. P. (2009). County-level estimates of mental health professional shortage in the United States. *Psychiatric Services, 60*(10), 1323–1328.

Tiwari, S. K., & Wang, J. (2008). Ethnic differences in mental health service use among White, Chinese, South Asian and South East Asian populations living in Canada. *Social Psychiatry and Psychiatric Epidemiology, 43*(11), 866–871.

United States Department of Health and Human Services. (2001). *Mental health: Culture, race, and ethnicity: A supplement to mental health: A report of the surgeon general*. Washington, DC: Author.

van Ryn, M., & Burke, J. (2000). The effect of patient race and socio-economic status on physicians' perceptions of patients. *Social Science & Medicine, 50*(6), 813–828.

Wafula, E. G., & Snipes, S. A. (2013). Barriers to health care access faced by Black immigrants in the US: Theoretical considerations and recommendations. *Journal of Immigrant and Minority Health, 16*, 689–698.

Wang, P. S., Lane, M., Olfson, M., Pincus, H. A., Wells, K. B., & Kessler, R. C. (2005). Twelve-month use of mental health services in the United States: Results from the National Comorbidity Survey Replication. *Archives of General Psychiatry, 62*(6), 629–640.

Wendler, D., Kington, R., Madans, J., Van Wye, G., Christ-Schmidt, H., Pratt, L. A., ... & Emanuel, E. (2006). Are racial and ethnic minorities less willing to participate in health research? *PLoS Medicine, 3*(2), e19.

White, K., Haas, J. S., & Williams, D. R. (2012). Elucidating the role of place in health care disparities: The example of racial/ethnic residential segregation. *Health Services Research, 47*(3), 1278–1299.

Williams, D. R., Priest, N., & Anderson, N. (2016). Understanding associations between race, socio-economic status and health: Patterns and prospects. *Health Psychology, 35*(4), 407–411.

Williams, D. R., Yu, Y., & Jackson, J. (1997). Racial differences in physical and mental health: Socio-economic status, stress and discrimination. *Journal of Health Psychology, 2*(3), 335–351.

Wong, C., Hosotani, H., & Her, J. (2012). *Information on small populations with significant health disparities: A report on data collected on the health of Asian Americans in Massachusetts.* Boston, MA: Institute for Asian American Studies.

Zuckerman, S., & Holahan, J. (2012). *Despite criticism, the Affordable Care Act does much to contain health care costs.* Washington, DC: The Urban Institute.

CHAPTER 2

Barriers to Mental Health Treatment for African Americans

APPLYING A MODEL OF TREATMENT INITIATION TO REDUCE DISPARITIES

Erlanger A. Turner,
University of Houston–Downtown

Celeste M. Malone,
Howard University

Courtland Douglas,
Texas Southern University

Introduction

Mental health disparities are a serious public health issue that continues to require attention. Decades of research document the high rates of mental health problems but low rates of seeking mental health treatment (Belgrave & Allison, 2014; Caldwell, Assari, & Breland-Noble, 2016; Turner, Camarillo, Daniel, Otero, & Parker, 2017). Among ethnic and racial groups, data show that these populations are significantly less likely to seek mental health treatment (Turner et al., 2016), as discussed in chapter 1. Data collected from the Substance Abuse and Mental Health Administration (SAMHSA, 2015) between 2008 and 2012 indicated that compared to Whites, individuals from other ethnic and racial groups were less likely to use outpatient mental health treatment (Blacks, 4.7 percent; Hispanics and Latinx, 3.8 percent; and Asians, 2.5 percent versus 7.8 percent for Whites). Among clinical and community samples, data suggest that differences in mental health across ethnic groups are often due to sociocultural factors such as experiences of discrimination, as opposed to clinical bias or social processes (Belgrave & Allison, 2014).

One of the challenges with understanding mental health diagnoses and prevalence rates among African Americans is that the literature often groups all people of African descent into one broad category. However, several authors have documented the importance of how prevalence rates and cultural differences influence mental health disparities across African Americans born in the United States and those who have immigrated, such as Blacks from Africa or the Caribbean (Caldwell et al. 2016; Turner et al., 2016). In this chapter, we will use the term "African American" broadly to describe Blacks living in the United States. Although African American and Black are often used interchangeably, it is important to recognize that these terms are different concepts. Womack (2010) provides a simple explanation: "Black" refers to everybody who is Black (of African ancestry), while "African American" refers to Blacks living in the United States. The focus of this chapter is to discuss how historical factors such as racism and discrimination have contributed to mental health disparities for African Americans, to provide an overview of barriers to treatment initiation, and to discuss evidence-based strategies for improving cultural sensitivity, addressing these barriers, and eliminating mental health disparities.

Racism and Mental Health

The mental health of African Americans must be understood within a social-historical context (see chapter 5, "The Impact of Racism on the Mental Health of People of Color," for more details). For many African Americans, the slave trade and its subsequent influence on race relations in the United States has contributed to African Americans' negative perceptions of mental health providers (Pieterse, Todd, Neville, & Carter, 2012; US Department of Health and Human Services [USDHHS], 2001). Scholars note that African people were brought as slaves to the United States more than two hundred years ago (Hall, 2010; Poussaint & Alexander, 2000). Although slavery ended decades ago, the oppression of African Americans has continued at varying degrees, and psychology has occasionally contributed to injustice and marginalization of this group (e.g., Grier & Cobbs, 1968; Hall, 2010; Pieterse et al., 2012; Suite, La Bril, Primm, & Harrison Ross, 2007).

Some of the early psychological research in the nineteenth and twentieth century was published under the premise of advancing science and knowledge, but was what we "now see was a misuse of science" (Sinclair, 2017, p. 21). In the nineteenth century, a number of psychologists made a series of studies utilizing sensory measurement devices producing a vast array of impressive statistical tables, curves, ranges, and distributions, which gave credibility to the inferiority myth of Black Americans (Guthrie, 1976). This early work by psychologists into racial differences provided inaccurate data that led to racist conclusions and also called into question the intentions of psychological researchers (e.g., Guthrie, 1976; Vasquez, 2012). Furthermore, psychology played a significant role in the eugenics movement. According to Guthrie (1976), researchers at the American

Breeders Association adopted a policy to use science for the practice of eugenics. According to the literature, the role of psychology was to use science to establish standards and practices for identifying those individuals that were perceived to have a mental defect and the information was to be used for sterilization (Guthrie, 1976).

African American history in the United States is painted with dismal shades, colored by centuries of slavery, decades of Jim Crow laws, dehumanization, human experimentation, racism, devaluing of Black life, and inequality. One of the clearest instance of devaluing Black life following emancipation was perhaps delivered in the form of the Tuskegee Syphilis Study, in which Black men were relegated to subjects for experimentation and were considered expendable (e.g., Suite et al., 2007). Taking into account historical injustices and daily bouts with racial prejudice and discrimination, it is understandable that African Americans have come to recognize the perceivably White institutions of mental health as having oppressive values reflective of the larger society. Furthermore, it is unsurprising that the African American community maintains a healthy paranoia in the form of cultural mistrust, exhibiting behaviors aimed at protecting their psychological well-being.

Mistrust of Mental Health Treatment

There are certain expectations that one maintains when contemplating seeking mental health services. Among these are competence, quality of care, and genuine concern for one's well-being. Members of ethnic minority groups are burdened with the concern of considering how their racial identity might impact the overall quality of care they will receive when visiting mental health providers. A cursory glance at the majority White make-up of mental health providers gives people of color cause for concern given the rocky history between European Americans—and the institutions they occupy, by extension—and ethnic minorities in the United States. Heinous historical events remain etched in the memory of older people of color and are passed down to the generational cohorts of their communities. Thus, a culture of caution and skepticism in approaching predominantly White institutions often results in reluctance to seek treatment, despite their services and goodwill (e.g., Turner, Jensen-Doss, & Heffer, 2015). This phenomenon is better known as cultural mistrust, a construct based on the work of Grier and Cobbs (1968). Cultural mistrust is a concept of cultural paranoia, in which suspicious attitudes toward White people are developed and maintained as barriers to protect against the deleterious psychological consequences associated with race-based persecution and discrimination (Whaley, 2001a). Cultural mistrust is evident in various communities of color and has implications for whether and how they interact with institutions of mental health, as well as how providers of these institutions respond to them as clients.

It is important to consider the influence of cultural mistrust on African Americans. This factor is increasingly concerning since African Americans' use of mental health services is more likely to be under emergency, coerced, or mandated conditions rather than the voluntary conditions as seen in their White counterparts (Hu, Snowden, Jerrell, & Nguyen, 1991; Takeuchi & Cheung, 1998). This mistrust results in the underutilization of mental health services by African Americans, lowered expectations for mental health treatment, and misdiagnoses of Black clients by clinicians when this mistrust is conceptualized as psychopathology (Austin, Carter, & Vaux, as cited in Townes, Chavez-Korell, & Cunningham, 2009; Watkins & Terrell, 1988). Aside from the history of cultural mistrust, we must also understand how healthy paranoia is maintained and how expressions of cultural mistrust affect therapeutic outcomes. What must then be assessed are the expectations African Americans have regarding mental health systems and practitioners, clinician responses that perpetuate cultural mistrust, and the reactions of clinicians toward distrustful African American clients.

As African Americans acknowledge institutions of mental health as reflective of the larger societal context, the expectations may be that systems will be White and inundated with toxic values that perpetuate discrimination and persecution (Sue & Sue, 2003; Townes et al., 2009). As this becomes the prevailing expectation, African Americans wonder whether their experiences will be validated in therapy and whether they will be subjected to the very same slights faced in the outside world during therapy. Negative attitudes toward mental health treatment are compounded when African American clients are provided with White counselors. Mistrustful African Americans assigned to White counselors are more likely to expect less from mental health treatment than if they are paired with Black counselors, expecting White counselors to be less accepting and trustworthy (Belgrave & Allison, 2014; Watkins & Terrell, 1988). Furthermore, African American clients may view White counselors as agents of the same institution that seeks to oppress them with solutions that reject their cultural values or practices that serve as instruments of oppression (Townes et al., 2009). Black counselors, however, are not exempt from the suspicions of same-race clients (Grier & Cobbs, 1968; Goode-Cross & Grim, 2016; Terrell & Terrell, 1984). Despite their shared racial identity with African American clients, Black counselors may also be viewed as agents of a White-oriented context (Terrell & Terrell, 1984). Thus, what is demonstrated is a generalized mistrust of people and settings belonging to systems associated with oppression.

African Americans must contend with modern-day racism, both overt and subtle. Displays of racism and acts of oppression have changed forms throughout the years to present as more systemic or appear socially justifiable. As a result, actions influenced by racist ideology have become more nuanced, including those actions that seem to be harmless or acceptable. Microaggressions are the intentional or unintentional slights that psychologically impact individuals from marginalized groups. Due to their subtle nature, the impact of microaggressions is often minimized, and they are viewed as harmless incidents to which African Americans overreact. In reality, microaggressions are a type of stressor, or trauma in some instances, for African Americans. As continuous stressors, the cumulative impact of microaggressions could over time serve as chronic trauma, as individuals are repeatedly slighted, invalidated, and erased and may endure negative impacts to their psychological well-being (Sue, Capodilupo, & Holder, 2008;

Williams, Kanter, & Ching, 2018). The conversation on microaggressions is necessary when discussing cultural mistrust, as it illuminates a factor that keeps African Americans away from therapy settings and increases their probability of premature termination.

As wary African American clients undergo therapy or evaluation, their actions or inactions may be misconstrued. Cautious responses and restricted self-disclosure in the presence of White clinicians or clinicians perceived as agents of White-oriented contexts can be erroneously appraised as maladaptive paranoia (e.g., Grier & Cobbs, 1968). Adaptive paranoia stemming from cultural mistrust functions as a means to protect African Americans in a context they perceive as harmful, as it is reflective of the greater US context, in which they are abused and devalued (Ridley, 1984). To the culturally encapsulated clinician, these responses may lead to an unwarranted diagnosis such as schizophrenia (Turner et al., 2016; Whaley, 2001b). Chapter 9, "Culturally Responsive Assessment and Diagnosis for Clients of Color," provides more information to help avoid this issue. Clinicians are susceptible to these errors if they are unaware that African American clients may exhibit cultural paranoia as a protective response (Grier & Cobbs, 1968; Whaley, 2001a). Thus, African Americans' mistrust, which functions to protect them, may become a double-edged sword in mental health settings, leading to a reduction in or cessation of help-seeking behaviors.

Barriers to Receiving Treatment

The literature notes numerous barriers to mental health treatment for individuals from ethnic and racial groups. Models of mental health treatment-seeking often identify barriers to care such as stigma, affordability of services, and lack of providers from racial backgrounds (Andersen, 1995; Hobbs, Dixon, Johnston, & Howie, 2013). These models are helpful to conceptualize treatment barriers but they often lack the ability to understand the complexity of variables that influence treatment decisions. Recently, we (Turner et al., 2016) proposed a conceptual Model of Treatment Initiation (MTI) to provide an alternative way of exploring the multiple factors that help explain mental health disparities. The MTI builds upon the Behavioral Model of Health Service Use (Andersen, 1995; Bradley et al., 2002) by capturing how predisposing factors, enabling factors, and perceptions of need influence individuals from ethnic and racial groups to seek mental health treatment. The MTI (Turner et al., 2016) contains four major areas: accessibility (structural variables that may influence an individual's ability to access treatment), availability (access to culturally competent services), appropriateness (how individuals view mental health problems as requiring treatment), and acceptability (capturing variables such as stigma and cultural mistrust). The acceptability domain, not represented in Andersen's model, allows for examining how attitudinal factors related to historical racism may represent additional barriers to treatment that interact with the other factors. See figure 2.1 for the Model of Treatment Initiation.

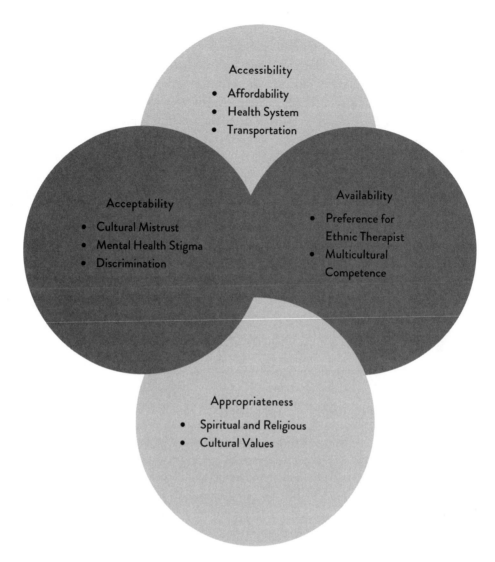

Figure 2.1. Model of Treatment Initiation for African Americans

One factor that may impact treatment use is expectations of therapy, which are consistent with appropriateness factors. Client expectations about therapy are broadly defined in two categories: outcome expectations and role expectations. Outcome expectations are clients' expectations that psychotherapy, as well as specific aspects of psychotherapy (i.e., therapist, therapeutic modality used, therapeutic setting, and therapy duration) will lead to change (Dew & Bickman, 2005; Glass, Arnkoff, & Shapiro, 2001). Role expectations are the patterns of behavior viewed as appropriate or expected by people who occupy certain professions. In a therapeutic relationship, clients have role expectations for both their therapist and for themselves (Dew & Bickman, 2005; Glass et al., 2001). Several studies have noted that these expectations can influence psychotherapy outcomes. Specifically, positive outcome expectations are associated with more positive psychotherapy results, and both congruent role expectations and positive outcome expectations are associated with more positive perceptions of the therapeutic alliance (Dew & Bickman, 2005). Because discrepancies between the client's role expectations and their actual experiences may hurt the therapeutic process, it is important for therapists to discuss both outcome and role expectations to ensure that the therapist knows what the client expects and wants from therapy and to clarify role expectations. For example, if a client is seeking a therapist that has similar religious beliefs or that will approach treatment by integrating religiosity, the client may terminate treatment when these expectations are not met.

For African Americans, their limited access to and use of mental health services and general distrust of therapists, coupled with previous experiences of discrimination and stereotyping, have likely shaped their outcome and role expectations and, in turn, their experiences once they enter therapy (Earl, Alegría, Mendieta, & Linhart, 2011). For example, using data from the National Comorbidity Survey, Diala and colleagues (2000) found that African Americans held positive behavioral and emotional attitudes toward mental health services prior to treatment, but those who received treatment reported more negative attitudes and were less likely to enter treatment in the future. This suggests that their expectations were not met in therapy or that there was something aversive about the therapy experience. Within the MTI model, factors such as cultural mistrust and perceived discrimination by providers may hinder the therapeutic relationship.

African Americans may also have expectations that their therapist feel comfortable discussing issues related to race, ethnicity, and culture. Consistent with MTI availability factors, African American clients may prefer same-race providers. They may avoid discussing sensitive topics such as racism in therapy if they believe that the therapist is not culturally sensitive (Thompson, Bazile, & Akbar, 2004). Chapter 8, "Becoming an Antiracist White Clinician," provides additional information on accepting rather than avoiding these difficult conversations. Pope-Davis and colleagues (2002) found that clients who defined themselves and their presenting problems using cultural constructs (i.e., race, ethnicity, gender) seemed to prefer racially or gender-similar therapists. However, many African Americans envision therapists as older White males who cannot understand them or their problems, and they may also question their therapists' ability to be unbiased (Thompson et al., 2004). Consequently, it should be no surprise that many studies have reported African Americans' preference for therapists of the same race.

A systematic review of studies on racial and ethnic matching in therapy found that African Americans had a very strong preference for racial and ethnic matching and that their perceptions of the therapists varied significantly as a function of that matching (Cabral & Smith, 2011). Moreover, African Americans' outcomes tended to be mildly better when paired with an African American therapist (Cabral & Smith, 2011). Similarly, Thompson and colleagues (2004) found that African American clients assigned to racially matched therapists reported greater self-understanding, acceptance, and belief in the utility of treatment strategies than did those assigned to White therapists. These examples highlight that African Americans often find same-race providers to be more culturally sensitive.

Regarding appropriateness of services, another potential barrier to seeking treatment for African Americans is their religious or spiritual beliefs. Research indicates that prayer is an important coping strategy for many African Americans, especially those with lower incomes, females, and adults over age 55 (Belgrave & Allison, 2014). As a result, African Americans may rely more on traditional support networks (e.g., relatives, spiritual advisors, friends) rather than professional psychological services (Turner et al., 2016). Consistent with the MTI appropriateness factor, African Americans may not perceive mental health treatment as a primary source of coping. Therefore, it is necessary to continue exploring how adherence to religious and spiritual beliefs serves as a barrier to treatment seeking.

Some scholars have reported that US-born African Americans may differ on treatment seeking barriers compared to immigrant Africans or Caribbean Blacks (Caldwell et al., 2016; Villatoro & Aneshensel, 2014). Although there may be general within-group differences, as noted previously, African Americans underutilize treatment compared to Whites (Broman, 2012; SAMHSA, 2015; Turner et al., 2016). For example, S. L. L. Williams (2014) reported data from the National Survey of American Life (NSAL), indicating that 28 percent of African Americans met criteria for a DSM diagnosis but only approximately 5 percent considered seeking treatment. Given these findings, it is incumbent upon all therapists to have the cultural awareness, knowledge, and skills to work effectively with clients of all racial backgrounds to ensure that clients from racial and ethnic groups feel comfortable, listened to, and respected by their providers (Earl et al., 2011).

Evidence-Based Strategies to Enhance Cultural Competence

A recurrent theme in African Americans' reluctance to utilize mental health services is the perception that providers do not understand cultural issues and will be biased against them (e.g., Earl et al., 2011; Newhill & Harris, 2007; Thompson et al., 2004). To alleviate these concerns, it is important for therapists to engage in culturally competent practices. Culturally competent therapists are aware of and sensitive to their own cultural heritage and are comfortable with the differences that may exist across the client-therapist dyad. When providers are culturally sensitive, they hold specific knowledge about diverse racial and ethnic minority groups, understand the generic characteristics of counseling and therapy, and possess the skills and abilities to generate a wide variety of verbal and non-verbal responses within the counseling relationship (Sue et al., 1982). To change African Americans' negative perceptions of mental health services, numerous steps should be considered, such as increased outreach in African American communities, making therapy more culturally relevant, and increased access to culturally competent therapists regardless of the therapists' ethnic identification. As noted in the MTI (see Figure 2.1), multiple variables may interact to influence treatment decisions and premature termination. To reduce these barriers, we must work as a field to increase our use of proven strategies to engage African American clients.

Assessment and Evaluation of African Americans

Psychological assessment and evaluation are important components of mental health treatment. One way to enhance treatment is to be open to understanding the clients' identity and environment. The Multicultural Guidelines, published by the American Psychological Association (APA), recommends that mental health providers invite their clients to describe their identities rather than relying on preconceived conceptualizations (APA, 2017). This is particularly important when working with African American clients that may have within-group differences related to cultural and ethnic identity (Turner et al., 2016; Williams et al., 2014). Research on assessment and diagnosis with African Americans often discuss racial biases when mental health providers make inadequate or inaccurate judgments about their clients (Turner & Mills, 2016; Whaley, 1997). Clinicians may overlook how context influences the clients' behaviors or neglect to consider how cultural mistrust prevents African Americans from developing rapport with their treatment providers. Racial differences across the client-therapist dyad may differentially impact provider bias. According to Grier and Cobbs (1968), White clinicians may avoid gathering information from African American clients regarding their social status or racial experiences because of the discomfort that occurs while acknowledging the clients' experiences. Furthermore, clinicians that identify as African American may have difficulties since the mental health discipline and training often occurs from a White perspective (Grier & Cobbs, 1968). These MTI acceptability factors such as discrimination and cultural mistrust should be explored early in the treatment process. One of the ways to limit bias and improve competence is to use structured clinical interviews. However, studies indicate that clinicians tend to use unstructured interviews during the assessment phase of treatment (Turner & Mills, 2016).

Cultural beliefs and practices affect all aspects of treatment including assessment, help-seeking, expectations about treatment, and interactions between the patient and provider (Weiss, 1997). Turner and Mills (2016) note that under- and overdiagnosis among African Americans may be related to providers' lack of cultural sensitivity and failure to use evidence-based assessment methods. Using explanatory models and interview approaches can reduce biases in assessment and treatment (e.g., Kleinman, 1978; Weiss, 1997). Explanatory models are connected to social, political, and historical factors that shape our knowledge and understanding of health and mental health care systems. Explanatory models contain an explanation of etiology, symptom presentation, pathophysiology, course of illness, and treatment approaches (Kleinman, 1978). When the client-therapist dyad is from the same ethnic or racial background, providers may fail to appreciate or inquire about the significance of their patients' ideas and experiences; therefore, it is necessary to use explanatory models to help guide the assessment and therapy experience (Weiss, 1997). Utilizing explanatory models assists providers in understanding and addressing MTI acceptability and appropriateness factors.

The recent version of the *Diagnostic and Statistical Manual of Mental Disorders* (DSM-5; American Psychiatric Association, 2013) includes a semi-structured interview called the DSM-5 Cultural Formulation Interview (CFI), which helps the provider to understand how the client's culture and environment relate to their mental health (Aggarwal, Nicasio, DeSilva, Boiler, & Lewis-Fernández, 2013). According to Weiss (1997), it is important that, when using instruments such as the CFI, the provider introduces the interview as a method to acquire information and clarify to the client that their responses will not be judged as right or wrong. Studies have documented that the CFI improves clinicians' cultural sensitivity, reduces bias in judgments, and improves therapy outcomes (e.g., Aggarwal et al., 2013; La Roche, Fuentes, & Hinton, 2015; Owen et al., 2016). Chapter 9, "Culturally Responsive Assessment and Diagnosis for Clients of Color," provides more information.

Outreach to African American Communities

Although African Americans believe psychotherapy and mental health treatment can be effective, they may be less likely to utilize these services because they may not understand the types of problems for which they should seek mental health treatment (Thompson et al., 2004) and believe that these problems will resolve themselves without intervention (Anglin, Alberti, Link, & Phelan, 2008). Moreover, African Americans may be more reluctant to address certain topics, particularly those related to cultural issues, out of fear that the therapist would not understand (Thompson et al., 2004). One method to address MTI availability factors is through targeted outreach to African American communities to promote the value of psychotherapy and increase utilization. Culturally appropriate community education is needed to explain the course of and potentially chronic nature of mental illness, the types of problems psychotherapy can address, and how psychotherapy can promote overall well-being (Anglin et al., 2008; Newhill & Harris, 2007; Thompson et al., 2004). This can help African Americans get a better sense of when situations merit mental health intervention and can also help to create a better cultural fit between psychotherapy and the African American community. Additionally, it is important to orient African American clients to the therapeutic process and provide a warm and welcoming clinical environment (Earl et al., 2011; Thompson et al., 2004).

Therapists should also disseminate information about mental health and mental health services in the settings where people naturally congregate. For example, therapists can consider partnering with churches, community centers, and schools to disseminate information about mental health and information about how to access mental health services (Newhill & Harris, 2007). In addition to sharing information, therapists can also consider providing some services (e.g., community-based support groups, mental health screening) in these locations to remove one of the barriers to accessing mental health services. As noted in the MTI, this could help reduce accessibility barriers. Furthermore, having multiple outlets for increased interaction between therapists and African American communities may result in community members having more accurate and positive images of therapists and being more willing to seek out mental health services.

Culturally Competent Psychotherapy

While targeted outreach can promote more positive attitudes about mental health treatment and increase the likelihood that African Americans will access mental health services, it is important that African Americans encounter culturally competent therapists with whom they can develop a strong therapeutic alliance and trusting relationship to foster positive client preferences and perceptions (Cabral & Smith, 2011). It is especially important to African American clients that therapists demonstrate they are sensitive to cultural issues and willing to discuss them in therapy (Pope-Davis et al., 2002). Therapists who address cultural issues in therapy are perceived by clients to have greater cultural competence and general competence than therapists who do not address those issues (Coleman, 1998). However, it is important that therapists understand when and how to address these issues in therapy. Cardemil and Battle (2003) provided six recommendations for discussing race and ethnicity in psychotherapy: (1) suspend preconceptions about clients' race or ethnicity and that of their family members; (2) recognize that clients may be different from other members of their racial and ethnic group; (3) consider how racial and ethnic differences between the therapist and client might affect psychotherapy; (4) acknowledge that power, privilege, and racism might affect interactions with clients; (5) err on the side of discussion when in doubt about the importance of race and ethnicity in treatment; and (6) continue to receive ongoing professional development on culturally competent practices (also see chapter 7, "Cultural Competence 101: Teaching about Race and Racism"). Aside from the information included in these sections, it is always important for providers to monitor their own competency and seek the necessary consultation.

In addition to providing culturally competent psychotherapy, providers should apply a social justice framework to their practice. Justice and fairness are concepts included in the general principles of the Ethics Code that serve as the basis for fair treatment in the assessment process, education, research, and therapy (Vasquez, 2012). Many of the issues for which African Americans seek psychotherapy are exacerbated by institutional and systemic factors such as racism, discrimination, ongoing poverty, and lack of institutional and community resources (Newhill & Harris, 2007). African Americans may avoid discussing these issues with White therapists out of fear that the therapist will not understand these concerns or judge them (Thompson et al., 2004). Within a social justice framework, therapists are called upon to be advocates to address institutional and systemic barriers that may limit their African American clients' ability to move toward optimal mental health. In addition to considering how culture impacts the therapeutic relationship, therapists should also consider the various ways in which oppression and social inequities manifest themselves at the individual and societal levels and be cognizant of the negative influences of oppression on mental health and well-being (Constantine, Hage, Kindaichi, & Bryant, 2007; Ratts, Singh, Nassar-McMillan, Butler, & McCullough, 2016).

Conclusion

For African Americans, numerous variables contribute to psychological difficulties and treatment decisions. Regarding utilization of mental health treatment, the literature has identified variables that influence treatment seeking such as perceived stigma related to mental illness, costs, insurance coverage, and levels of distress (e.g., Turner et al., 2016). Furthermore, clinicians may engage in behaviors that invalidate African American clients' experiences or disregard cultural factors (e.g., family connectedness and religion), resulting in ruptures in the therapeutic relationship. Mental health professionals must strive to become culturally sensitive and develop knowledge of African Americans' attitudes and reactions toward the mental health system. Clinicians must remain cognizant of the power differential that exists in the therapeutic relationship and the power they hold to create, affirm, or reject the realities of African American clients. Limited encounters with competent clinicians will not erase years of injustice or immediately dispel cultural mistrust. However, in practicing cultural sensitivity and maintaining a heightened level of awareness, we can continue to reduce barriers to providing care to ethnic and racial minority groups.

KEY POINTS FOR CLINICIANS

After reading this chapter, readers will:

- Better understand barriers to treatment for African Americans

- Recognize the influence of racism and historical oppression on mental health use

- Be more aware of therapists' racial bias and how therapists' actions influence clients' behaviors

- Recognize the implications of healthy cultural paranoia in African Americans during assessment and treatment

- Be more knowledgeable about intervening to reduce barriers to treatment engagement and retention.

References

Aggarwal, N. K., Nicasio, A. V., DeSilva, R., Boiler, M., & Lewis-Fernández, R. (2013). Barriers to implementing the DSM-5 cultural formulation interview: a qualitative study. *Culture, Medicine, and Psychiatry, 37*(3), 505–533.

American Psychological Association (2017). *Multicultural guidelines: An ecological approach to context, identity, and intersectionality.* Retrieved from http://www.apa.org/about/policy/multicultural-guidelines.pdf

Andersen, R. M. (1995). Revisiting the behavioral model and access to medical care: does it matter? *Journal of Health and Social Behavior, 36*(1), 1–10.

Anglin, D. M., Alberti, P. M., Link, B. G., & Phelan, J. C. (2008). Racial differences in beliefs about the effectiveness and necessity of mental health treatment. *American Journal of Community Psychology, 42,* 17–24.

Austin, N. L., Carter, R. T., & Vaux, A. (1990). The role of racial identity in Black students' attitudes toward counseling and counseling centers. *Journal of College Student Development, 31,* 237–244.

Belgrave, F. Z., & Allison, K. W. (2014). Psychosocial adaptation and mental health. In *African American psychology: From Africa to America.* (pp. 409–444). Thousand Oaks, CA: Sage.

Bradley, E. H., McGraw, S. A., Curry, L., Buckser, A., King, K. L., Kasl, S. V., & Andersen, R. (2002). Expanding the Andersen model: The role of psychosocial factors in long-term care use. *Health Services Research, 37*(5), 1221–1242.

Broman, C. L. (2012). Race differences in the receipt of mental health services among young adults. *Psychological Services, 9*(1), 38–48.

Burkard, A. W., & Knox, S. (2004). Effect of therapist color-blindness on empathy and attributions in cross-cultural counseling. *Journal of Counseling Psychology, 51,* 387–397.

Cabral, R. R., & Smith, T. B. (2011). Racial/ethnic matching of clients and therapists in mental health services: A meta-analytic review of preferences, perceptions, and outcomes. *Journal of Counseling Psychology, 58*(4), 537–554.

Caldwell, C. H., Assari, S., & Breland-Noble, A. M. (2016). The epidemiology of mental disorders in African American children and adolescents. In A. M. Breland-Noble, C. S. Al-Mateen, & N. N. Singh (Eds.), *Handbook of Mental Health in African American Youth* (pp. 3–20). New York, NY: Springer.

Cardemil, E. V., & Battle, C. L. (2003). Guess who's coming to therapy? Getting comfortable with conversations about race and ethnicity in psychotherapy. *Professional Psychology: Research and Practice, 34*(3), 278–286.

Coleman, H. L. (1998). General and multicultural counseling competency: Apples and oranges? *Journal of Multicultural Counseling and Development, 26*(3), 147–156.

Constantine, M. G. (2007). Racial microaggressions against African American clients in cross-racial counseling relationships. *Journal of Counseling Psychology, 54*(1), 1–16.

Constantine, M. G., Hage, S. M., Kindaichi, M. M., & Bryant, R. M. (2007). Social justice and multicultural issues: Implications for the practice and training of counselors and counseling psychologists. *Journal of Counseling and Development, 85,* 24–29.

Dew, S. E., & Bickman, L. (2005). Client expectancies about therapy. *Mental Health Services Research, 7*(1), 21–33.

Diala, C., Muntaner, C., Walrath, C., Nickerson, K. J., LaVeist, T. A., & Leaf, P. J. (2000). Racial differences in attitudes toward professional mental health care and in the use of services. *American Journal of Orthopsychiatry, 70*(4), 455–464.

Earl, T. R., Alegría, M., Mendieta, F., & Linhart, Y. D. (2011). "Just be straight with me": An exploration of Black patient experiences in initial mental health encounters. *American Journal of Orthopsychiatry, 81*(4), 519–525.

Glass, C. R., Arnkoff, D. B., & Shapiro, S. J. (2001). Expectations and preferences. *Psychotherapy: Theory, Research, Practice, Training, 38*(4), 455–461.

Goode-Cross, D. T., & Grim, K. A. (2016). "An unspoken level of comfort": Black therapists' experiences working with black clients. *Journal of Black Psychology, 42*(1), 29–53.

Grier, W. H., & Cobbs, P. M. (1968). *Black rage*. New York, NY: Basic Books.

Guthrie, R. V. (1976) *Even the rat was White: A historical view of psychology*. New York, NY: Harper & Row.

Hall, G. N. (2010). African Americans. In *Multicultural Psychology* (2nd Edition) (pp. 143–163). Boston, MA: Prentice Hall.

Hobbs, N., Dixon, D., Johnston, M., & Howie, K. (2013). Can the theory of planned behaviour predict the physical activity behaviour of individuals? *Psychology & Health, 28*(3), 234–249.

Hu, T. W., Snowden, L. R., Jerrell, J. M., & Nguyen, T. D. (1991). Ethnic populations in public mental health: Service choice and level of use. *American Journal of Public Health, 81*, 1429–1434.

Kearney, L. K., Draper, M., & Baron, A. (2005). Counseling utilization by ethnic minority college students. *Cultural Diversity and Ethnic Minority Psychology, 11*, 272–285.

Kleinman, A. (1978). Concepts and a model for the comparison of medical systems as cultural systems. *Social Science & Medicine. Part B: Medical Anthropology, 12*, 85–93.

La Roche, M. J., Fuentes, M. A., & Hinton, D. (2015). A cultural examination of the DSM-5: Research and clinical implications for cultural minorities. *Professional Psychology: Research and Practice, 46*(3), 183–189.

Neville, H. A., Lilly, R. L., Duran, G., Lee, R. M., & Browne, L. (2000). Construction and initial validation of the Color-Blind Racial Attitudes Scale (CoBRAS). *Journal of Counseling Psychology, 47*(1), 59–70.

Newhill, C. E., & Harris, D. (2007). African American consumers' perceptions of racial disparities in mental health services. *Social Work in Public Health, 23*(2–3), 107–124.

Owen, J., Tao, K. W., Drinane, J. M., Hook, J., Davis, D. E., & Kune, N. F. (2016). Client perceptions of therapists' multicultural orientation: Cultural (missed) opportunities and cultural humility. *Professional Psychology: Research and Practice, 47*(1), 30–37.

Pieterse, A. L., Todd, N. R., Neville, H. A., & Carter, R. T. (2012). Perceived racism and mental health among Black American adults: A meta-analytic review. *Journal of Counseling Psychology, 59*(1), 1–9.

Pope-Davis, D. B., Toporek, R. L., Ortega-Villalobos, L., Ligiéro, D. P., Brittan-Powell, C. S., Liu, W. M., … & Liang, C. T. (2002). Client perspectives of multicultural counseling competence: A qualitative examination. *The Counseling Psychologist, 30*(3), 355–393.

Poussaint, A. F., & Alexander, A. (2000). *Lay my burden down: Unraveling suicide and the mental health crisis among African-Americans*. Boston, MA: Beacon Press.

Ratts, M. J., Singh, A. A., Nassar-McMillan, S., Butler, S. K., & McCullough, J. R. (2016). Multicultural and social justice counseling competencies: Guidelines for the counseling profession. *Journal of Multicultural Counseling and Development, 44*, 28–48.

Ridley, C. R. (1984). Clinical treatment of the nondisclosing black client: A therapeutic paradox. *American Psychologist, 39*, 1234–1244.

Sinclair, C. (2017). Ethics in psychology: Recalling the past, acknowledging the present, and looking to the future. *Canadian Psychology/Psychologie canadienne, 58*(1), 20–29.

Substance Abuse and Mental Health Services Administration (2015). *Racial/ethnic differences in mental health service use among adults*. HHS Publication No. SMA-15-4906. Rockville, MD.

Sue, D. W., Bernier, J. E., Durran, A., Feinberg, L., Pederson, P., Smith, E. J., & Vasquez-Nuttall, E. (1982). Position paper: Cross cultural counseling competencies. *The Counseling Psychologist, 10*, 45–52. doi:10.1177/0011000082102008

Sue, D. W, Capodilupo, C. M., & Holder, A. M. B. (2008). Racial microaggressions in the life experience of Black Americans. *Professional Psychology: Research and Practice, 39 (3),* 329–336.

Sue, D. W., & Sue, D. (2003). Counseling the culturally diverse: Theory and practice. New York, NY: Wiley.

Suite, D. H., La Bril, R., Primm, A., & Harrison-Ross, P. (2007). Beyond misdiagnosis, misunderstanding and mistrust: relevance of the historical perspective in the medical and mental health treatment of people of color. *Journal of the National Medical Association, 99*(8), 879–885.

Takeuchi, D. T., & Cheung, M. K. (1998). Coercive and voluntary referrals: How ethnic minority adults get into mental health treatment. *Ethnicity and Health, 3,* 149–158.

Terrell, F., & Terrell, S. (1981). An inventory to measure cultural mistrust among Blacks. *The Western Journal of Black Studies, 5*(3), 180–185.

Terrell, F., & Terrell, S. (1984). Race of counselor, client sex, cultural mistrust level, and premature termination from counseling among Black clients. *Journal of Counseling Psychology, 31,* 371–375.

Thompson, V. L. S., Bazile, A., & Akbar, M. (2004). African Americans' perceptions of psychotherapy and psychotherapists. *Professional Psychology: Research and Practice, 35*(1), 19–26.

Townes, D. L., Chavez-Korell, S., & Cunningham, N. J. (2009). Reexamining the relationships between racial identity, cultural mistrust, help-seeking attitudes, and preference for a Black counselor. *Journal of Counseling Psychology, 56*(2), 330–336.

Turner, E. A., Jensen-Doss, A., & Heffer, R. W. (2015). Ethnicity as a moderator of how parents' attitudes and perceived stigma influence intentions to seek child mental health services. *Cultural Diversity and Ethnic Minority Psychology, 21*(4), 613–618.

Turner, E. A., & Mills, C. (2016). Culturally relevant diagnosis and assessment of mental illness. In A. Breland-Noble, C. Al-Mateen, & N. Singh (Eds.), *Handbook of Mental Health in African American Youth* (pp. 21–35). New York, NY: Springer.

Turner, E. A., Camarillo, J., Daniel, S., Otero, J., & Parker, A. (2017) Correlates of psychotherapy use among ethnically diverse college students. *Journal of College Student Development, 58*(2), 300–307.

Turner, E. A., Cheng, H., Llamas, J., Tran, A. T., Hill, K., Fretts, J. M., & Mercado, A. (2016). Factors impacting the current trends in the use of outpatient psychiatric treatment among diverse ethnic groups. *Current Psychiatry Reviews, 12*(2), 199–220.

U.S. Department of Health and Human Services. (2001). *Mental health: Culture, race, and ethnicity (a supplement to Mental health: A report of the surgeon general).* Rockville, MD.

Vasquez, M. J. (2012). Psychology and social justice: Why we do what we do. *American Psychologist, 67*(5), 337–346.

Villatoro, A. P., & Aneshensel, C. S. (2014). Family influences on the use of mental health services among African Americans. *Journal of Health and Social Behavior, 55*(2), 161–180.

Watkins, C. E., Jr., & Terrell, F. (1988). Mistrust level and its effects on counseling expectations in Black client–White counselor relationships: An analogue study. *Journal of Counseling Psychology, 35* (2), 194–197.

Weiss, M. (1997). Explanatory Model Interview Catalogue (EMIC): framework for comparative study of illness. *Transcultural Psychiatry, 34*(2), 235–263.

Whaley, A. L. (1997). Ethnicity/race, paranoia, and psychiatric diagnoses: Clinician bias versus sociocultural differences. *Journal of Psychopathology and Behavioral Assessment, 19,* 1–20.

Whaley, A. L. (2001a). Cultural mistrust of White mental health clinicians among African Americans with severe mental illness. *American Journal of Orthopsychiatry, 71,* 252–256.

Whaley, A. L. (2001b). Cultural Mistrust: An important psychological construct for diagnosis and treatment of African Americans. *Professional Psychology: Research and Practice, 32*(6), 555–562.

Williams, M. T., Kanter, J. W., & Ching, T. H. W. (2018). Anxiety, stress, and trauma symptoms in African Americans: Negative affectivity does not explain the relationship between microaggressions and psychopathology. *Journal of Racial and Ethnic Health Disparities, 5*(5), 919–27. doi:10.1007/s40615-017-0440-3.

Williams, M. T., Malcoun, E., Sawyer, B. A., Davis, D. M., Nouri, L. B., & Bruce, S. L. (2014). Cultural adaptations of prolonged exposure therapy for treatment and prevention of posttraumatic stress disorder in African Americans. *Behavioral Sciences, 4*(2), 102–124.

Williams, S. L. L. (2014). Mental health service use among African-American emerging adults, by provider type and recency of use. *Psychiatric Services, 65*(10), 1249–1255.

Womack, Y. L. (2010). *Post Black: How a new generation is redefining African American identity.* Chicago, IL: Lawrence Hill Books.

CHAPTER 3

The Science of Clinician Biases
and (Mis)Behavior

John F. Dovidio,
Yale University

Ava T. Casados,
Yale University

Previous chapters in this volume have described the problem of minority exclusion from mental health treatment outcome research studies and reviewed the literature concerning why some communities of color mistrust clinical care. In part as a consequence of such concerns, members of traditionally disadvantaged groups, particularly Black and Latinx individuals, are less likely to utilize psychological services available to them and are more likely than are White persons to delay seeking mental health treatment (Jackson, Knight, & Rafferty, 2010). Greater mistrust of mental health clinicians is based, in part, in negative historical treatment of such groups by the health care community generally (Byrd & Clayton, 2002) or with the generalization of everyday experiences of discrimination to health care settings (Penner et al., 2009). However, some of the mistrust and suspicion experienced by members of these groups is rooted in the behavior (or misbehavior) of mental health professionals specifically in clinical settings (Thompson, Bazile, & Akbar, 2004).

This chapter provides a contextual psychological perspective on the intrapersonal variables that influence clinical behavior and prevent the formation of effective therapeutic relationships and culturally responsive care. These processes can adversely affect the quality of mental health care that members of racial and ethnic minority groups receive relative to members of the social majority group—in the United States, White Americans.

In the next section, we review racial and ethnic disparities in two main aspects of mental health care, assessment and treatment. After that, we consider evidence of the role of personal biases of health care professionals generally and the effects of these biases on treatment, proposing the need for more direct investigation of such effects specifically among mental health professionals. We then discuss how understanding the influences these biases may have on clinical interactions can provide insight into why members of racial and ethnic minority groups remain underserved with respect to mental health care.

Racial and Ethnic Disparities in Psychological Assessment and Intervention

Research on the quality of mental health care has revealed systematic disparities in access, use, and quality of care across racial and ethnic groups. Two comprehensive reports, *Mental Health: A Report of the Surgeon General* (US Department of Health and Human Services, 1999) and *Mental Health: Culture, Race, and Ethnicity* (US Department of Health and Human Services, 2001) noted that members of traditionally disadvantaged racial and ethnic groups have less access to mental health services than do Whites, are less likely to receive the care they need, and receive poorer quality of care when treated. Moreover, little progress has been made toward eliminating disparities in mental health care since those reports (Miranda, McGuire, Williams, & Wang, 2008).

Racial and ethnic biases of clinical psychologists and other mental health professionals can affect the quality of care that members of racial and ethnic minorities receive at a number of key stages of clinical treatment. In this section, we first discuss how racial and ethnic bias can enter into clinical judgments made in both psychodiagnostic and neuropsychological assessment, and then we review racial and ethnic disparities in treatment planning and service delivery.

Disparities and Bias in Assessment

When an individual seeks or is first referred into clinical care, certain characteristics of both the patient and the clinician can affect how the patient's symptoms will be interpreted. Although disparities based on race or ethnicity can, and often do, have multiple causes, clinician bias may be one contributor. Even well-meaning clinicians may be vulnerable to bias when tasked with assessing and clarifying the often complex and nuanced psychological profiles their clients present.

PSYCHODIAGNOSTIC ASSESSMENT

Establishing a diagnosis is often the first priority of most clinicians, and this process may also be one of the first sources of race- and ethnicity-related mental health service disparities. Clinical bias can result in both the underdiagnosis of some disorders and overdiagnosis of other disorders for ethnic minority patients. Black, Latinx, and Asian patients are all less likely than White patients to have their depression detected or diagnosed (Hahm, Cook, Ault-Brutus, & Alegría, 2015). These findings persist even when controlling for symptom severity and level of functioning, indicating that some other feature of the patient's presentation must be influencing clinician judgments (Gallo, Bogner, Morales, & Ford, 2005). Even when Black psychiatric patients are rated as having equally significant affective symptoms as White patients in race-blind ratings, Black patients are less likely to receive a mood disorder diagnosis (Gara et al., 2012). At the same time, ethnic minorities, and Black individuals especially, are disproportionately likely to receive a diagnosis of schizophrenia (Fearon et al., 2006; Neighbors, Trierweiler, Ford, & Muroff, 2003). While Black patients' mood symptoms appear to be under-weighted, their psychotic symptoms may be over-weighted relative to individuals from other groups.

The exact reason for these discrepancies is unclear. On one hand, there may be true differences in the prevalence rates of certain symptoms. On the other hand, it is also possible that many clinicians are not prepared to assess—or accept—the symptoms that their ethnic minority patients present, relying instead on racial stereotypes when evaluating these patients (Rosenthal, 2004). Both the manifestation of symptoms and the language used to describe symptoms can vary across racial and ethnic groups, so clinicians who are not specifically trained to identify the mental health needs of ethnic minority patients may have trouble accurately assessing culture-specific symptom profiles (Alegría & McGuire, 2003). Clinicians' use of standardized symptom checklists may also produce a source of bias, because the language used and symptoms included in these measures may not align with the typical experiences of ethnic minority patients (e.g., Williams, Turkheimer, Schmidt, & Oltmanns, 2005; Williams, Turkheimer, Magee, & Guterbock, 2008). In the case of Black patients, clinicians may also be less prone to trust their patients' descriptions of their own symptoms. Clinician distrust or suspicion surrounding Black patients' ability to recognize and accurately report their own symptoms may explain some of the aforementioned disparities in mood and schizophrenia diagnoses among Black patients (Eack, Bahorik, Newhill, Neighbors, & Davis, 2012).

Notably, differences in symptom perception are related to clinician race as well as patient race. Black clinicians are more likely to perceive Black patients' negative symptoms (e.g., blunt affect, apathy) as indicative of mood disorder, while non-Black clinicians are more likely to perceive those negative symptoms as indicative of a psychotic disorder (Gara et al., 2012; Trierweiler et al., 2006). These findings suggest that clinicians themselves, and their own culturally based perspectives, may be a source of bias when it comes to making psychodiagnostic assessments.

NEUROPSYCHOLOGICAL ASSESSMENT

Race-based bias can also influence the process of neuropsychological assessment, and the results of these biased assessments can have significant ramifications on educational, psychological, and forensic outcomes. There is consistent, substantive evidence that many of the instruments and procedures used in neuropsychological assessment may be culturally biased and do not have "acceptable diagnostic accuracy" within ethnic minority populations (see Manly 2008; Reynolds & Suzuki, 2013). Black and Latinx individuals tend to perform lower than Whites on measures of intelligence and cognitive ability, and are disproportionately diagnosed with cognitive impairment (e.g., Jencks & Phillips, 1998).

Whether or not any individual test is biased, however, it is also possible that clinicians may themselves be contributing to disparities in assessment and diagnosis. Bias can emerge even before testing begins if clinicians select instruments or batteries that are inappropriate for their patients. For example, test language and degree of English profi-ciency impact IQ scores for Latinx children and Alzheimer's detection for Latinx older adults, but when working with bilingual patients, most clinicians use the standard English version of tests or, occasionally, non-validated Spanish verbatim translations. They will rarely use the more appropriate published Spanish tests (Echemendia & Harris, 2004). As with the problem with standardized symptom checklists for psychodiagnostic assess-ment (see Williams et al., 2005, 2008), it is possible that clinicians, perhaps in a genuine attempt to be colorblind in their treatment, may choose particular, commonly used stan-dardized tests that may be less accurate in neurological assessments of non-White, com-pared to White, patients.

Racial and ethnic stereotypes, activated on the part of both clinicians and patients, may also substantially affect the validity of the results of neuropsychological assessment. Personal stereotypes of a social group could lead clinicians to differentially interpret ambiguous test responses. Patients' awareness of negative stereotypes of their group in the domain in which they are being tested (e.g., IQ), even though they do not personally endorse the stereotype, can adversely affect their performance through the experience of stereotype threat. Stereotype threat occurs when a situation makes negative stereotypes of one's group salient, and there is awareness that one's performance will confirm those stereotypes (Steele, 2010). Stereotype threat creates anxiety and cognitive interference that erode performance. Such possibilities are, at this point, plausible but hypothetical, and more research is needed in order to understand the scope and implications of clini-cian bias in both neuropsychological and psychodiagnostic assessment.

Disparities and Bias in Treatment Planning and Service Delivery

Bias in assessment can result in corresponding disparities in treatment planning and service delivery. Just as certain racial or ethnic groups are less likely to have their depres-sion detected, they are also less likely to have their depression appropriately treated (Hahm et al., 2015). Even in the absence of observable bias at the assessment level, however, bias can emerge in other stages of care. Black and Latinx patients are signifi-cantly less likely than Whites to receive minimally adequate care, and these disparities in treatment quality persist even when diagnostic differences are removed (Alegría et al., 2008; Stockdale, Lagomasino, Siddique, McGuire, & Miranda, 2008).

One stark example of unequal treatment is the disproportionate rate of psychiatric medication prescribed by clinicians. Compared to White patients, Black and Latinx patients are significantly less likely to receive psychiatric medications, and when medica-tions are prescribed, Black patients are less likely to receive the most effective medica-tions for their condition (González et al., 2008; McGuire & Miranda, 2008). Although symptom severity is correlated with antidepressant use for White Americans, no such association was found for Black Americans (González et al., 2008).

These discrepancies may be due in part to structural issues (e.g., medication costs) or reluctance on the part of Black patients to use medication; however, the differences emerge not only at the treatment adherence level but also earlier, at the treatment recommendation and prescription level. Clinician biases or stereotypes of Black patients, whether explicit or implicit, may influence the types of treatment they select for these patients. In the domain of medical treatment, for example, doctors' and medical students' beliefs that Black patients experience less pain than do White patients substantially explained the less effective pain treatment they prescribed for Black, compared to White, patients (Hoffman, Trawalter, Axt, & Oliver, 2016). In mental health treatment, the documented minimization of Black depressive symptoms by White clinicians (Gara et al., 2012), for example, may be leading clinicians to view Black patients as less in need of antidepressants relative to White patients.

In addition to receiving lower quality or less appropriate services, patients from racial or ethnic minority groups often experience negative treatment in the form of racial microaggressions, which are everyday subtle and often automatic insults directed toward members of racial and ethnic minority groups (Pierce, 1970; Sue et al., 2007) by mental health providers (Ridley, 2005). Emphasis on race- or ethnicity-based stereotypes in therapy discussions, even when mentioned without ill-will or explicit prejudice, may have a serious impact on the comfort and trust patients feel (see Sue et al., 2007). As Sue et al. (2007) note, the power dynamics between clinician and patient are such that patients are generally unable to directly confront clinician microaggresions. These misbehaviors on the part of clinicians may therefore serve as a distraction, offense, or even as a barrier to continued treatment.

Clinician Bias: Explicit and Implicit

Despite the evidence of disparities in assessment, treatment planning, and service, which appears to implicate clinician bias, the literature directly linking the personal prejudices of individual clinicians to their treatment of patients is surprisingly limited. The paucity of literature on this particular topic could suggest that clinicians' racial and ethnic attitudes do not actually influence their clinical practice. However, there is a growing body of literature relating to physical health care professionals that suggests that further examination of mental health professionals' personal biases may account, at least in part, for racial and ethnic disparities in assessment and treatment. The provocative findings of clinician bias in physical health care suggests that this is a particularly promising area for understanding the dynamics or racial and ethnic disparities in mental health care, implicating the role of biases among clinical psychologists and therapists, at least in part, in these outcomes.

The literature on the biases of medical professionals draws upon the fundamental distinction in the social psychological literature between explicit and implicit biases (for a review, see Dovidio, Schellhaas, & Pearson, 2018). Explicit biases are consciously held and overtly expressed attitudes toward a group (e.g., racial or ethnic minority groups) and its members. These explicit biases have traditionally been assessed with self-reported measures of racial or ethnic prejudice. In addition to explicit prejudices, people may harbor racial and ethnic biases implicitly, often unconsciously. Implicit biases, which are automatically activated responses that occur often without conscious awareness, tend to form from repeated exposure to positive or negative information about a group, either through socialization or direct experience, and can be resistant to change in response to new information. Currently, implicit biases are most commonly measured using the Implicit Association Test (IAT; Greenwald, Poehlman, Uhlmann, & Banaji, 2009).

People higher in education, socioeconomic status, and in occupations representative of helping professions tend to exhibit relatively low levels of explicit bias (Sidanius & Pratto, 1999). However, because implicit attitudes may form through general socialization experiences and without intention, even highly educated individuals in helping professions, such as medicine and clinical psychology, may exhibit systematic implicit racial and ethnic bias (Kuppens & Spears, 2014). Indeed, in the medical domain, there is evidence that, on average, although they appear low in prejudice explicitly, physicians and nurses harbor significant implicit biases, and at a level comparable to the general public (Sabin, Nosek, Greenwald, & Rivara, 2009). For example, physicians harbor implicit stereotypes of Blacks as less compliant, less trustworthy patients, and as more likely than Whites to engage in risky behaviors (Moskowitz et al., 2011).

There is only limited evidence that medical practitioners' explicit biases lead to lower-quality care for racial and ethnic minorities than for Whites or less motivation to involve the patient in medical decision making (Penner, Phelan, Earnshaw, Albrecht, & Dovidio, 2018). One reason is that when people are aware of their own bias, they can readily inhibit its expression in contexts where they perceive differential treatment as inappropriate. Health care is obviously one such context. By contrast, because people are often unaware of their implicit biases, which are automatically activated, the implicit biases of medical care professionals do play a significant role in the quality of care racial and ethnic minority patients receive.

In their review of the literature on medical care, Hall et al. (2015; see also Dehon et al., 2017) reported that in approximately 20 percent of the studies they reviewed, physicians higher in implicit bias recommended less effective treatments to racial and ethnic minority patients (see also Sabin & Greenwald, 2012). Although physicians offered treatments of comparable quality in over 80 percent of the cases, the systematic nature of the physician bias in care can have long-term cumulative negative effects on the health of racial and ethnic minorities. In over 40 percent of studies reviewed concerning the quality of the medical interactions between physicians and patients, the quality of communication and the degree of rapport with racial and ethnic minority patients were lower when the physician was higher in implicit bias. One reason for this greater impact is that physician implicit bias is manifested in subtle verbal, nonverbal, and paraverbal behaviors, which often occur spontaneously, that affect the quality of communication (Dovidio & LaFrance, 2013), and consequently interpersonal perceptions, in medical interactions with racial or ethnic minority patients (for a review, see Penner et al., 2018). For example,

Cooper et al. (2012), who analyzed physician-patient interactions, reported that physicians higher in implicit racial bias had shorter visits, spoke less and faster, and were less patient-centered with their Black patients (see also Penner et al., 2016).

In addition, racial and ethnic minority patients detect these physician behaviors associated with implicit racial bias and react negatively (Cooper et al., 2012; Penner et al., 2013). One study of medical interactions (Blair et al., 2013), for example, found that Black patients viewed more implicitly racially biased physicians as being lower in patient centeredness. However, the comparable effect was not significant for Latinx patients. Black patients also perceive physicians higher in implicit bias as less trustworthy, and they experience less satisfaction in their medical interactions with them. Lower levels of patient satisfaction and trust in their physician predict, in turn, less adherence to physicians' recommendations, less likelihood of returning for further treatment, and, ultimately, more subsequent health problems for patients. In addition, Black patients with physicians higher in implicit bias are more hesitant to pursue treatments recommended by the physician, even when the recommended treatment is for a life-threatening condition (e.g., for cancer; Penner et al., 2016).

Unfortunately, little parallel research has been conducted for mental health professionals specifically (Boysen, 2010). Peris, Teachman, and Nosek (2008) compared the explicit and implicit attitudes of almost seven hundred clinical psychology graduate students and professional mental health clinicians to members of the general public and individuals involved in other health or social service professions. These authors, however, did not examine participants' racial or ethnic biases; instead, they studied biases toward "mentally ill" people. Overall, participants involved in mental health training or practice displayed the least negative explicit and implicit attitudes toward people with mental illness. Moreover, both the level of explicit and implicit biases of the mental health sample had significant effect on mental health treatment outcomes (based on vignettes), but in different ways. Graduate students and professional clinicians higher in explicit bias had more negative prognoses of patients displaying signs of mental illness; those higher in implicit bias tended to attribute greater mental illness to the patient, overdiagnosing the symptoms. Peris et al. (2008) concluded that explicit and implicit attitudes can uniquely relate to clinical biases, and thus both types of attitudes need to be considered for understanding the effects of clinician stigma or prejudice.

A meta-analysis of implicit attitudes in health care professionals by FitzGerald and Hurst (2017) further suggests the relevance of work on bias in medical care to clinical treatment for mental health. These researchers found similar effects for the implicit biases of mental health professionals as for those in medical care. Over two-thirds of the studies investigated implicit racial bias, but those that examined other forms of implicit bias (e.g., based on weight or disability) showed similar results. Overall, FitzGerald and Hurst found that across the range of areas of practice, health care professionals display levels of implicit bias similar to those exhibited by the general public and that implicit bias systematically relates to the quality of care provided by the health care professions. Specifically, the authors concluded that the influence of implicit bias "was evident either in the diagnosis, the treatment recommendations, the number of questions asked of the patient, the number of tests ordered, or other responses indicating bias against the characteristic of the patient under examination" (FitzGerald & Hurst, 2017, p. 13).

Implications of Clinicians' Implicit Bias

In this section, drawing on the evidence of racial and ethnic disparities and potential biases in health care, we identify both practical and research implications for both patients and mental health clinicians. Based on the research showing that when physicians are higher in implicit bias, Black patients perceive them as less trustworthy and their medical care as less satisfactory (see Dovidio, Penner, & Pachankis, 2016), future research in mental health care might thus investigate not only the degree to which clinicians' explicit and implicit prejudices affect their behavior toward racial and ethnic minority patients but also the way patients experience their therapeutic interactions. Effective treatment in clinical psychology, like effective medical care, requires the trust of an individual to seek and continue care. However, members of the racial and ethnic minority groups similarly display mistrust and have concerns about the quality of mental health care they receive. For example, many Blacks display general mistrust for psychotherapy and psychotherapists and believe that psychologists are insensitive to the Black experience, which may reduce their motivation to seek psychological assistance (Thompson et al., 2004). Several studies have found that Blacks are more trusting of a therapist of the same race than of a different race and evaluate the care they receive from a clinician of their own race more positively than the quality of care from a therapist of a different race (for a review, see Cabral & Smith, 2011).

This mistrust of the mental health community (Whaley, 2001) has a range of detrimental effects on racial and ethnic minorities. As noted earlier, members of traditionally disadvantaged groups, particularly Black and Latinx individuals, are less likely to utilize psychological services available to them and are more likely than Whites to delay or fail to seek mental health treatment, in part because of greater mistrust of the mental health community (Masuda, Anderson, & Edmonds, 2012). For example, Blacks are less likely to seek psychological treatment and complete treatment for depression than Whites (Fortuna, Alegría, & Gao, 2010), and Latinxs are less likely to seek psychological services for depression than Blacks (Nadeem et al., 2007).

The greater mistrust exhibited by members of racial and ethnic minority groups, particularly Blacks and Native Americans, has been attributed to historical trauma related to systematic, unethical mistreatment by the medical community (e.g., the Tuskeegee syphilis research; Byrd & Clayton, 2002). Another explanation is that racial and ethnic minority individuals may generalize from their everyday experiences with discrimination in other spheres of life (Penner et al., 2009). We propose another potential contributor, and a direction for future research: we recommend that future research focus as well on the degree to which experiences with clinicians who are explicitly or implicitly biased contribute directly to these perceptions and responses of racial and ethnic minorities in need of psychological assistance.

Another important direction for future research might further address how clinicians' concerns about subtly expressing bias affect their clinical treatment of racial and ethnic minority patients. For instance, even though people may not be fully aware of their implicit racial or ethnic biases, people who are higher in implicit bias often express greater concern about acting inappropriately with racial and ethnic biases (Perry, Murphy, & Dovidio, 2015). These concerns, which are associated with greater feelings of intergroup anxiety, can affect both whether and how clinicians engage in therapeutic interactions with racial and ethnic minority patients. Just as calling attention to a patient's race or ethnicity in a stereotyped way may be damaging to the therapeutic relationship, being overly anxious about avoiding offense may also have a deleterious effect.

Intergroup anxiety relates to the decisions people make about engaging with members of another group, both informally and formally. Greater experience of interracial anxiety leads people at an interpersonal level to avoid interactions with members of the other group (Plant & Devine, 2003). Professionally, medical students who have greater concerns about appearing biased and who consequently experience higher levels of intergroup anxiety are less motivated to practice medicine with underserved populations (Perry, Dovidio, Murphy, & van Ryn, 2015). Thus, the attitudes, both explicit and implicit, of mental health professionals can affect the accessibility of mental health services to members of racial and ethnic minority groups.

Concerns about appearing biased can also interfere with the effectiveness of communication between a therapist and a patient. People who have such concerns focus more strongly on how they appear to others rather than on being attuned to the interest and needs of minority-group members with whom they are interacting (Migacheva & Tropp, 2013). This self-focused orientation interferes with the development of perspective taking and empathy, key elements in forming a therapeutic bond with a patient (Moyers & Miller, 2013). Individuals who are self-focused and anxious display less fluent communicative behavior (Pearson & Dovidio, 2014), which impedes the development of rapport and trust. Moreover, when racial or ethnic minority individuals anticipate experiencing bias (as has historically occurred in health care settings), they tend to interpret disfluent behavior as an indication that others hold negative attitudes toward them and their group (Shelton, Dovidio, Hebl, & Richeson, 2009). These attributions confirm general feelings of mistrust and undermine the effectiveness of therapy.

Another potential consequence—one meriting further systematic study—of clinicians experiencing intergroup anxiety due to insecurities about their own cultural competence or abilities to appear unbiased is that clinicians may be hesitant to acknowledge cultural differences between themselves and their patients, adopting a "colorblind" strategy in their clinical interactions and treatment. A colorblind interpersonal strategy involves acting in a way that attempts to minimize the salience of race or ethnicity in these interactions. This orientation involves attempts to deny the possibility that one could be acting in a racially biased way in these interactions, because the minority partner's "color" is perceived to be irrelevant. However, in medical care, attempts of physicians to be colorblind may actually exacerbate racial mistrust and impair the quality of medical interactions with Black patients (Penner & Dovidio, 2016). In clinical treatment for mental health, beyond its negative impact on the relationship between a clinician and patient, colorblindness can directly undermine the quality of treatment, for example, by limiting the extent to which a clinician will probe about the patient's own cultural experiences (see Terwilliger, Bach, Bryan, & Williams, 2013). As Williams (2011) explained, in psychotherapy "such an approach hinders the exploration of conflicts related to race, ethnicity, and culture. The therapist doesn't see the whole picture.... This approach ignores the incredibly salient experience of being stigmatized by society and represents an empathetic failure on the part of the therapist. Colorblindness does not foster equality or respect; it merely relieves the therapist of his or her obligation to address important racial differences and difficulties."

Discussion of race and ethnicity is considered a necessary component of treatment with racial and ethnic minority patients (see Cardemil & Battle, 2003). Failure to initiate these types of conversations can impact mental health care in at least three specific ways, which have important practical therapeutic implications and merit further research. First, it can impede the clinician's ability to gain a full understanding of their patient's social stressors or strengths or of how the patient is functioning within the relevant social systems in which they operate (Lakes, López, and Garro, 2006). Without these conversations, a clinician may also be unable to identify culture-specific manifestations of symptomology necessary to developing a thorough case formulation (Mezzich, Caracci, Fabrega, & Kirmayer, 2009). Limited knowledge or appreciation for the patient's own cultural norms and social context can thus affect diagnosis and treatment planning.

Second, the overall ability of clinicians to listen to and validate their patients' perspectives and experiences is important in promoting a positive therapeutic relationship. Clinician displays of respect, interest, exploration, accurate interpretation, and attendance of patient experiences are directly related to the strength of alliance between clinician and patient (Ackerman & Hilsenroth, 2003). Acknowledgment of a patient's racial, ethnic, or cultural identity plays a critical role in conveying this respect; exhibiting instead a colorblind perspective, which actively avoids acknowledgment of race or ethnicity, is often perceived by members of racial and ethnic minority groups as disrespectful and interpreted as a clinical microaggression (Sue et al., 2007) or as overt evidence of racial or ethnic prejudice (Apfelbaum, Norton, & Sommers, 2012). There is a vast research literature establishing that therapeutic alliance is consistently associated with patients' continued treatment engagement and positive clinical outcomes (e.g., Priebe & McCabe, 2006).

Third, when clinicians adopt a colorblind perspective in their interactions with racial or ethnic minority patients, they are likely to provide lower-quality care.

Employing a "colorblind" approach to therapy is associated with lower levels of clinician empathy and higher rates of clinicians attributing personal responsibility to Black patients (Burkard & Knox, 2004). Disregarding a patient's racial or ethnic background also thwarts the possibility of providing the most culturally appropriate services. Group- and culturally tailored adaptations can often be readily made to evidence-based treatments to enhance outcomes for ethnic minority patients (Huey, Tilley, Jones, & Smith, 2014), but such treatment decisions rely on clinicians' willingness to acknowledge and incorporate a patient's racial or ethnic background in treatment planning and delivery. The overall quality of care for racial and ethnic minority patients may be compromised when clinicians feel that they are not culturally competent or are concerned and anxious about appearing racially or ethnically biased.

Conclusion

Subtle and typically unintentional biases of clinicians can prevent the formation of effective therapeutic relationships and culturally responsive care and can ultimately adversely affect the quality of mental health care that members of racial and ethnic minority groups experience. We reviewed evidence of the role of personal biases of health care professionals generally and the effects of these biases on treatment, identifying implications for practice and directions for future research.

Table 1 highlights six key points developed in this chapter, reflecting what is currently known about clinician bias and highlighting productive avenues for future research. There is clear documentation of the existence of disparities, but the reason for disparities and the part that clinicians may be playing are still far from clear. Systematic racial and ethnic disparities in mental health treatment implicate clinician bias (points 1 and 2 in the column Clinician Bias Findings in table 1). Clinicians who may appear relatively unprejudiced on explicit measures and believe that they are unbiased are likely to still harbor implicit, unconscious negative attitudes and stereotypes, which can adversely affect their interactions with patients and the quality of care they provide (points 3, 4, and 5). Moreover, in an effort to reassert their nonbiased self-concept, clinicians may adopt a colorblind strategy, which limits their ability to understand the particular stressors that members of underrepresented racial and ethnic groups experience (point 6).

Recognizing potential clinician biases, the various ways it may manifest, and the consequences it can have in psychotherapy can help guide new strategies, training, and interventions to ensure high quality, equitable mental health care across members of different racial and ethnic groups. As illustrated in table 1 (in the Potential Interventions column), these new initiatives may involve greater awareness of potential clinician bias in clinical training and assessment (points 1, 2, and 3), as well as in a more vigorous research focus on the effects of implicit bias, subtle and unintentional expressions of clinician bias, and, ultimately, on ways to combat the negative effects of bias in clinical treatment (points 4, 5, and 6). Particularly when viewed in the context of the rapidly expanding literature on medical provider bias in physical health care, aggressively pursuing a research agenda illuminating the science of clinician bias and (mis)behavior is timely and critical for ensuring equitable mental treatment in an increasingly diverse society.

Table 1. Key Findings, Points, and Conclusions

Clinician Bias Findings	Potential Interventions
1. Systematic racial and ethnic disparities, which implicate clinician bias, appear in both the psychodiagnostic and neuropsychological assessment of racial and ethnic minority clients.	*1. Appropriate measures and norming standards should be developed for use with ethnic minority populations.*
2. Even when controlling for differences in assessment, racial and ethnic minority clients tend to receive less effective mental health care and are less likely to receive medications that can alleviate their conditions than do White clients.	*2. Clinician awareness regarding treatment disparities can be improved. Further research is needed to determine which biases or stereotypes might be most impacting treatment practices.*
3. Health care workers, in general, often display less racial and ethnic prejudice explicitly but harbor implicit racial and ethnic biases at a level comparable to the general public.	*3. Clinicians should receive training about the role of implicit bias in treatment, with emphasis on tools to proactively address implicit bias.*
4. Despite a growing literature that directly documents the adverse effects of bias, particularly implicit biases, among medical professionals on the quality of medical treatment and the effectiveness of physician-patient interaction, there is a paucity of similar work on clinician explicit or implicit bias on mental health care.	*4. Lines of research matching and elaborating on those existent in medical treatment bias should be developed for the study of mental health treatment bias.*
5. Clinician implicit bias, like physician bias, can potentially undermine the trust, confidence, and satisfaction of racial and ethnic minority clients.	*5. As the above-mentioned line of research evolves, corresponding tools to combat the negative effects of bias can be developed.*
6. Clinician concerns about appearing biased can increase intergroup anxiety and lead to less effective approaches to therapy with racial and ethnic minority clients, such as adopting a colorblind perspective, that can impede the clinician's ability to gain a full understanding of their patient's social stressors, strengths, and culture-specific manifestations of symptomology.	*6. Education about the risks of "colorblind" therapy should be provided in training programs; alternative approaches that emphasize increased contact and open communication with ethnic minority patient populations should be developed and integrated into practice.*

KEY POINTS FOR CLINICIANS

- Bias against racial and ethnic minority clients is found in diagnostic determinations and neuropsychological assessments, and standards should be developed to address these biases.

- Racial and ethnic minority clients receive less effective mental health and psychiatric care, and improved clinician awareness of these processes is needed.

- Health care workers display implicit biases at the level of the general public and effective bias-reduction training interventions are needed.

- Less is known about implicit bias in mental health care specifically, and more research is needed.

References

Ackerman, S. J., & Hilsenroth, M. J. (2003). A review of therapist characteristics and techniques positively impacting the therapeutic alliance. *Clinical Psychology Review, 23*, 1–33.

Alegría, M., Canino, G., Shrout, P. E., Woo, M., Duan, N., Vila, D., … & Meng, X. L. (2008). Prevalence of mental illness in immigrant and non-immigrant US Latino groups. *The American Journal of Psychiatry, 165*, 359–369.

Alegría, M., & McGuire, T. (2003). Rethinking a universal framework in the psychiatric symptom-disorder relationship. *Journal of Health and Social Behavior, 44*, 257–274.

Apfelbaum, E. P., Norton, M. I., & Sommers, S. R. (2012). Racial color blindness: Emergence, practice, and implications. *Current Directions in Psychological Science, 21*, 205–209.

Blair, I. V., Steiner, J. F., Fairclough, D. L., Hanratty, R., Price, D. W., Hirsh, H. K., … & Havranek, E. P. (2013). Clinicians' implicit ethnic/racial bias and perceptions of care among Black and Latino patients. *Annals of Family Medicine, 11*(1), 43–52.

Boysen, G. A. (2010). Integrating implicit bias into counselor education. *Counselor Education and Supervision, 49*, 210–227.

Burkard, A. W., & Knox, S. (2004). Effect of therapist colorblindness on empathy and attributions in cross-cultural counseling. *Journal of Counseling Psychology, 51*, 387–397.

Byrd, W. M., & Clayton, L. A. (2002). *An American health dilemma: A medical history of African Americans and the problem of race*. New York, NY: Routledge.

Cabral, R. R., & Smith, T. B. (2011). Racial/ethnic matching of clients and therapists in mental health services: A meta-analytic review of preferences, perceptions, and outcomes. *Journal of Counseling Psychology, 58*, 537–554.

Cardemil, E. V., & Battle, C. L. (2003). Guess who's coming to therapy? Getting comfortable with conversations about race and ethnicity in psychotherapy. *Professional Psychology: Research and Practice, 34*, 278–286.

Cooper, L. A., Roter, D. L., Carson, K. A., Beach, M. C., Sabin, J. A., Greenwald, A. G., & Inui, T. S. (2012). The associations of clinicians' implicit attitudes about race with medical visit communication and patient ratings of interpersonal care. *American Journal of Public Health, 102*, 979–987.

Dehon, E., Weiss, N., Jones, J., Faulconer, W., Hinton, E., & Sterling, S. (2017). A systematic review of the impact of physician implicit racial bias on clinical decision making. *Academic Emergency Medicine, 24*, 895–904.

Dovidio, J. F., & LaFrance, M. (2013). Race, ethnicity, and nonverbal behavior. In J. A. Hall & M. Knapp (Eds.), *Nonverbal communication* (pp. 671–696). The Hague, Netherlands: DeGruyter -Mouton.

Dovidio, J. F., Penner, L. A., & Pachankis, J. E. (2016). Promoting diversity and inclusiveness. In J. C. Norcross, G. R. VandenBos, D. K. Freedheim, & N. Pole (Eds.), *APA handbook of clinical psychology* (Vol. 4, pp. 583–596). Washington, DC: American Psychological Association.

Dovidio, J. F., Schellhaas, F. M. H., & Pearson, A. R. (2018). The role of attitudes in intergroup relations. In D. Albarracín, & B. T. Johnson (Eds.), *The handbook of attitudes* (pp. 419–354). New York, NY: Psychology Press.

Eack, S. M., Bahorik, A. L., Newhill, C. E., Neighbors, H. W., & Davis, L. E. (2012). Interviewer-perceived honesty as a mediator of racial disparities in the diagnosis of schizophrenia. *Psychiatric Services, 63*, 875–880.

Echemendia, R. J., & Harris, J. G. (2004). Neuropsychological test use with Hispanic/Latin populations in the United States: Part II of a national survey. *Applied Neuropsychology, 11*, 4–12.

Fearon, P., Kirkbride, J. B., Morgan, C., Dazzan, P., Morgan, K., Lloyd, T., ... & Mallett, R. (2006). Incidence of schizophrenia and other psychoses in ethnic minority groups: Results from the MRC AESOP Study. *Psychological Medicine, 36*, 1541–1550.

FitzGerald, C., & Hurst, S. (2017). Implicit bias in healthcare professionals: A systematic review. *BMC Medical Ethics, 18*, 19, https://doi.org/10.1186/s12910-017-0179-8

Fortuna, L. R., Alegría, M., & Gao, S. (2010). Retention in depression treatment among ethnic and racial minority groups in the United States. *Depression and Anxiety, 27*, 485–494.

Gallo, J. J., Bogner, H. R., Morales, K. H., & Ford, D. E. (2005). Patient ethnicity and the identification and active management of depression in late life. *Archives of Internal Medicine, 165*, 1962–1968.

Gara, M. A., Vega, W. A., Arndt, S., Escamilla, M., Fleck, D. E., Lawson, W. B., ... & Strakowski, S. M. (2012). Influence of patient race and ethnicity on clinical assessment in patients with affective disorders. *Archives of General Psychiatry, 69*, 593–600.

González, H. M., Croghan, T. W., West, B. T., Tarraf, W., Williams, D. R., Nesse, R., ... & Jackson, J. S. (2008). Antidepressant use among Blacks and Whites in the United States. *Psychiatric Services, 59*, 1131–1138.

Greenwald, A. G., Poehlman, T. A., Uhlmann, E. L., & Banaji, M. R. (2009). Understanding and using the Implicit Association Test: III. Meta-analysis of predictive validity. *Journal of Personality and Social Psychology, 97*, 17–41.

Hahm, H. C., Cook, B. L., Ault-Brutus, A., & Alegría, M. (2015). Intersection of race-ethnicity and gender in depression care: Screening, access, and minimally adequate treatment. *Psychiatric Services, 66*, 258–264.

Hall, W. J., Chapman, M. V., Lee, K. M., Merino, Y. M., Thomas, T. W., Payne, B. K., ... & Coyne-Beasley, T. (2015). Implicit racial/ethnic bias among health care professionals and its influence on health care outcomes: A systematic review. *American Journal of Public Health, 105*, e60–e76.

Hoffman, K. M., Trawalter, S., Axt, J. R., & Oliver, N. (2016). Racial bias in pain assessment and treatment recommendations, and false beliefs about Blacks and Whites. *Proceedings of the National Academy of Sciences (PNAS), 113*, 4296–4301.

Huey, S. J., Jr., Tilley, J. L., Jones, E. O., & Smith, C. A. (2014). The contribution of cultural competence to evidence-based care for ethnically diverse populations. *Annual Review of Clinical Psychology, 10*, 305–338.

Jackson, J. S., Knight, K. M., & Rafferty, J. A. (2010). Race and unhealthy behaviors: Chronic stress, the HPA axis, and physical and mental health disparities over the life course. *American Journal of Public Health, 100*, 933–939.

Jencks, C., & Phillips, M. (1998). The black-white test scope gap: Why it persists and what can be done. *The Brookings Review, 16,* 24–27.

Kuppens, T., & Spears, R. (2014). You don't have to be well-educated to be an aversive racist, but it helps. *Social Science Research, 45,* 211–223.

Lakes, K., López, S. R., & Garro, L. C. (2006). Cultural competence and psychotherapy: Applying anthropologically informed conceptions of culture. *Psychotherapy: Theory, Research, Practice, Training, 43,* 380–396.

Manly, J. J. (2008). Critical issues in cultural neuropsychology: Profit from diversity. *Neuropsychology Review, 18,* 179–183.

Masuda, A., Anderson, P. L., & Edmonds, J. (2012). Help-seeking attitudes, mental health stigma, and self-concealment among African American college students. *Journal of Black Studies, 43,* 773–786.

McGuire, T. G., & Miranda, J. (2008). New evidence regarding racial and ethnic disparities in mental health: Policy implications. *Health Affairs, 27,* 393–403.

Mezzich, J. E., Caracci, G., Fabrega, H., Jr., & Kirmayer, L. J. (2009). Cultural formulation guidelines. *Transcultural Psychiatry, 46,* 383–405.

Migacheva, K., & Tropp, L. R. (2013). Learning orientation as a predictor of positive intergroup contact. *Group Processes & Intergroup Relations, 16,* 426–444.

Miranda, J., McGuire, T. G., Williams, D. R., & Wang, P. (2008). Mental health in the context of health disparities. *American Journal of Psychiatry, 165,* 1102–1108.

Moskowitz, D., Thom, D. H., Guzman, D., Penko, J., Miaskowski, C., & Kushel, M. (2011). Is primary care providers' trust in socially marginalized patients affected by race? *Journal of General Internal Medicine, 26,* 846–851.

Moyers, T. B., & Miller, W. R. (2013). Is low therapist empathy toxic? *Psychology of Addictive Behaviors, 27,* 878–884.

Nadeem, E., Lange, J. M., Edge, D., Fong, M., Belin, T., & Miranda, J. (2007). Does stigma keep poor young immigrant and US-born Black and Latina women from seeking mental health care? *Psychiatric Services, 58,* 1547–1554.

Neighbors, H. W., Trierweiler, S. J., Ford, B. C., & Muroff, J. R. (2003). Racial differences in DSM diagnosis using a semi-structured instrument: The importance of clinical judgment in the diagnosis of African Americans. *Journal of Health and Social Behavior, 44,* 237–256.

Pearson, A. R., & Dovidio, J. F. (2014). Intergroup fluency: How processing experiences shape intergroup cognition and communication. In J. P. Forgas, J. Laszlo, & O. Vincze (Eds.), *Social cognition and communication* (pp. 101–120). New York, NY: Psychology Press.

Penner, L. A., & Dovidio, J. F. (2016). Racial colorblindness and Black-White health disparities. In H. A. Neville, M. E. Gallardo & D. W. Sue (Eds.), *The myth of racial color blindness: Manifestation, dynamics, and impact* (pp. 275–293). Washington, DC: American Psychological Association.

Penner, L. A., Dovidio, J. F., Edmondson, D., Dailey, R. K., Markova, T., Gaertner, S. L., & Albrecht, T. (2009). Subtle racism, perceptions of discrimination, and Black-White health disparities. *Journal of Black Psychology, 35,* 180–203.

Penner, L. A., Dovidio, J. F., Gonzalez, R., Albrecht, T. L. … & Eggly, S. (2016). The effects of oncologist implicit racial bias in racially discordant oncology interactions. *Journal of Clinical Oncology, 24,* 2874–2880.

Penner L. A., Hagiwara, N., Eggly, S., Gaertner, S. L., Albrecht, T. L., & Dovidio, J. F. (2013). Racial healthcare disparities: A social psychological analysis. *European Review of Social Psychology, 24,* 70–122.

Penner, L. A., Phelan, S. M., Earnshaw, V., Albrecht, T. L., & Dovidio, J. F. (2018). Patient stigma, medical interactions, and healthcare disparities: A selective review. In B. Major, J. F. Dovidio, &

B. G. Link (Eds.), *The Oxford handbook of stigma and health* (pp. 183–201). New York, NY: Oxford University Press.

Peris, T. S., Teachman, B. A., & Nosek, B. A. (2008). Implicit and explicit stigma of mental illness: Links to clinical care. *The Journal of Nervous and Mental Disease, 196,* 752–760.

Perry, S. P., Dovidio, J. F., Murphy, M. C., & van Ryn, M. (2015). The joint effect of bias awareness and self-reported prejudice on intergroup anxiety and intentions for intergroup contact. *Cultural Diversity and Ethnic Minority Psychology, 21,* 89–96.

Perry, S. P., Murphy, M. C., & Dovidio, J. F. (2015). Modern prejudice: Subtle, but unconscious? The role of bias awareness in Whites' perceptions of personal and others' biases. *Journal of Experimental Social Psychology, 61,* 64–78.

Pierce, C. (1970). Offensive mechanisms. In F. Barbour (Ed.), *In the Black seventies* (pp. 265–282). Boston, MA: Porter Sargent.

Plant, E. A., & Devine, P. G. (2003). The antecedents and implications of interracial anxiety. *Personality and Social Psychology Bulletin, 29,* 790–801.

Priebe, S., & McCabe, R. (2006). The therapeutic relationship in psychiatric settings. *Acta Psychatrica Scandinavica, 113,* 69–72.

Reynolds, C. R., & Suzuki, L. (2013). Bias in psychological assessment: An empirical review and recommendations. In J. R. Graham, J. A. Naglieri, & I. B. Weiner (Eds.), *Handbook of psychology, Vol. 10: Assessment psychology* (2nd ed., pp. 82–113). Hoboken, NJ: Wiley.

Ridley, C. R. (2005). *Overcoming unintentional racism in counseling and therapy* (2nd ed.). Thousand, Oaks, CA: Sage.

Rosenthal, D. A. (2004). Effects of client race on clinical judgment of practicing European American vocational rehabilitation counselors. *Rehabilitation Counseling Bulletin, 47,* 131–141.

Sabin, J. A., & Greenwald, A. G. (2012). The influence of implicit bias on treatment recommendations for 4 common pediatric conditions: Pain, urinary tract infection, attention deficit hyperactivity disorder, and asthma. *American Journal of Public Health, 102,* 988–995.

Sabin, J. A., Nosek, B. A., Greenwald, A. G., & Rivara, F. P. (2009). Physicians' implicit and explicit attitudes about race by MD race, ethnicity, and gender. *Journal of Healthcare for the Poor and Underserved, 20,* 896–913.

Shelton, J. N., Dovidio, J. F., Hebl, M., & Richeson, J. A. (2009). Prejudice and intergroup interaction. In S. Demoulin, J.-P. Leyens, & J. F. Dovidio (Eds.), *Intergroup misunderstandings: Impact of divergent social realities* (pp. 21–38). New York, NY: Psychology Press.

Sidanius, J., & Pratto, F. (1999). *Social dominance: An intergroup theory of social hierarchy and oppression.* New York, NY: Cambridge University Press.

Steele, C. M. (2010). *Whistling Vivaldi: And other clues how stereotypes affect us.* New York, NY: Norton.

Stockdale, S. E., Lagomasino, I. T., Siddique, J., McGuire, T., & Miranda, J. (2008). Racial and ethnic disparities in detection and treatment of depression and anxiety among psychiatric and primary health care visits, 1995–2005. *Medical Care, 46,* 668–677.

Sue, D. W., Capodilupo, C. M., Torino, G. C., Bucceri, J. M., Holder, A. M. B., Nadal, K. L., & Esquilin, M. (2007). Racial microaggressions in everyday life: Implications for clinical practice. *American Psychologist, 62,* 271–286.

Terwilliger, J. M., Bach, N., Bryan, C., & Williams, M. T. (2013). Multicultural versus colorblind ideology: Implications for mental health and counseling. In A. Di Fabio (Ed.), *Psychology of counseling* (pp. 111–122). New York, NY: Nova Science Publishers.

Thompson, V. L. S., Bazile, A., & Akbar, M. (2004). African Americans' perceptions of psychotherapy and psychotherapists. *Professional Psychology: Research and Practice, 35,* 19–26.

Trierweiler, S. J., Neighbors, H. W., Munday, C., Thompson, E. E., Jackson, J. S., & Binion, V. J. (2006). Differences in patterns of symptom attribution in diagnosing schizophrenia between African American and non-African American clinicians. *American Journal of Orthopsychiatry, 76,* 154–160.

US Department of Health and Human Services (1999). *Mental Health: A report of the Surgeon General.* Rockville, MD: US Department of Health and Human Services, Substance Abuse and Mental Health Services Administration, Center for Mental Health Services, National Institutes of Health, National Institutes of Mental Health.

US Department of Health and Human Services (2001). *Mental health: Culture, race, and ethnicity— A supplement to Mental Health: A report of the Surgeon General.* Rockville, MD: US Department of Health and Human Services, Public Health Service, Office of the Surgeon General.

Whaley, A. L. (2001). Cultural mistrust and mental health services for African Americans: A review and meta-analysis. *The Counseling Psychologist, 29,* 513–531.

Williams, M. T. (2011, December 27). Colorblind ideology is a form of racism. *Psychology Today, 27.* Retrieved from https://colouredjustice.wordpress.com/2015/09/24/colorblind-ideology-is-a-form -of-racism/

Williams, M. T., Turkheimer, E., Magee, E., & Guterbock, T. (2008). The effects of race and racial priming on self-report of contamination anxiety. *Personality and Individual Differences, 44,* 746–757.

Williams, M. T., Turkheimer, E., Schmidt, K. M., & Oltmanns, T. F. (2005). Ethnic identification biases responses to the Padua Inventory for obsessive-compulsive disorder. *Assessment, 12,* 174–185.

CHAPTER 4

Strategies for Promoting Patient Activation, Self-Efficacy, and Engagement in Treatment for Ethnic and Racial Minority Clients

Margarita Alegría,
Harvard Medical School and Massachusetts General Hospital

Naomi Ali,
Massachusetts General Hospital

Larimar Fuentes,
Massachusetts General Hospital

The persistence of mental health care disparities over time and across racial and ethnic groups is greater than nearly all other areas of the health care system (AHRQ, 2008). The problem appears to be most stubborn in the area of access disparities in improving mental health care for racial and ethnic minorities. In 2016, Cook and colleagues reported a continuing trend in mental health access disparities detected for the three major US racial-ethnic minority groups compared with Whites (Cook, Trinh, Li, Hou, & Progovac, 2016). Their results showed that Black-White disparities (Blacks having 10.8 percent less access) and Latinx-White disparities (Latinxs having 10.9 percent less access than Whites) had increased over time. Non-Latinx White mental health care use is approximately twice the level of that of racial and ethnic minorities in many analyses of mental health service disparities (Cook, McGuire, & Miranda, 2007; Lê Cook, McGuire, Lock, & Zaslavsky, 2010), underscoring the need for strategies that actually target the reduction of these disparities as opposed to simply offering continued research on their identification. For example, disparities in overall mental health care expenditures were found to be almost entirely driven by disparities in entering mental health care as opposed to expenditures after entering treatment (Lê Cook et al., 2010). This suggests that engaging minorities in care and facilitating their better experiences during care is a critical task for disparities reduction.

In this chapter, we extract and build upon lessons learned from our efforts to identify factors underlying mental health care disparities that are amenable to change, highlighting how to assist practitioners in grappling with these seemingly intractable disparities and pointing the way toward developing creative solutions to these problems. We delve into the findings in two main areas that focus specifically on patients: patient engagement and patient activation and self-efficacy.

Why focus on these areas? Research shows that providers communicate differently with ethnic and racial minority patients, particularly in racial and ethnic discordant encounters (Alegría, Atkins, Farmer, Slaton, & Stelk, 2010; Street, O'Malley, Cooper, & Haidet, 2008). According to Street et al., provider's communication and rapport in clinical sessions may be influenced by the patient's race or ethnicity. In analyzing audiotapes of outpatient visits, providers demonstrated more patient-centered communication and efforts in engagement when they assessed the patient to be a fine communicator who displayed more positive affect and appeared less argumentative. Providers appear to engage in less rapport building with minority patients as compared to non-Latinx White patients (Shapiro & Saltzer, 1981) and to display more verbal dominance and less positive affect with African American patients than with their non-Latinx White counterparts (Cooper et al., 2003; Ghods et al., 2008; Johnson, Roter, Powe, & Cooper, 2004).

Studies show that in consults around depression, providers tend to minimize the emotional suffering of African American patients as compared to non-Latinx Whites and that Black patients are more likely to receive care that focuses on biomedical aspects of care, neglecting discussion of psychosocial factors (Cooper et al., 2012; Johnson et al., 2004). Not surprisingly, racial and ethnic minority patients have also been found to be assessed as less verbal, less assertive, and less effective in consultations with providers, and consequently less satisfied with their care (LaVeist & Nuru-Jeter, 2002).

Yet for treatments to be effective, minority clients must be willing to enter and remain in care and establish a collaborative relationship with their providers. Optimal patient-provider communication is integral to effective health care delivery (Green et al., 2010; Perloff, Bonder, Ray, Ray, & Siminoff, 2006). Indeed, effective communication is thought to facilitate the development of the therapeutic bond between patient and provider and enhance information exchange and encourage patient participation in decision making (Green et al., 2010), all tenets of high-quality patient-centered care. The failure to communicate important information may result in delays in diagnosis or misdiagnosis, unnecessary tests, undertreatment, and higher medical costs (Duffy, Gordon, Whelan, Cole-Kelly, & Frankel, 2004; Kirmayer, Groleau, Guzder, Blake, & Jarvis, 2003; Levinson, Lesser, & Epstein, 2010). This may require more time during the clinical visit for tackling ethnic and racial differences in treatment preferences, relational style with the provider, and expectations about mental health care as an approach to improve the patient-provider therapeutic connection and to achieve treatment goals (Lakes, López, & Garro, 2006). Ignoring the complexity of differences in culture and ethnic and racial identity between the patient and the provider may result only in poor patient-provider interaction, which has been linked to persistent racial and ethnic disparities in health care access and outcomes (Schnittker & Liang, 2006). In addition, lack of resources in community health clinics to deal with high-quality service delivery (e.g., paperwork and patient referrals to other services) in the context of increasing demands (e.g., productivity, determination of patient eligibility in services) may lead providers to focus on getting things done, with limited opportunities to truly listen to their minority patients. Thus, activating patients, facilitating their illness self-management, and having the provider focus on patient engagement are ways to improve the clinical encounter.

The recommendations of this chapter, in part, are derived from an innovative research study we conducted, the Patient-Provider Encounter Study (Alegría et al., 2008), which examined racial and ethnic disparities in the clinical encounter. The study focused on a key clinical decision point, the intake session—the brief time in which a provider must determine which information will help to diagnose the problem and identify a treatment plan, and when patients determine the likelihood of entering care. Videotaped intake sessions between forty-seven providers and 129 multicultural patients and post-diagnostic interviews with all participants resulted in a nuanced understanding of how clinical, cultural, environmental, and institutional factors influence one another; shape expectations, behaviors, and communication patterns during the clinical encounter; and result in significant disparities (Katz & Alegría, 2009). A growing body of evidence suggests the importance of addressing diversity issues in psychotherapy as a way to enhance the therapeutic relationship and to accomplish treatment goals (Vasquez, 2007). Acknowledging the complexity of culture and ethnic and racial identity may result in more accurate diagnosis and treatment (Comas-Diaz, 2006; Lakes et al., 2006; Lewis-Fernández et al., 2002). This chapter emphasizes the difficulties of intercultural encounters, where the provider and patient do not share the same culture or background.

Racial and ethnic concordance exerts a strong influence on retention in care—particularly among Latinx patients as compared to non-Latinx Whites (Alegría et al., 2013). Similar findings have been shown for African American and Asian patients (Meyer & Zane, 2013). Research to identify why and for whom ethnic and racial concordance matters is called for, though it has been suggested that the construct itself touches upon notions of perceived patient-provider similarity that may prove essential to enhancing patient-provider communication, such as mutual understanding of the problem(s) that brought the patient into care (Street et al., 2008). Providers who do not share the same background with their patients may not be sensitive to how the content of information exchanged with a provider and the style in which it is exchanged differ by patient race or ethnicity (Mulvaney-Day, Earl, Diaz-Linhart, & Alegría, 2011), or to the mutually binding nature of stereotypes that constrain communication between patient and provider and affect the course of the diagnostic interview (Katz & Alegría, 2009).

An examination of Black patients' interactions with providers (Earl, Alegría, Mendieta, & Linhart, 2011) suggest that achieving good, patient-centered interactions in racially discordant patient-provider relationships is possible and is consistent with evidence that multiple demographic and interpersonal variables underlie effective patient-provider interactions (Rosen, Miller, Nakash, Halperin, & Alegría, 2012). Differences in social identities can be overcome by a strong interpersonal connection early in the therapeutic relationship. Providers must develop a capacity for reflection and engagement—particularly in navigating personal interactions with patients from different cultures. They must recognize and actively work to transform assumptions of the other, to take note of "surprises," and to elicit what really matters to patients in their care and treatment (Katz & Alegría, 2009).

The Role of Patient Activation

Patients who take an active role in their health care (Post, Cegala, & Miser, 2002) have increased likelihood of positive treatment outcomes, including greater satisfaction with services and greater probability of achieving their treatment goals (Linhorst & Eckert, 2003). The growth of the consumer movement has renewed interest in patient activation strategies to better match patients' needs with services and to transform treatment plans by including patients in their disease management, but strategies to do so are missing. Patient activation could generally be defined as a patient "understanding one's role in the care process and having the knowledge, skill, and confidence to manage one's health and health care" (Hibbard & Greene, 2013; Hibbard, Mahoney, Stockard, & Tusler, 2005 p. 207). The term "patient activation" has been often considered synonymous with "patient engagement" (Chen, Mullins, Novak, & Thomas, 2016), but it is best understood as one of the components of patient engagement (Hibbard & Greene, 2013) and interdependent with patient empowerment (Fumagalli, Radaelli, Lettieri, & Masella, 2015). Activating patients involves developing their skills with question formulation and information seeking to increase collaboration with the health care provider. Ideally, patients are able to tell their concerns to health care providers; to manage symptoms (emotional or mental health); to get information to make decisions about treatment; to take an active role in care (such as contacting the provider if they are not feeling well); to discuss treatment options with the provider; and to discuss side effects of medication (Hibbard, Stockard, Mahoney, & Tusler, 2004). We specifically focus on empowering patients and building capacity whereby individuals increase their belief that they play an active role in their care (such as taking action to solve their problems), participate in decision making (seeing themselves as capable in making decisions and feeling confident of the decisions they make) and manage their care to achieve a greater measure of control over their health and their health care process (such as being able to accomplish what they set out to do, making their plan work).

The importance of patient activation in mental health cannot be emphasized enough. Higher levels of patient activation may be positively associated with both decreasing severity of depressive symptoms and reported quality of life (Magnezi, Glasser, Shalev, Sheiber, & Reuveni, 2014). Among patients with moderate to severe depression, higher patient activation before treatment has shown to predict lower depression severity and a higher likelihood of symptom remission and increases in healthy behaviors, like reducing weight and taking preventive screening tests (Sacks, Greene, Hibbard, & Overton, 2014). Additionally, patients with mental disorders who reported greater activation also reported better illness self-management, positive recovery attitudes, higher levels of hope, and less emotional discomfort (Kukla, Salyers, & Lysaker, 2013; Salyers et al., 2009). Increasing patient activation has also been associated with augmenting patient-perceived quality of mental health care in studies conducted with female veterans (Kimerling, Pavao, & Wong, 2016) and racial and ethnic minorities (Alegría et al., 2018). It has also been associated with therapeutic processes in mental health care, like shared decision making (Fukui et al., 2014) and therapeutic alliance (Allen et al., 2017), and peer support for those with the same illness (Firmin, Luther, Lysaker, & Salyers, 2015), as well as being motivated and goal-directed toward recovery (Oles, Fukui, Rand, & Salyers, 2015).

To assess patient-reported activation in patients participating in general medical care, several measures have been developed, with the Patient Activation Measure (PAM) already adapted for various ethnic groups, as well as tailored to mental health patients (Green et al., 2010). Levels of patient activation appear to vary by race, with White patients in national samples and in Medicaid scoring significantly higher on the PAM than African Americans in both samples (Hibbard et al., 2008). Similarly, recent studies have suggested that racial and ethnic minorities tend to report lower activation levels than White patients (Eliacin et al., 2018; Lubetkin, Zabor, Brennessel, Kemeny, & Hay, 2014). Therefore, augmenting and monitoring activation in ethnic and racial minority clients should be an important strategy to decrease disparities in mental health care.

Despite the known benefits of patient activation, known racial and ethnic disparities in activation, and solid frameworks to guide these efforts, the mental health system has maintained a passive, paternalistic approach, whereby patient involvement implies being a passive recipient of health care decisions, with few attempts to change this traditionally passive role (Barello, Graffinga, Vegni, Bosio & Bosio, 2014). Thus, it is important for providers to recognize this problematic status quo and to make explicit efforts to focus on and support patient activation and empowerment, and help patients maximize their time spent with the provider. Being receptive to patients becoming more activated and focusing on incremental changes in activation is integral to the growth of strong, supportive relationships with patients, especially racial and ethnic minority patients who are more likely to start treatment at lower activation levels (Alegría et al., 2018; Alvarez, Greene, Hibbard, & Overton, 2016; Hibbard, 2017). Several empirically supported patient-activation interventions exist, providing important tools and resources to shape providers' efforts. These efforts require providers to think outside the box of the usual one-on-one clinical encounter and consider the necessity of additional resources and programs to increase patient activation, including peer support and coaching interventions.

Some Models for Improving Patient Activation

Chen et al. (2016) proposed a multilevel framework for culturally sensitive patient activation and empowerment among racial and ethnic minorities based on the Personalized

Patient Activation and Empowerment (P-PAE) model, with the ultimate goal of reducing health disparities (Chen et al., 2016). In their framework, patient activation and empowerment efforts must be tailored to the patient's race or ethnicity, culture, and language, in addition to sociodemographic factors and clinical needs. When executed at multiple levels, patient activation and empowerment interventions may lead to improvements in patient-provider relationships, increased community engagement, improvements in patient health, and overall reductions in health disparities. Furthermore, activating patients may be a necessary part of promoting other integral components of patient-centered care, like shared decision making, by increasing patients' self-efficacy to advocate for themselves in care (Thomas et al., 2018).

Several studies have concluded that patients may benefit from peer-support efforts to increase activation, rather than simply relying on the provider. For example, Lara-Cabrera and colleagues (2016) developed an intervention facilitated by both peers and clinicians that led to increases in patient activation, patient satisfaction, and treatment retention. To develop more collaborative primary care among elders with serious mental illness and cardiovascular health risks, Bartels et al. (2013) similarly developed a peer co-facilitated intervention to improve patient activation, and included a brief educational program for providers to increase their receptivity to increased patient activation. While these studies have primarily been conducted among White patients, Druss et al. (2010) conducted a peer-led educational intervention with primarily African American patients and also found improvements in patient activation. Thus, integrating peer support as an integral resource in mental health care should be considered to increase patient activation among racial and ethnic minorities.

In addition to peer-led educational programs, providers should consider individualized coaching to activate patients by helping them develop the knowledge and skills to participate in their care (Cabassa et al., 2018; McCusker et al., 2016). Cabassa et al. (2018) adapted a previous health care manager intervention for Latinx individuals with serious mental illness and at risk for cardiovascular disease that focused on physical health and improving care coordination between primary care services and mental health services, as well as patient activation specifically for physical health issues. The health care manager intervention consisted of three phases over the course of twelve months: phase 1 involved getting to know the patients, providers, and their goals and developing trust; phase 2 involved developing and putting an action plan into practice based on patient goals, as well as promoting problem-solving skills and enhancing activation skills; and phase 3 involved reinforcement of skills learned. Cabassa et al. also identified important strategies to overcome potential barriers for Latinx minorities to engage in their intervention (Cabassa et al., 2014). These strategies included using bilingual health care managers, incorporating cultural competency in the care-manager training, providing health education materials in Spanish, and using the DSM-5 Cultural Formulation Interview to collect cultural information tied to health status of patients. The importance of linguistic and racial and ethnic concordance is reflected in the P-PAE model, which recommends matching providers and patients by linguistic and racial and ethnic background to overcome cultural barriers to increasing patient activation and empowerment (Chen et al., 2016). However, the evidence is inconclusive, and we have some evidence that communicating with patients according to their cultural norms could promote patient activation (Alegría et al., 2013; Eliacin et al., 2018). Visit http://www.newharbinger.com/41962 to download an outline of these programs.

Similarly, other studies (Alegría et al., 2008; Cortes, Mulvaney-Day, Fortuna, Reinfeld, & Alegría, 2009) have specifically developed a care-manager intervention for racial and ethnic minorities in behavioral health care to improve patient activation. The manualized intervention across three to four sessions is offered by care managers, who, through discussion and reflection, communication skills training, and role play, help patients develop knowledge of resources and skills to actively participate and collaborate with their providers. Care managers encourage patients to take an active role in their care by identifying their questions and concerns and developing related questions to ask their provider during their visits. Consistent with such care-manager interventions, providers themselves may improve communication with patients by emphasizing the importance of preparing for visits and collaboratively setting an agenda at the beginning of each session (Eliacin, Rollins, Burgess, Salyers, & Matthias, 2016), a practice not ubiquitous across mental health care settings (Frankel, Salyers, Bonfils, Oles, & Matthias, 2013). Actively and consistently encouraging patients to prepare for sessions with questions and concerns and subsequently beginning sessions by setting session agendas based on those questions and concerns creates an environment in which patients are an equal partner in their mental health and treatment (Eliacin et al., 2016). This reciprocal process may be especially important for racial and ethnic minorities whose cultural backgrounds may incline them to view the provider as the director of their care (Cortes et al., 2009).

Some Approaches to Improving Patient Engagement

Limited patient engagement continues to be a chief constraint on the effectiveness of available treatments (Alegría, 2017; Barello, 2014;Hettema, Steele, & Miller, 2005) and multiple strategies have been identified to help providers increase patient engagement. Dixon, Holoshitz, and Nossel (2016) emphasize more focus on the therapeutic alliance, addressing patients' immediate needs in mental health services, fast access to care, and use of recovery-oriented strategies. They also recommend that providers be open to and flexible in trying and integrating new approaches. Similarly, Aggarwal and colleagues (2016) recommend integrating patient outlooks of their illness (by using the Cultural Formulation), tackling patient stigma, employing plain language, addressing patient preferences, conversing about their differences, and showing positive affect. Because engaging patients in their care is so critical, several models like the Chronic Care Model (Bodenheimer, Wagner, & Grumbach, 2002) and patient-centered medical homes

(Rittenhouse & Shortell, 2009) have been exponentially growing to promote patient engagement, augment adherence, and reduce costs. However, how much they contribute to patient engagement remains unknown.

Electronic health care mediums, like the Internet and smartphone programs, text messaging, and telepsychiatry also hold promise as mechanisms to engage patients in mental health services (Clarke & Yarborough, 2013). Graffigna and colleagues highlight how to improve engagement around patients' understanding of their condition (Graffigna, Barello, & Riva, 2013; Graffigna et al., 2014; Wiederhold & Riva, 2013). By using technological applications, patients can access information about their illness and identify existing resources to better manage it (Graffigna et al., 2013; Graffigna et al., 2014; Wiederhold & Riva, 2013). Websites like Big White Wall in the United Kingdom have received financial support from local National Health Services (NHS) affiliates and have been made available by various public and private employers to serve as a mental health community where people gain support in managing their care from peers, family, friends, and clinicians (Laurance et al., 2014). In addition, there are novel technologies for communication that enable providers to engage patients in mental health services at a distance either by video chat or teleHealth. eHealth technologies make it possible for patients to participate in their treatment and, consequently, engage more in care (Neuhauser & Kreps, 2003). Providers may consider their own use of such strategies when working with racial and ethnic minority patients to increase engagement, including not automatically assuming patients are noncompliant if they have difficulty engaging and also employing more flexible use of the internet and Smartphone applications when patients may be unable to attend live visits.

The Patient Health Engagement (PHE) Model describes the patients' inner psychological experiences of engagement with their disease or problem as a continuum, and providers may benefit from assessing where a patient is on this continuum as they consider the patient's level of engagement in treatment (Graffigna & Barello, 2018; Graffigna, Barello, Bonanomi, & Lozza, 2015). In stage 1 (blackout), the patient is largely in denial and frozen about their problem and has yet to accept their new illness condition. In stage 2 (arousal), the patient has superficial knowledge of the problem, may be in a state of high alert and disorganization around it, and needs to reframe their understanding of the physical and psychological embodiment of the changes they are undergoing because of their illness. In this phase, it is critical that the provider understands the patient's experience. In the third stage (adhesion), the patient is accepting their condition, developing emotional strength to cope with it, and demonstrating adherence to treatment. The patient is emotionally connected to their loss and impacted by the failure to exert control over their body and reactions, so they feel that they have limited self-efficacy over the disease and daily circumstances. Providers during this third stage can engage patients by giving them skills that make patients' feel confident when managing their health, such as prioritizing their goals in treatment, recognizing barriers to effective actions, and developing a trusting relationship with their provider. In the fourth stage (eudiamonic project), the patient is fully accepting, activated, and engaged in the process.

Providers should focus on maintaining a strong therapeutic alliance, especially for patients at the latter stages of the engagement process. According to Poleshuck et al. (2015), participants identified the patient-therapist relationship as a primary barrier to treatment engagement, and Thompson and McCabe, in a systematic review of the literature, also found that clinician-patient alliance and communication are connected with more positive patient adherence (Thompson & McCabe, 2012). Foo and colleagues (2017) recommend training providers on how to avoid the loss of empathy with their minority patients and how to ensure paying attention to the time allotted to mental health topics in the visit. Attending to patients' preferences for treatment has also been demonstrated to be a significant factor for engagement in care. For example, when there is a mismatch between the preferred and actual treatment, there is an increased odds of patient dropout, a worse alliance between patient and provider, fewer sessions attended, and worse depression outcomes in patients with major depressive disorder (Kwan, Dimidjian, & Rizvi, 2010). Thus, providers should assess patients for the symptoms that are most relevant and problematic to them and use language that fits with their concerns, rather than encouraging them to accept a diagnosis, to facilitate building rapport and improving engagement in treatment.

Providers may also consider integrating patient-reported and patient-defined outcomes into their care to engage patients in treatment (Lavallee et al., 2016). This allows for enhanced patient engagement and shared decision making, because it incorporates the patient's experience of illness, how the patient feels about their functioning, health, quality of life, or general well-being. Focusing on patient-reported outcomes also provides the opportunity to support patient-provider engagement by helping patients decide on the priorities for the visit, identifying treatment decisions, and adjusting care, if necessary.

Finally, we discuss motivational enhancement therapies (METs) and related motivational interviewing (MI), which have also been proposed as approaches to improve patient engagement (Westra, Aviram, & Doell, 2011). MI centers around client-centered communication that builds patient awareness of internal motivation for positive behavioral change. At its core, MI involves providers demonstrating respect for patients' goals and values, and a willingness to meet patients where they are in their process of change (Rollnick & Miller, 1995). Evidence supports the usefulness of adding MI to existing therapies for increasing engagement with treatment and in improving clinical outcomes. But results seem to suggest that MI works only with some clients and not others. For example, study results demonstrate that MI appears to increase engagement for those who exhibit high worry severity but not moderate worry severity (Westra, Arkowitz, & Dozois, 2009), or for people with social anxiety disorder (Buckner & Schmidt, 2009), PTSD (Murphy, 2008), or eating disorders (Cassin, von Ranson, Heng, Brar, & Wojtowicz, 2008). In their systematic review, Romano and Peters (2015) found that in most studies, clients who were in the MI condition participated more in treatment as compared to those in the control condition. Their results suggest that MI has a stronger effect for patients with anxiety, mood, or psychotic disorders but less so for those with eating disorders. When explaining results of the mechanisms by which MI might operate, they found that therapist behaviors of empathy, collaboration, evocation, and autonomy appear to happen more often in MI conditions as compared to comparison conditions.

MI-based interventions combined with preventive approaches for depression have also shown promise. For example, Van Voorhees and colleagues (2009) demonstrated that MI combined with an Internet behavior change program could lessen the probability of having a depressive episode. MI has also been employed to decrease resistance to PTSD treatment among Vietnam veterans (Murphy, Thompson, Murray, Rainey, & Uddo, 2009). Because combat veterans may interpret their problematic behaviors (e.g., anger, hyper-vigilance, mistrust, and social isolation) as adequate coping strategies to deal with an uncertain and dangerous world, they might be resistant to treatment. In a motivation-enhancement group, participants demonstrated greater willingness to believe they needed to change and more responsibility for attending to their problems (Murphy et al., 2009). As a result, veterans in the motivation-enhancement group showed greater readiness to change, increased perceived treatment relevance, and PTSD program attendance as compared to a psychoeducation-only group. In parallel, Aviram and Westra (2011) report that getting four sessions of MI significantly lessens resistance to cognitive behavioral therapy (CBT), as contrasted to just receiving CBT only in patients with generalized anxiety by augmenting client engagement with treatment (Aviram & Alice Westra, 2011).

Previous meta-analytic reviews of MI have shown that MI may be even more effective to engage racial and ethnic minority patients compared to their White counterparts, but these effects may differ across racial and ethnic groups, and research assessing the differential benefits of MI according to race and ethnicity is limited (Hettema et al. 2005; Lundahl, Kunz, Brownell, Tollefson, & Burke, 2010). Studies utilizing MI as a technique to improve treatment, including patient engagement, for racial and ethnic minority patients in mental health services have examined cultural adaptation as a means to improve the process of individually tailoring care for these populations (Oh & Lee, 2016).

Previous work with American Indian and Alaskan Native youth (AI/ANs) finds greater patient satisfaction when providers' utilize MI to actively elicit opinions and concerns from patients about their mental health, and thus reinforcing the collaborative nature of their relationships with patients (Dickerson, Brown, Johnson, Schweigman, & D'Amico, 2016). In fact, a randomized trial comparing culturally adapted treatment modalities for substance use disorder among AI/AN adults found that those receiving an MI-based treatment experienced significantly greater improvement in substance use (Venner et al., 2016). These cultural adaptations included matching counselors in AI/AN background, emphasizing spirituality and the role of family and community to enhance motivation for change in substance use behaviors, and using greetings and introductions concordant to the patient's social and cultural norms (Venner et al., 2016). While these strategies reflect the potential importance of linguistic and ethnic concordance between patient and provider, providers treating patients from differing backgrounds could still adopt a culturally grounded MI approach to improve patient engagement. Venner, Feldstein, and Tafoya (2007) offer additional cultural adaptations to MI techniques for providers to utilize with AI/AN patients, including the provider disclosing more personal information; using humor, metaphors, myths, and storytelling; acknowledging the historical trauma of AI/AN groups; avoiding stereotypes and reflecting on their own biases; and focusing on patient strengths.

Studies with Latinx patients have suggested similar cultural adaptations to MI, including providers discussing cultural factors and the role of familial relationships in their substance use behavior, as well as greater probing of how friends and family could better support substance use behavior change (Lee et al., 2011). In a current randomized trial, the authors compare regular MI to culturally adapted MI, the latter of which emphasizes adapting commonly used MI techniques like building discrepancy and intrinsic motivation, to reflect on stressors related to social and cultural dynamics that impact the behavioral health of Latinx individuals (Lee et al., 2016). Building discrepancy refers to separating patients from where they are and where they want to be (Lee et al., 2011). In building discrepancy and intrinsic motivation, the authors present the example of providers probing patients to reflect on differences between familial cultural values and their current substance use (Dickerson et al., 2016). Along with these targeted improvements in patient-provider communication and rapport, cultural adaptation to MI techniques could be directly linked to engaging Latinx people in mental health services through open communication of relevant cultural beliefs. Añez, Silva, Paris, and Bedregal (2008) recommend that providers openly discuss concepts of *personalismo*, *respeto*, and *confianza* with patients to gauge how important these values are to them and how they may affect their relationship with the patient.

Conclusion

This chapter has reviewed strategies that providers may employ for increasing racial and ethnic minority patients' activation and engagement in treatment. Regarding activation, a first step is recognizing that disparities exist in how empowered and activated patients are in managing their care, including talking to their providers about concerns, getting information to make informed decisions, taking an active role in contacting the provider as needed, and discussing treatment options. An initial position of this chapter is that the status quo of one-on-one visits between a patient and provider may not be sufficient for racial and ethnic minority patients, who may not demonstrate the activation skills necessary to maximize visit productivity. Supplementing the visit with peer support, coaching, or care manager resources may be important options for clinics that are committed to improving these important health care disparities.

Regarding both increased patient activation and engagement, recognizing barriers that exist at the provider level is also crucial. For example, providers who are not of the same background of the patient may have difficulties with cultural competency and with forming the strong therapeutic alliances that are necessary. Providers may benefit from increasing flexibility around trying new approaches; incorporating the patient's preferences, perspective, and language into treatment; developing patient-centered outcome assessments that prioritize the patient's goals rather than the provider's; and using electronic health care mediums to address difficulties with engagement. Providers may benefit from trainings that improve their abilities to demonstrate empathy, take the patient's perspective, and demonstrate genuine warmth and positive affect with patients who are ethnically and culturally different. Increased attention to the patient's relationship to her illness and how that may be affecting engagement in treatment may be beneficial. Motivational enhancement therapies and motivational interviewing may be approaches that help providers attune to the motivation, engagement, and needs of patients who are racially and ethnically different.

In conclusion, patient activation and engagement strategies among ethnic and racial minority clients can lead to improving the patient's experience in treatment. Interventions to improve patient activation among racial and ethnic minorities are available with evidence of their effectiveness such as the Personalized Patient Activation and Empowerment (P-PAE) model, peer co-led collaborative activation trainings, peer-led educational programs and interventions, and individualized coaching to activate patients, as well as culturally adapted health care manager interventions for racial and ethnic minorities in behavioral health. Augmenting activation and engagement in ethnic and racial minority clients can improve the quality of the patient-provider relationships in clinical encounters and consequently increase opportunities for patients of color to voice their preferences and objectives in the clinical visit. Strategies of patient engagement can also strengthen therapeutic alliances, address patients' needs, improve access to care, and lead to recovery-oriented strategies for patients to better manage their conditions. There is a lot to gain with the many approaches, supported by research, to augment patients' positive experiences in entering and remaining in treatment. The opportunity to train providers in patient activation, self-efficacy, and engagement has never been better.

KEY POINTS FOR CLINICIANS

- Patient-provider communication is integral to the effective delivery of health care services.

- Research has shown significant differences in how providers interact with racial and ethnic minority patients as compared to non-Latinx Whites; this leads to persisting disparities in health care.

- The traditional model of care supports the idea of patients taking a passive role in their health care despite evidence that patients who take an active role have an increased likelihood of positive treatment outcomes.

- Models of treatment involving patient activation and engagement strategies have been tested and have been shown to be efficacious in improving the quality of the patient-provider relationship and clinical encounter.

References

Aggarwal, N. K., Pieh, M. C., Dixon, L., Guarnaccia, P., Alegría, M., & Lewis-Fernández, R. (2016). Clinician descriptions of communication strategies to improve treatment engagement by racial/ethnic minorities in mental health services: a systematic review. *Patient Education and Counseling, 99*(2), 198–209.

AHRQ. (2008). *National Healthcare Disparities Report.* Retrieved from http://archive.ahrq.gov/research/findings/nhqrdr/nhdr08/index.html

Alegría, M., Alvarez, K., & Falgas-Bague, I. (2017). Clinical care across cultures: What helps, what hinders, what to do. *JAMA Psychiatry, 74*(9), 865–866.

Alegría, M., Atkins, M., Farmer, E., Slaton, E., & Stelk, W. (2010). One size does not fit all: taking diversity, culture and context seriously. *Administration and Policy in Mental Health and Mental Health Services Research, 37*(1–2), 48–60.

Alegría, M., Nakash, O., Johnson, K., Ault-Brutus, A., Carson, N., Fillbrunn, M., … Polo, A. (2018). Effectiveness of the DECIDE Interventions on shared decision making and perceived quality of care in behavioral health with multicultural patients: A randomized clinical trial. *JAMA Psychiatry, 75*(4), 325–335.

Alegría, M., Polo, A., Gao, S., Santana, L., Rothstein, D., Jimenez, A., … Normand, S.-L. (2008). Evaluation of a patient activation and empowerment intervention in mental health care. *Medical Care, 46*(3), 247.

Alegría, M., Roter, D. L., Valentine, A., Chen, C.-n., Li, X., Lin, J., … Larson, S. (2013). Patient–clinician ethnic concordance and communication in mental health intake visits. *Patient Education and Counseling, 93*(2), 188–196.

Allen, M. L., Cook, B., Carson, N., Interian, A., La Roche, M., & Alegría, M. (2017). Patient-provider therapeutic alliance contributes to patient activation in community mental health clinics. *Administration and Policy in Mental Health and Mental Health Services Research, 44*(4), 431–440.

Alvarez, C., Greene, J., Hibbard, J., & Overton, V. (2016). The role of primary care providers in patient activation and engagement in self-management: a cross-sectional analysis. *BMC Health Services Research, 16*(1), 85.

Añez, L. M., Silva, M. A., Paris Jr, M., & Bedregal, L. E. (2008). Engaging Latinos through the integration of cultural values and motivational interviewing principles. *Professional Psychology: Research and Practice, 39*(2), 153.

Aviram, A., & Alice Westra, H. (2011). The impact of motivational interviewing on resistance in cognitive behavioural therapy for generalized anxiety disorder. *Psychotherapy Research, 21*(6), 698–708.

Barello, S., Graffigna, G., Vegni, E., Bosio, A., & Bosio, A. C. (2014). The challenges of conceptualizing patient engagement in health care: a lexicographic literature review. *Journal of Participatory Medicine, 6*(11).

Barello, S., Graffinga, G., Vegni, E., Bosio, A., & Bosiol, A. C. (2014). The challenges of conceptualizing patient engagement in health care: a lexicographic literature review. *Journal of Participatory Medicine, 6*(11).

Bartels, S. J., Aschbrenner, K. A., Rolin, S. A., Hendrick, D. C., Naslund, J. A., & Faber, M. J. (2013). Activating older adults with serious mental illness for collaborative primary care visits. *Psychiatric Rehabilitation Journal, 36*(4), 278.

Bodenheimer, T., Wagner, E. H., & Grumbach, K. (2002). Improving primary care for patients with chronic illness. *JAMA, 288*(14), 1775–1779.

Buckner, J. D., & Schmidt, N. B. (2009). A randomized pilot study of motivation enhancement therapy to increase utilization of cognitive–behavioral therapy for social anxiety. *Behaviour Research and Therapy, 47*(8), 710–715.

Cabassa, L. J., Gomes, A. P., Meyreles, Q., Capitelli, L., Younge, R., Dragatsi, D., ... & Lewis-Fernández, R. (2014). Using the collaborative intervention planning framework to adapt a health-care manager intervention to a new population and provider group to improve the health of people with serious mental illness. *Implementation Science, 9*(1), 178.

Cabassa, L. J., Manrique, Y., Meyreles, Q., Camacho, D., Capitelli, L., Younge, R., ... & Lewis-Fernández, R. (2018). Bridges to better health and wellness: An adapted health care manager intervention for Hispanics with serious mental illness. *Administration and Policy in Mental Health and Mental Health Services Research, 45*(1), 163–173.

Cassin, S. E., von Ranson, K. M., Heng, K., Brar, J., & Wojtowicz, A. E. (2008). Adapted motivational interviewing for women with binge eating disorder: A randomized controlled trial. *Psychology of Addictive Behaviors, 22*(3), 417.

Chen, J., Mullins, C. D., Novak, P., & Thomas, S. B. (2016). Personalized strategies to activate and empower patients in health care and reduce health disparities. *Health Education & Behavior, 43*(1), 25–34.

Clarke, G., & Yarborough, B. J. (2013). Evaluating the promise of health IT to enhance/expand the reach of mental health services. *General Hospital Psychiatry, 35*(4), 339–344.

Comas-Diaz, L. (2006). Latino healing: The integration of ethnic psychology into psychotherapy. *Psychotherapy: Theory, Research, Practice, Training, 43*(4), 436.

Cook, B. L., McGuire, T., & Miranda, J. (2007). Measuring trends in mental health care disparities, 2000–2004. *Psychiatric Services, 58*(12), 1533–1540.

Cook, B. L., Trinh, N.-H., Li, Z., Hou, S. S.-Y., & Progovac, A. M. (2016). Trends in racial-ethnic disparities in access to mental health care, 2004–2012. *Psychiatric Services, 68*(1), 9–16.

Cooper, L. A., Gonzales, J. J., Gallo, J. J., Rost, K. M., Meredith, L. S., Rubenstein, L. V., ... & Ford, D. E. (2003). The acceptability of treatment for depression among African-American, Hispanic, and white primary care patients. *Medical Care, 41*(4), 479–489.

Cooper, L. A., Roter, D. L., Carson, K. A., Beach, M. C., Sabin, J. A., Greenwald, A. G., & Inui, T. S. (2012). The associations of clinicians' implicit attitudes about race with medical visit communication and patient ratings of interpersonal care. *American Journal of Public Health, 102*(5), 979–987.

Cortes, D. E., Mulvaney-Day, N., Fortuna, L., Reinfeld, S., & Alegría, M. (2009). Patient—provider communication: understanding the role of patient activation for Latinos in mental health treatment. *Health Education & Behavior, 36*(1), 138–154.

Dickerson, D. L., Brown, R. A., Johnson, C. L., Schweigman, K., & D'Amico, E. J. (2016). Integrating motivational interviewing and traditional practices to address alcohol and drug use among urban American Indian/Alaska Native youth. *Journal of Substance Abuse Treatment, 65*, 26–35.

Dixon, L. B., Holoshitz, Y., & Nossel, I. (2016). Treatment engagement of individuals experiencing mental illness: review and update. *World Psychiatry, 15*(1), 13–20.

Druss, B. G., Zhao, L., Silke, A., Bona, J. R., Fricks, L., Jenkins-Tucker, S., ... & Lorig, K. (2010). The health and recovery peer (HARP) program: a peer-led intervention to improve medical self-management for persons with serious mental illness. *Schizophrenia Research, 118*(1), 264–270.

Duffy, F. D., Gordon, G. H., Whelan, G., Cole-Kelly, K., & Frankel, R. (2004). Assessing competence in communication and interpersonal skills: the Kalamazoo II report. *Academic Medicine, 79*(6), 495–507.

Earl, T. R., Alegría, M., Mendieta, F., & Linhart, Y. D. (2011). "Just be straight with me": An exploration of black patient experiences in initial mental health encounters. *American Journal of Orthopsychiatry, 81*(4), 519.

Eliacin, J., Coffing, J. M., Matthias, M. S., Burgess, D. J., Bair, M. J., & Rollins, A. L. (2018). The relationship between race, patient activation, and working alliance: Implications for patient engagement in mental health care. *Administration and Policy in Mental Health and Mental Health Services Research, 45*(1), 186–192.

Eliacin, J., Rollins, A. L., Burgess, D. J., Salyers, M. P., & Matthias, M. S. (2016). Patient activation and visit preparation in African American veterans receiving mental health care. *Cultural Diversity and Ethnic Minority Psychology, 22*(4), 580.

Firmin, R. L., Luther, L., Lysaker, P. H., & Salyers, M. P. (2015). Self-initiated helping behaviors and recovery in severe mental illness: Implications for work, volunteerism, and peer support. *Psychiatric Rehabilitation Journal, 38*(4), 336.

Foo, P. K., Frankel, R. M., McGuire, T. G., Zaslavsky, A. M., Lafata, J. E., & Tai-Seale, M. (2017). Patient and physician race and the allocation of time and patient engagement efforts to mental health discussions in primary care: An observational study of audiorecorded periodic health examinations. *The Journal of Ambulatory Care Management, 40*(3), 246–256.

Frankel, R. M., Salyers, M. P., Bonfils, K. A., Oles, S. K., & Matthias, M. S. (2013). Agenda setting in psychiatric consultations: An exploratory study. *Psychiatric Rehabilitation Journal, 36*(3), 195.

Fukui, S., Salyers, M. P., Matthias, M. S., Collins, L., Thompson, J., Coffman, M., & Torrey, W. C. (2014). Predictors of shared decision making and level of agreement between consumers and providers in psychiatric care. *Community Mental Health Journal, 50*(4), 375–382.

Fumagalli, L. P., Radaelli, G., Lettieri, E., & Masella, C. (2015). Patient empowerment and its neighbours: clarifying the boundaries and their mutual relationships. *Health Policy, 119*(3), 384–394.

Ghods, B. K., Roter, D. L., Ford, D. E., Larson, S., Arbelaez, J. J., & Cooper, L. A. (2008). Patient–physician communication in the primary care visits of African Americans and whites with depression. *Journal of General Internal Medicine, 23*(5), 600–606.

Graffigna, G., & Barello, S. (2018). Spotlight on the Patient Health Engagement model (PHE model): a psychosocial theory to understand people's meaningful engagement in their own health care. *Patient Preference and Adherence, 12*, 1261–1271. doi:10.2147/PPA.S145646

Graffigna, G., Barello, S., Bonanomi, A., & Lozza, E. (2015). Measuring patient engagement: development and psychometric properties of the patient health engagement (PHE) scale. *Frontiers in Psychology, 6*, 274.

Graffigna, G., Barello, S., & Riva, G. (2013). Technologies for patient engagement. *Health Affairs, 32*(6), 1172.

Graffigna, G., Barello, S., Triberti, S., Wiederhold, B. K., Bosio, A. C., & Riva, G. (2014). Enabling eHealth as a pathway for patient engagement: a toolkit for medical practice. *Studies in Health Technology and Informatics, 199*, 13–21.

Green, C. A., Perrin, N. A., Polen, M. R., Leo, M. C., Hibbard, J. H., & Tusler, M. (2010). Development of the patient activation measure for mental health. *Administration and Policy in Mental Health and Mental Health Services Research, 37*(4), 327–333.

Hettema, J., Steele, J., & Miller, W. R. (2005). Motivational interviewing. *Annual Review of Clinical Psychology, 1*, 91–111.

Hibbard, J. H. (2017). Patient activation and the use of information to support informed health decisions. *Patient Education and Counseling, 100*(1), 5–7.

Hibbard, J. H., & Greene, J. (2013). What the evidence shows about patient activation: better health outcomes and care experiences; fewer data on costs. *Health Affairs, 32*(2), 207–214.

Hibbard, J. H., Greene, J., Becker, E. R., Roblin, D., Painter, M. W., Perez, D. J., & Tusler, M. (2008). Racial/ethnic disparities and consumer activation in health. *Health Affairs, 27*(5), 1442–1453.

Hibbard, J. H., Mahoney, E. R., Stockard, J., & Tusler, M. (2005). Development and testing of a short form of the patient activation measure. *Health Services Research, 40*(6p1), 1918–1930.

Hibbard, J. H., Stockard, J., Mahoney, E. R., & Tusler, M. (2004). Development of the patient activation measure (PAM): conceptualizing and measuring activation in patients and consumers. *Health Services Research, 39*(4p1), 1005–1026.

Johnson, R. L., Roter, D., Powe, N. R., & Cooper, L. A. (2004). Patient race/ethnicity and quality of patient-physician communication during medical visits. *American Journal of Public Health, 94*(12), 2084–2090.

Katz, A. M., & Alegría, M. (2009). The clinical encounter as local moral world: Shifts of assumptions and transformation in relational context. *Social Science & Medicine*, 68(7), 1238–1246.

Kimerling, R., Pavao, J., & Wong, A. (2016). Patient activation and mental health care experiences among women veterans. *Administration and Policy in Mental Health and Mental Health Services Research*, 43(4), 506–513.

Kirmayer, L. J., Groleau, D., Guzder, J., Blake, C., & Jarvis, E. (2003). Cultural consultation: A model of mental health service for multicultural societies. *The Canadian Journal of Psychiatry*, 48(3), 145–153.

Kukla, M., Salyers, M. P., & Lysaker, P. H. (2013). Levels of patient activation among adults with schizophrenia: Associations with hope, symptoms, medication adherence, and recovery attitudes. *The Journal of Nervous and Mental Disease*, 201(4), 339–344.

Kwan, B. M., Dimidjian, S., & Rizvi, S. L. (2010). Treatment preference, engagement, and clinical improvement in pharmacotherapy versus psychotherapy for depression. *Behaviour Research and Therapy*, 48(8), 799–804.

Lakes, K., López, S. R., & Garro, L. C. (2006). Cultural competence and psychotherapy: Applying anthropologically informed conceptions of culture. *Psychotherapy: Theory, Research, Practice, Training*, 43(4), 380.

Lara-Cabrera, M. L., Salvesen, Ø., Nesset, M. B., De las Cuevas, C., Iversen, V. C., & Gråwe, R. W. (2016). The effect of a brief educational programme added to mental health treatment to improve patient activation: A randomized controlled trial in community mental health centres. *Patient Education and Counseling*, 99(5), 760–768.

Laurance, J., Henderson, S., Howitt, P. J., Matar, M., Al Kuwari, H., Edgman-Levitan, S., & Darzi, A. (2014). Patient engagement: four case studies that highlight the potential for improved health outcomes and reduced costs. *Health Affairs*, 33(9), 1627–1634.

Lavallee, D. C., Chenok, K. E., Love, R. M., Petersen, C., Holve, E., Segal, C. D., & Franklin, P. D. (2016). Incorporating patient-reported outcomes into health care to engage patients and enhance care. *Health Affairs*, 35(4), 575–582.

LaVeist, T. A., & Nuru-Jeter, A. (2002). Is doctor-patient race concordance associated with greater satisfaction with care? *Journal of Health and Social Behavior*, 43(2), 296–306.

Lê Cook, B., McGuire, T. G., Lock, K., & Zaslavsky, A. M. (2010). Comparing methods of racial and ethnic disparities measurement across different settings of mental health care. *Health Services Research*, 45(3), 825–847.

Lee, C. S., Colby, S. M., Magill, M., Almeida, J., Tavares, T., & Rohsenow, D. J. (2016). A randomized controlled trial of culturally adapted motivational interviewing for Hispanic heavy drinkers: Theory of adaptation and study protocol. *Contemporary Clinical Trials*, 50, 193–200.

Lee, C. S., López, S. R., Hernández, L., Colby, S. M., Caetano, R., Borrelli, B., & Rohsenow, D. (2011). A cultural adaptation of motivational interviewing to address heavy drinking among Hispanics. *Cultural Diversity and Ethnic Minority Psychology*, 17(3), 317.

Levinson, W., Lesser, C. S., & Epstein, R. M. (2010). Developing physician communication skills for patient-centered care. *Health Affairs*, 29(7), 1310–1318.

Lewis-Fernández, R., Guarnaccia, P. J., Martínez, I. E., Salmán, E., Schmidt, A., & Liebowitz, M. (2002). Comparative phenomenology of ataques de nervios, panic attacks, and panic disorder. *Culture, Medicine and Psychiatry*, 26(2), 199–223.

Linhorst, D. M., & Eckert, A. (2003). Conditions for empowering people with severe mental illness. *Social Service Review*, 77(2), 279–305.

Lubetkin, E. I., Zabor, E. C., Brennessel, D., Kemeny, M. M., & Hay, J. L. (2014). Beyond demographics: Differences in patient activation across new immigrant, diverse language subgroups. *Journal of Community Health*, 39(1), 40–49.

Lundahl, B. W., Kunz, C., Brownell, C., Tollefson, D., & Burke, B. L. (2010). A meta-analysis of motivational interviewing: Twenty-five years of empirical studies. *Research on Social Work Practice*, *20*(2), 137–160.

Magnezi, R., Glasser, S., Shalev, H., Sheiber, A., & Reuveni, H. (2014). Patient activation, depression and quality of life. *Patient Education and Counseling*, *94*(3), 432–437.

McCusker, J., Lambert, S. D., Cole, M. G., Ciampi, A., Strumpf, E., Freeman, E. E., & Belzile, E. (2016). Activation and self-efficacy in a randomized trial of a depression self-care intervention. *Health Education & Behavior*, *43*(6), 716–725.

Meyer, O. L., & Zane, N. (2013). The influence of race and ethnicity in clients' experiences of mental health treatment. *Journal of Community Psychology*, *41*(7), 884–901.

Mulvaney-Day, N. E., Earl, T. R., Diaz-Linhart, Y., & Alegría, M. (2011). Preferences for relational style with mental health clinicians: A qualitative comparison of African American, Latino and non-Latino white patients. *Journal of Clinical Psychology*, *67*(1), 31–44.

Murphy, R. T. (2008). Enhancing combat veterans' motivation to change posttraumatic stress disorder symptoms and other problem behaviors. In H. Arkowitz, H. A. Westra, W. R. Miller, & S. Rollnick (Eds.), *Applications of motivational interviewing: Motivational interviewing in the treatment of psychological problems* (pp. 57–84). New York, NY: Guliford Press.

Murphy, R. T., Thompson, K. E., Murray, M., Rainey, Q., & Uddo, M. M. (2009). Effect of a motivation enhancement intervention on veterans' engagement in PTSD treatment. *Psychological Services*, *6*(4), 264.

Neuhauser, L., & Kreps, G. L. (2003). Rethinking communication in the e-health era. *Journal of Health Psychology*, *8*(1), 7–23.

Oh, H., & Lee, C. (2016). Culture and motivational interviewing. *Patient Education and Counseling*, *99*(11), 1914–1919.

Oles, S. K., Fukui, S., Rand, K. L., & Salyers, M. P. (2015). The relationship between hope and patient activation in consumers with schizophrenia: Results from longitudinal analyses. *Psychiatry Research*, *228*(3), 272–276.

Perloff, R. M., Bonder, B., Ray, G. B., Ray, E. B., & Siminoff, L. A. (2006). Doctor-patient communication, cultural competence, and minority health: Theoretical and empirical perspectives. *American Behavioral Scientist*, *49*(6), 835–852.

Poleshuck, E., Wittink, M., Crean, H., Gellasch, T., Sandler, M., Bell, E., … & Cerulli, C. (2015). Using patient engagement in the design and rationale of a trial for women with depression in obstetrics and gynecology practices. *Contemporary Clinical Trials*, *43*, 83–92.

Post, D. M., Cegala, D. J., & Miser, W. F. (2002). The other half of the whole: Teaching patients to communicate with physicians. *Family Medicine-Kansas City*, *34*(5), 344–352.

Rittenhouse, D. R., & Shortell, S. M. (2009). The patient-centered medical home: Will it stand the test of health reform? *JAMA*, *301*(19), 2038–2040.

Rollnick, S., & Miller, W. R. (1995). What is motivational interviewing? *Behavioural and cognitive Psychotherapy*, *23*(4), 325–334.

Romano, M., & Peters, L. (2015). Evaluating the mechanisms of change in motivational interviewing in the treatment of mental health problems: A review and meta-analysis. *Clinical Psychology Review*, *38*, 1–12.

Rosen, D. C., Miller, A. B., Nakash, O., Halperin, L., & Alegría, M. (2012). Interpersonal complementarity in the mental health intake: A mixed-methods study. *Journal of Counseling Psychology*, *59*(2), 185.

Sacks, R. M., Greene, J., Hibbard, J. H., & Overton, V. (2014). How well do patient activation scores predict depression outcomes one year later? *Journal of Affective Disorders*, *169*, 1–6.

Salyers, M. P., Matthias, M. S., Spann, C. L., Lydick, J. M., Rollins, A. L., & Frankel, R. M. (2009). The role of patient activation in psychiatric visits. *Psychiatric Services*, *60*(11), 1535–1539.

Schnittker, J., & Liang, K. (2006). The promise and limits of racial/ethnic concordance in physician-patient interaction. *Journal of Health Politics, Policy and Law, 31*(4), 811–838.

Shapiro, J., & Saltzer, E. (1981). Cross-cultural aspects of physician-patient communications patterns. *Urban Health, 10*(10), 10–15.

Street, R. L., O'Malley, K. J., Cooper, L. A., & Haidet, P. (2008). Understanding concordance in patient-physician relationships: personal and ethnic dimensions of shared identity. *The Annals of Family Medicine, 6*(3), 198–205.

Thomas, K. C., Owino, H., Ansari, S., Adams, L., Cyr, J. M., Gaynes, B. N., & Glickman, S. W. (2018). Patient-centered values and experiences with emergency department and mental health crisis care. *Administration and Policy in Mental Health and Mental Health Services Research*, 1–12.

Thompson, L., & McCabe, R. (2012). The effect of clinician-patient alliance and communication on treatment adherence in mental health care: a systematic review. *BMC Psychiatry, 12*(1), 87.

Van Voorhees, B. W., Fogel, J., Reinecke, M. A., Gladstone, T., Stuart, S., Gollan, J., … & Ross, R. (2009). Randomized clinical trial of an internet-based depression prevention program for adolescents (Project CATCH-IT) in primary care: 12-week outcomes. *Journal of Developmental & Behavioral Pediatrics, 30*(1), 23–37.

Vasquez, M. J. (2007). Cultural difference and the therapeutic alliance: An evidence-based analysis. *American Psychologist, 62*(8), 878.

Venner, K. L., Feldstein, S. W., & Tafoya, N. (2007). Helping clients feel welcome: Principles of adapting treatment cross-culturally. *Alcoholism Treatment Quarterly, 25*(4), 11–30.

Venner, K. L., Greenfield, B. L., Hagler, K. J., Simmons, J., Lupee, D., Homer, E., … & Smith, J. E. (2016). Pilot outcome results of culturally adapted evidence-based substance use disorder treatment with a southwest tribe. *Addictive Behaviors Reports, 3*, 21–27.

Westra, H. A., Arkowitz, H., & Dozois, D. J. (2009). Adding a motivational interviewing pretreatment to cognitive behavioral therapy for generalized anxiety disorder: A preliminary randomized controlled trial. *Journal of Anxiety Disorders, 23*(8), 1106–1117.

Westra, H. A., Aviram, A., & Doell, F. K. (2011). Extending motivational interviewing to the treatment of major mental health problems: current directions and evidence. *The Canadian Journal of Psychiatry, 56*(11), 643–650.

Wiederhold, B. K., & Riva, G. (2013). *Annual Review of Cybertherapy and Telemedicine 2013: Positive Technology and Health Engagement for Healthy Living and Active Ageing* (Vol. 191). Amsterdam, Netherlands: Ios Press.

CHAPTER 5

The Impact of Racism on the Mental Health of People of Color

Shawn C. T. Jones,
University of Pennsylvania

Enrique W. Neblett Jr.,
University of North Carolina at Chapel Hill

But racism, his real foe, had gutted and decapitated his existence without his ever being able to draw a bead on even its most salient manifestations.... Buttressed by powers a thousand times more formidable than his, racism had ensured that his mind would construe the world in a fashion that would put him on a course toward self-destruction.

—Camara Jules Harrell, *Manichean Psychology*

Introduction

In his shrewd and insightful treatise, *Manichean Psychology: Racism and the Minds of People of African Descent*, clinical psychologist Camara Jules P. Harrell (1999) describes the impact of racism on the mind of a twenty-something "drug kingpin" found guilty of all charges related to drug distribution. He described racism as a protracted and power-based social phenomenon that saturates society and compromises the core consciousness, mindset, and cognitive framework of the oppressed. Twenty years later, racism remains an ever-relevant and ubiquitous force—whether named or unnamed—that impacts everyday life for many people of color.

Recent data suggest that racial discrimination is a common experience for people of color in the United States, with 93 percent of African Americans, 78 percent of Latinx Americans, and 61 percent of Asian Americans reporting that their racial and ethnic group experiences discrimination (National Public Radio, 2017). The health impacts of racism are profound and vexing, with people of color in the United States generally experiencing poorer health, including mental health, relative to their White, advantaged counterparts, even after adjustment for socioeconomic status (D. R. Williams, 2012).

The goal of this chapter is to summarize and provide perspective on the conceptual and empirical literature addressing the impact of racism on the mental health of people of color. We begin by providing an overview of the various forms of racism and presenting several models that can explain the racism–mental health link. The primary thrust of the chapter summarizes literature regarding that link, discussing both mental health disorders as well as other indicators of psychological health. We also consider often overlooked institutional and cultural forms of racism and how they may impact the mental health of people of color. Finally, we provide a summary statement highlighting the significance of this important topic, as well as implications for improving the mental health suffering of people of color who experience racism.

Defining Racism in Its Multiple Forms

According to James Jones's (1997) seminal work on racism and prejudice, racism refers to "the exercise of power against a racial group defined as inferior" (p. 280) and consists of *prejudice*—negative attitudes and beliefs toward racial out-groups—and *discrimination*—differential treatment of members of such out-groups, either by individuals or social institutions. An example of racial prejudice is the internal belief that Whites are superior to other races and ethnicities, while discrimination could take the form of someone being denied a job because of an "ethnic" sounding name (Nunley, Pugh, Romero, & Seals, 2015).

Jones further suggested that racism manifests in three primary forms. *Individual racism* is the belief that another racial group is inferior and the interpersonal behavioral enactments that maintain these beliefs. This form of racism can be either *overt and blatant* (such as use of a racial slur) or *covert and subtle* (such as being mistaken for someone who serves others). The latter has also been termed "microaggressions"—"innocuous, preconscious or unconscious degradations and putdowns" (Pierce, 1995; p. 281; Sue et al., 2007). Recent scholarship has increasingly recognized the subtler nature of racism-related stress experiences as compared to more overt acts of racism (Dovidio & Gaertner, 2000; Merritt, Bennett, Williams, Edwards, & Sollers, 2006; Neblett, Gaskin, Lee, & Carter, 2011; Tynes & Markoe, 2010). A second type of racism is *institutional racism*, which is the manipulation of societal institutions in ways that achieve racist objectives or limit the access and rights of a group. Examples of institutional racism include racial profiling, predatory lending, and race-related disparities in access to mental health care services (Rostain, Ramsay, & Waite, 2015; Smedley, Stith, & Nelson, 2003) or quality mental health care. Third, *cultural racism* is a broader "racialized" worldview reflective of beliefs in the race-based superiority of one group's cultural heritage over another (Jones, 1997). Cultural racism often manifests in "images and ideas in contemporary culture" (Williams & Mohammed, 2013a, p. 1155), such as negative depictions and stereotypes of people of color in television programs, books, and newspapers (Mutz & Goldman, 2010; D. R. Williams & Mohammed, 2013a) and the systematic exclusion or erasure of the contributions of people of color in textbooks, course curricula, and other media. C. P. Jones (2000) argued that cultural racism can lead to *internalized racism*, defined as acceptance by members of stigmatized racial groups of negative messages from the mainstream about their groups. Internalized racism includes messages about a people's ability, value, or worth, and is conceptualized to manifest as an embracing of "Whiteness," self-devaluation, and persistent hopelessness and helplessness (C. P. Jones, 2000). As definitions of racism have evolved, scholars have increasingly recognized racism as an organized system (i.e., *structural* racism; Bonilla-Silva, 1997) in which individual beliefs, institutional practices, and cultural representations combine to reinforce and perpetuate racial group inequity.

Shelly Harrell (2000) articulated several ways in which "race-related transactions between individuals or groups and their environment that emerge from the dynamics of racism" (p. 44), or *racism-related stress*, can impact the psychological well-being of people of color. Although many of Harrell's dimensions of racism-related stress fit within the three types of racism offered by C. P. Jones, they are worth presenting for their nuance, specificity, and relevance to modern, twenty-first-century racism. *Racism-related life events* are time-limited, specific life experiences. *Vicarious racism* occurs through the observation and report of others' racism experiences and has become more frequent with social media, as individuals are presented and reexposed to a litany of highly publicized racial events (e.g., the arrest of two Black men in a Philadelphia Starbucks who were waiting for a friend; Dias, Eligon, & Oppel Jr., 2018). *Daily racism microstressors* are synonymous with the previously discussed microaggressions, with recent examples including #LivingWhileBlack (or other racial and ethnic minorities; Underhill, 2018; Victor, 2018): stressful racial encounters occurring during a number of seemingly mundane tasks (i.e., barbequing, swimming, walking, gaming, sleeping, moving in, mowing, and even "couponing"). *Chronic-contextual stress* and *collective experiences* are analogous to Jones's institutional and cultural forms, respectively. Finally, Harrell posited that racism-related stress is *transgenerational* and can be transmitted through the passing down of historical events (e.g., Native Americans recalling the lasting effects of the Trail of Tears). Importantly, these distinct types of racism-related stressors often co-occur. They also interact with other stressors, both those general in nature (e.g., financial) and those due to other social identities (e.g., sexism, heterosexism, Islamophobia). Though far from exhaustive, the aforementioned foundational definitions of racism and evolution of the racism concept have proved instructive in providing a framework and advancing our understanding of the profound, nuanced, and multilevel impacts of racism on the mental health of people of color.

Models Explaining Racism's Impact on Mental Health

Several informative frameworks and models have been offered to explain the impact of racism on health (Clark, Anderson, Clark, & Williams, 1999; Gee, Walsemann, and Brondolo, 2012; Harrell et al., 2011; Krieger, 2012; Williams & Mohammed, 2009; Williams & Mohammed, 2013a), though it is disappointing that few focus exclusively on mental health and psychological well-being. Although originally conceptualized in the context of African American experiences and extended to other populations of color (e.g., Kaholokula et al., 2017), Rodney Clark and colleagues' (1999) seminal *Biopsychosocial Model of Racism* suggested that the perception of environmental stimuli as racially discriminatory or prejudiced leads to amplified psychological (e.g., anger) and physiological responses. These perceptions are influenced by constitutional factors (e.g., skin tone), sociodemographic factors (e.g., socioeconomic status), and psychological and behavioral factors (e.g., anger expression) that also moderate the psychological outcomes that stem from exposure to racial discrimination. The model also defines mediating variables (i.e., coping responses and stress responses) that are thought to positively or negatively impact the relationship between perceived racism-related stressors and health outcomes.

The most recent models of racism and (mental) health are similar to Clark and colleagues' biopsychosocial model and other early models of racism and health in their use of stress and coping as a theoretical framework and their consideration of context (e.g., sociodemographic factors), psychological processes (e.g., worry and rumination; changes in affective states), and racism at the individual level (e.g., racial discrimination). But these models also are increasingly complex and distinct from earlier models. First, they highlight multiple levels of racism and include not only individual racism but also institutional and cultural racism as fundamental determinants of health (Williams & Mohammed, 2013a). Second, recent models delineate specific pathways by which racism might impact mental health. These mechanisms span multiple levels and domains of analysis and include cognitive factors (e.g., cognitive schema); neural mechanisms such as amygdala and prefrontal cortical activation and inhibition; structural and functional changes in neuroendocrine, autonomic, and immune physiological systems; cultural transmission via stereotypes; unhealthy behaviors (e.g., substance use); socioeconomic opportunities (e.g., education, employment, income and wealth); and societal resources (e.g., medical care, housing, neighborhood) (Harrell et al., 2011; Williams & Mohammed, 2009; Williams & Mohammed, 2013a). Third, the models incorporate life-course perspectives that consider not only how racism impacts health at a specific moment but also how the effects of racism on subsequent health can begin as early as the gestational period, with prenatal effects that extend throughout life (Gee et al., 2012; Harrell et al., 2011). These models are welcome additions for shaping future research in a field that has traditionally focused on individual racism and other oversimplified reductions of racism that fail to capture the complex and enduring ways in which racism impacts the mental health of people of color across multiple levels, ecologies, and contexts. Furthermore, the delineation of underlying mechanisms and pathways and relevant contexts will be a critical next step necessary to develop effective interventions that can reduce the health impact of multiple dimensions of racism (see Williams & Mohammed, 2013b) and produce large-scale improvement in mental health disparities.

"Under the Skin, into the Mind": Detailing the Impact of Racism on Mental Health

Scholars have long sought to understand the ways in which racism gets "under the skin," referring to physical health disparities related to diseases such as diabetes and cardiovascular disease. Consistent with C. J. P. Harrell's (1999) central premise, we further argue that it is equally important to understand how racism can get "into the mind" and impinge upon the mental health status of people of color. Though not a formal conceptual model, Harrell posited three regions of mental impact: (1) competence and efficacy; (2) standards of beauty and body image; and (3) views of culture and history. Briefly, Harrell argued that racism affects the "cognitive operations" of people of color by sowing seeds of doubt and dependency such that people of color begin to doubt their own competence. Second, the oppressed come to see the physical characteristics of the European (e.g., skin color, facial features, and hair texture) as exalted and the physical counterparts of people of color as ugly, evil, and in need of fixing (e.g., through skin bleaching, rhinoplasty). Third, racism "reinterprets, diminishes, or destroys the historical and cultural memory of the oppressed" (p. 23), such that the oppressed internalize distortions and derogatory evaluations of their history and culture, and contributions of their history and culture are minimized and seen as inferior. While the focus of work examining racism and mental health is often on psychological symptoms, Harrell's contribution is invaluable in its contribution of underlying cognitive factors that may mediate some of the negative mental health impacts of racism.

Before turning to the relevant empirical literature, it is important to acknowledge that race-related differences in mental health depend on the index under investigation. Epidemiological research from the Epidemiologic Catchment Area (ECA) Survey and the National Comorbidity Survey (NCS) and Replication (NCS-R) has suggested that the prevalence of most mental health disorders is lower for Hispanics and non-Hispanic Blacks relative to their White counterparts (Breslau et al., 2006; Breslau, Kendler, Su, Gaxiola-Aguilar, & Kessler, 2005; Suarez, Polo, Chen, & Alegría, 2009; Zhang & Snowden, 1999). Unfortunately, Native American and Asian American samples either were not included in these studies or were too small to draw meaningful conclusions on their responses (US Department of Health and Human Services [USDHHS], 2001). Despite findings of lower prevalence rates for diagnostically defined disorders, ethnic minority populations are consistently found to have higher *psychological distress*, which often includes psychological symptoms that make up these disorders (e.g., nervousness, hopelessness, aggression, substance use; Centers for Disease Control, 2016; USDHHS, 2001). In addition, populations of color are often found to report lower *psychological well-being*, which can include variables such as "mental health status" as well as happiness, life satisfaction, and self-esteem. Given that the majority of studies have examined the link between racism and distress and well-being factors, we present these, followed by studies that have examined the link between racism and specific mental health disorders.

Racism, Psychological Distress, and Well-Being

The literature regarding the psychological distress (e.g., Chae, Lincoln, & Jackson, 2011; Syed & Juan, 2012) and well-being correlates of racism is expansive, with an impressive number of reviews synthesizing these findings (e.g., Priest et al., 2013; Williams & Mohammed, 2009). For example, Williams, Neighbors, and Jackson (2003) reviewed fifty-three community studies exploring the link between racial and ethnic discrimination and health, accounting for eighty-six associations. Of these studies, more than half (thirty-two studies, forty-seven associations) contained at least one measure of mental health. Most of these studies included markers of psychological distress; however, studies exploring indices of psychological well-being, as well as diagnosable psychiatric disorders (e.g., major depression) were included. In total, thirty-eight of these studies found that higher endorsement of discrimination was associated with higher levels of mental health illness or risk. Williams and Mohammed (2009) identified forty-seven studies that could be related to mental health and discrimination in ethnic minority populations, with most studies evincing a negative discrimination–mental health link. Subsequent meta-analyses found significant associations between racial discrimination and poor mental health (e.g., Pascoe & Smart Richman, 2009; Pieterse, Todd, Neville, & Carter, 2012).

Regarding youth outcomes, Priest and colleagues (2013) determined that of 461 associations explored across 121 studies of multiethnic youth, more than half of these studies investigated the association between racism and mental health, with significant cross-sectional and prospective associations between racism-related stress and negative mental health (e.g., depression, anxiety) and behavioral problems (e.g., conduct problems, aggression), as well as decreases in indices of positive mental health (e.g., self-worth, self-esteem, resilience). Hope, Hoggard, and Thomas (2015) also reviewed the physiological, psychological, and sociopolitical consequences of racial discrimination for African American emerging adults.

In addition to these reviews and meta-analyses, more recent findings continue to extend our understanding of the pernicious ways in which racism impacts psychological distress and well-being. Tobler and colleagues (2013) determined that discrimination due to race and ethnicity was associated with increased depression as well as behavioral issues (e.g., physical aggression) and suicidal ideation, with a dose-response pattern such that being more disturbed by discriminatory experiences was associated with poorer outcomes. Kwate and Goodman (2015) explored both cross-sectional and longitudinal (two-month and one-year) associations between racism (measured using three different measures of discrimination) and psychological distress, depression symptoms, and poor mental health status among two Black neighborhoods in New York City. In addition to compelling cross-sectioning associations, findings suggested that increases in both daily experiences of discrimination and everyday discrimination over time were associated with increased reports of distress, depression, and poor mental health days. Moreover, the authors determined that these associations were stronger among those individuals who reported not thinking about race, a relevant finding given the promulgation of "post-racial" and "color-blind" ideologies that emerged during the presidency of Barack Obama (Bouie, 2014). Beyond individual racial discrimination, recent investigations have also examined Harrell's notion of collective transgenerational racism-related stress. Park, Du, Wang, Williams, and Alegría (2018) used Gee and colleagues' (2012) life course perspective of racism and health to explore the *linked lives* hypothesis within a Mexican-origin sample. Specifically, they assessed whether parents' experiences with discrimination impacted the association between youths' experiences of discrimination and psychological distress. Findings indicated that fathers' experiences with discrimination exacerbated the association between adolescents' discrimination and depressive symptoms. This study serves as one of the first to highlight the intergenerational impact of racism on mental health for communities of color.

Racism and Psychological Disorders

Conceptual and empirical work (see table 1 for recent examples) also link racism with specific psychological disorders and associated symptoms. For instance, a recent review paper (Berger & Sarnyai, 2015) offered a stress neurobiology framework for understanding how racial discrimination might lead to adverse mental health outcomes. Chronic racial discrimination experiences may activate stress hormones (e.g., cortisol) and neurotransmitters (e.g., dopamine), which impact functional brain networks (e.g., prefrontal cortex), in turn leading to structural and network activity changes and deleterious mental health outcomes (e.g., development of anxiety disorders). With respect to empirical studies, there are far fewer studies that have associated racism with specific psychiatric disorders relative to studies of the associations between racism and mental health symptoms (see Mouzon, Taylor, Keith, Nicklett, & Chatters, 2017). However, some studies examine both. Gee, Spencer, Chen, Yip, and Takeuchi (2007) found that Asian Americans' self-reported racial discrimination was associated with twelve-month prevalence of any disorder (assessed as the presence of at least one of the eleven most common psychiatric disorders), as well as depressive disorder and anxiety disorder, even after controlling for social desirability, other stressors, and socioeconomic status. Those experiencing discrimination were also two times as likely to meet criteria for one disorder in the past twelve months, and three times more likely to have two or more disorders.

Phillips and Lauterbach (2017) recently catalogued the extant literature on racism and mental health as it pertains to American Muslim immigrants, noting that individual forms of racism have been found to be associated with psychological disorders such as PTSD, as well as symptoms of stress, anxiety, and depression. Importantly, a recent investigation by Rodriguez-Seijas, Stohl, Hasin, and Eaton (2015) found direct associations between perceived discrimination and twelve common psychiatric disorders (e.g., MDD, GAD, PTSD); however, using structural equation modeling techniques, the investigators were able to determine that this relationship was either partially or completely (e.g., social anxiety, ADHD) mediated by factors that represented the shared variance among internalizing and externalizing disorders (termed "transdiagnostic factors"). As such, these findings may help to contextualize the prior research on the racism–psychiatric disorder link. Continued explorations of transdiagnostic variance may reveal that it is racism's relationship with this latent construct (e.g., underlying internalizing factors) that drives the racism–mental health link, rather than racism's relationship to any specific disorder (e.g., GAD).

In addition to cataloguing the impact of racism on mental health disorders, some scholars have argued for the unique inclusion of the traumatic nature of racism as a mental health consequence (or "psychological injury"). Indeed, *racist-incident trauma* and *race-based traumatic stress* have been used to describe the psychological and psychophysiological sequelae associated with racist incidents (for an extensive overview, see Carter, 2007). In this framing, racist encounters are seen as "cognitive/affective assaults" (Bryant-Davis & Ocampo, 2005, p. 480) and described as emotionally painful, sudden, and uncontrollable (Carlson, 1997). Per Carlson, these incidents must include intrusion, avoidance, arousal, or irritability, with psychological symptoms such as anxiety, depression, anger, low self-esteem, guilt, and shame. Carter (2007), moreover, conceptualized this traumatic criterion with respect to racialized experiences. Nevertheless, despite the extensive work by Carter and colleagues (e.g., Carter & Forsyth, 2009; Carter & Sant-Barket, 2015) and calls for the formal recognition of race-based traumatic stress (see also Holmes, Facemire, & Da Fonseca, 2016), as of the writing of this chapter, neither the diagnostic guidelines for psychology (DSM-5) nor medicine (ICD-10) formally includes racism-related trauma. As a whole, recent literature documents diverse and far-reaching mental health impacts (broadly defined) of racism (primarily racial discrimination).

Table 1. Recent Studies of Racism and Mental Health

Mental Health Condition and Symptoms	Racial and Ethnic Groups	Representative Studies
Generalized Anxiety Disorder	African Americans, Afro Caribbeans	Soto, Dawson-Andoh, & BeLue, 2011
Post-traumatic Stress Disorder	African Americans; Latinx; Mexican Americans	Cheng and Mallinckrodt, 2015; Flores et al., 2010; Williams et al., 2014

Major Depressive Disorder	African Americans, Latinx	Banks & Kohn-Wood, 2007; Torres et al., 2010; Umaña-Taylor & Updegraff, 2007
Psychotic Disorders	African Americans, US Multiethnic	Anglin et al., 2014; Oh et al., 2014
Obsessive Compulsive Disorder	African Americans	Williams et al., 2017
Eating Disorders	African Americans; Asian Americans; Multiethnic	Cheng et al., 2017; Hicken, Lee, & Hing, 2017
Alcohol Use Disorder	African Americans; US Multiethnic	Blume et al., 2012; Hurd et al., 2014
Substance Use Disorders	African Americans; Latinx	Acosta et al., 2015; Gerrard et al., 2012
Suicidal Ideation	African Americans	Hollingsworth et al., 2017; O'Keefe et al., 2015

Institutional Racism and Mental Health

The overwhelming emphasis on individual racism (i.e., racial discrimination) reflects a shortcoming of the extant literature in light of prior theoretical formulations of racism and empirical evidence suggesting that institutional and cultural racism also are important to consider in understanding the link between racism and mental health (Bécares, Nazroo, and Jackson, 2014; Cooper, McLoyd, Wood, & Hardaway, 2008; Williams & Mohammed, 2013a). Williams and Williams-Morris (2000) have suggested that institutional racism leads to truncated socioeconomic mobility, a known risk factor for psychological distress, psychiatric disorder, and illness (Gong, Xu, & Takeuchi, 2012; Kessler et al., 1994; Robins & Regier, 1991; Williams, Takeuchi, & Adair, 1992). Their analysis highlights *residential segregation*—physical separation of the races intersecting with vital institutions such as real estate, consumer banking, and housing policies—as a specific example of institutional racism that compromises access to quality education, employment, and overall quality of life (e.g., increased exposure to chronic and acute stress, poorer-quality housing and mental health care [Wang, Demler, & Kessler, 2002]), with implications for mental health.

First, given decreased access to resources and the presence of inflexible policies, residential segregation negatively impacts the school context. Challenges facing segregated schools include lower test scores, fewer students in advanced placement courses, more limited curricula, fewer qualified teachers, more deteriorated buildings, higher levels of teen pregnancy, and higher dropout rates. Second, residential segregation limits employment opportunities by decreasing access to low-skilled, entry-level high-paying jobs. Third, residential segregation perpetuates unequal access to social services and economic resources due to reduction in the urban tax base that supports these services because of out-migration of Whites and middle-class Blacks from cities to the suburbs. Finally, Williams and Williams-Morris suggested that segregation can affect socioeconomic status by isolating individuals from role models of stable employment and social networks that could provide leads about employment opportunities. Collectively, the lack of access to critical resources mediated by segregation leads to compromised socioeconomic mobility, which, in turn, increases risk for poor mental health. Moreover, several characteristics that are concomitant with highly segregated, economically impoverished neighborhoods, such as crime, violence, homicide, and other forms of personal victimization (e.g., assaults), are commonly associated with adverse mental health effects such as suicidal ideation and attempts, trauma exposure and symptoms, psychosomatic symptoms, depression, and drug and alcohol use (Vinkers, de Beurs, Barendregt, Rinne, & Hoek, 2011; Williams & Williams-Morris, 2000). While the underlying mechanisms responsible for these consequences still require further examination, scholars have suggested that, in some cases, the negative impact of segregation on mental health is mediated by not only racial differences in socioeconomic status and truncated socioeconomic mobility but also increased family stress (Charles, Dinwiddie, & Massey, 2004) or even the chronic experience of grief over the loss of loved ones in neighborhoods and communities that experience a disproportionate share of homicides (Williams & Williams-Morris, 2000).

In addition to segregation, scholars have suggested that unequal treatment in the criminal justice system may be a second form of institutional racism with implications for mental health. Disproportionate police surveillance (e.g., stop-and-frisk programs), combined with racial biases found in stand-your-ground states, might lead to increased stress and psychological (and physiological) arousal as a function of anticipatory coping and heightened vigilance due to fear of a humiliating or fatal encounter (Brunson & Miller, 2006; Nordberg, Twis, Stevens, & Hatcher, 2018; Purdie-Vaughns & Williams, 2015; Stewart, Baumer, Brunson, & Simons, 2009). The negative mental health impacts of incarceration—another commonly cited example of institutional racism involving the justice system—are also far-reaching, with implications for not only the incarcerated but also their families. Incarcerated individuals are often contending with serious mental illness (Leidenfrost et al., 2016) and may experience additional psychological distress as a result of being unable to provide social and economic support to their families, the strain of being separated, abuse from correctional officers and other inmates while imprisoned, and the negative stigma of being incarcerated. A criminal record upon reentry to society may further exacerbate adverse mental health (Begun, Early, & Hodge, 2016) due to the loss of previously enjoyed rights (e.g., temporary or permanent prohibition from voting following felony conviction) or the difficulty obtaining employment and accessing housing, financial aid, and social welfare programs because of the stigma attached to having a criminal record. These broad difficulties can lead to personal blame, disengagement, and psychological distress (Cooper et al., 2008), further amplifying risk factors associated with negative mental health (e.g., unemployment). Partners of the incarcerated may experience negative economic, social, and emotional impacts such as isolation and the demands of child rearing alone, while children of the incarcerated may experience rejection, guilt, depressive symptoms, discipline problems, antisocial behavior, and declines in school performance (Gaston, 2016; Miller, Browning, & Spruance, 2001; Murray, Farrington, & Sekol, 2012). Collectively, the available literature examining segregation and mass incarceration calls attention to the fact that a focus on racism at the individual level provides an incomplete picture of the psychological impacts of racism.

Cultural Racism and Mental Health

Even fewer empirical studies have examined the impact of cultural racism on mental health; however, scholars have argued that cultural racism, as mediated by negative images of people of color and negative stereotypes, may influence thoughts, feelings, and behaviors and impact mental health in several ways (Harrell, 1999; Williams, Gooden, & Davis, 2012; Williams & Mohammed, 2013a; Williams & Williams-Morris, 2000). First, repeated exposure to negative images of people of color may lead to acceptance of negative stereotypes or beliefs by stigmatized groups about their own race or perceptions of themselves as worthless and powerless (internalized racism). The negative self-cognitions associated with internalized racism have been found to be associated with negative mental health outcomes such as alcohol consumption (Taylor & Jackson, 1990), decreased marital satisfaction (Taylor, 1990), low self-esteem and psychological well-being (Williams & Mohammed, 2009), and, more recently, anxious arousal (Graham, West, Martinez, & Roemer, 2016) and depressive symptoms (Mouzon & McLean, 2017).

Second, the negative racial and ethnic stereotypes that permeate society may undergird implicit bias—cognitive associations that exist beyond conscious awareness (Banaji & Greenwald, 2013). Such biases are pervasive in books, newspapers, and other materials (Verhaegen, Aikman, & Van Gulick, 2011), and may be responsible, in part, for misdiagnosis (e.g., overdiagnosis of paranoid schizophrenia, underdiagnosis of affective disorders) and differential treatment of patients in the mental health system (Hall et al., 2015; Williams & Williams-Morris, 2000). Prior research suggests, for example, that unconscious discrimination by providers may lead to biased treatment recommendations and impact patient-provider communications and the overall quality of care provided (van Ryn et al., 2011; Williams & Mohammed, 2013a). Negative medical encounters may facilitate cultural mistrust in patients and lead to decreased engagement with treatment and utilization of services, further exacerbating negative mental health outcomes (Earl & Williams, 2009). The impact of negative stereotypes on mental health may also be mediated by stereotype threat (Steele, 1997), or fear of confirming stereotypes about one's group. Stereotype threat has been linked with increased anxiety and reduced self-regulation (Inzlicht & Kang, 2010), placing individuals who experience stereotype threat at risk for poorer mental health. Thus, cultural racism may lead to internalized racism or shape the thoughts, feelings, and behaviors of people of color and mental health service providers, with implications for well-being, distress, and the quality of mental health care. There is little question that, going forward, research examining racism and mental health will need to carefully examine how cultural representations of racism impact mental health and compromise the mental health functioning of people of color.

Conclusion

Racism, in all its forms, constitutes a significant risk to the mental health of people of color in the United States. In this chapter, we have named multiple forms of racism and briefly considered evidence suggesting their impact on the mental health of people of color. We reviewed several theoretical frameworks that support conceptualization of racism as a stressor that operates on multiple levels (i.e., individual, institutional, cultural) to influence mental health. Next, we provided a brief review of literature high-lighting the impact of individual racism as well as institutional and cultural racism on mental health. As residential segregation persists, and manifestations of institutional racism as mediated by differential treatment in the justice system are ongoing, it will be important to adopt a multipronged, multisystemic approach to addressing racism in our minds as a critical social determinant of mental health. As always, the most arduous work will be not only in documenting the link between racism and its multiple forms and mental health, but also in delineating underlying (and disrupting) pathways and mechanisms, and targeting and reshaping societal institutions and structures, which also, albeit indirectly, impact the mental health of people and communities of color in the United States. Through understanding the structural foundation and composition of racism and unpacking its undergirding mechanisms for people of color, we can chart a path forward that will lead to salutary outcomes for all.

KEY POINTS FOR CLINICIANS

- Racism poses a significant risk to the mental health of people of color.

- Racism is multidimensional and consists of not only individual racism but also institutional, cultural, and structural racism, all of which interact with non-race-related stressors to impact the mental health of people of color.

- It is important to understand clients' experiences with racism and discrimination, as well as their coping strategies, which can be both adaptive and maladaptive and can shape the health impacts of racism.

- Institutional racism may confer additional mental health risks above and beyond interpersonal experiences of racial discrimination through negatively influencing opportunities for socioeconomic mobility and increasing the co-occurrence of other known risk factors for negative mental health.

- Cultural racism may impact clients' trust of providers, the ways in which clients interface with the mental health system, and the quality of the mental health care that they receive.

References

Acosta, S. L., Hospital, M. M., Graziano, J. N., Morris, S., & Wagner, E. F. (2015). Pathways to drinking among Hispanic/Latino adolescents: perceived discrimination, ethnic identity, and peer affiliations. *Journal of Ethnicity in Substance Abuse, 14*(3), 270–286.

Anglin, D. M., Lighty, Q., Greenspoon, M., & Ellman, L. M. (2014). Racial discrimination is associated with distressing subthreshold positive psychotic symptoms among US urban ethnic minority young adults. *Social Psychiatry and Psychiatric Epidemiology, 49*(10), 1545–1555.

Banaji, M. R., & Greenwald, A. G. (2013). *Blindspot: Hidden biases of good people.* New York, NY: Delacorte Press.

Banks, K. H., & Kohn-Wood, L. P. (2007). The influence of racial identity profiles on the relationship between racial discrimination and depressive symptoms. *Journal of Black Psychology, 33*(3), 331–354.

Bécares, L., Nazroo, J., & Jackson, J. (2014). Ethnic density and depressive symptoms among African Americans: Threshold and differential effects across social and demographic subgroups. *American Journal of Public Health, 104*(12), 2334–2341.

Begun, A. L., Early, T. J., & Hodge, A. (2016). Mental health and substance abuse service engagement by men and women during community reentry following incarceration. *Administration and Policy in Mental Health and Mental Health Services Research, 43*(2), 207–218.

Berger, M., & Sarnyai, Z. (2015). "More than skin deep": Stress neurobiology and mental health consequences of racial discrimination. *Stress, 18*(1), 1–10.

Blume, A. W., Lovato, L. V., Thyken, B. N., & Denny, N. (2012). The relationship of microaggressions with alcohol use and anxiety among ethnic minority college students in a historically White institution. *Cultural Diversity and Ethnic Minority Psychology, 18*(1), 45.

Bonilla-Silva, E. (1997). Rethinking racism: Toward a structural interpretation. *American Sociological Review*, 62(3) 465–480.

Bouie, J. (2014). Why do millennials not understand racism? *Slate*. (May 16, 2014). Retrieved from http://www.slate.com/articles/news_and_politics/politics/2014/05/millennials_raci sm_and_mtv_poll_young_people_are_confused_about_bias_prejudice.html

Breslau, J., Aguilar-Gaxiola, S., Kendler, K. S., Su, M., Williams, D., & Kessler, R. C. (2006). Specifying race-ethnic differences in risk for psychiatric disorder in a USA national sample. *Psychological Medicine*, 36(1), 57–68.

Breslau, J., Kendler, K. S., Su, M., Gaxiola-Aguilar, S., & Kessler, R. C. (2005). Lifetime risk and persistence of psychiatric disorders across ethnic groups in the United States. *Psychological Medicine*, 35(3), 317–327.

Brunson, R. K., & Miller, J. (2006). Gender, race, and urban policing: The experience of African American youths. *Gender & Society*, 20(4), 531–552.

Bryant-Davis, T., & Ocampo, C. (2005). Racist incident–based trauma. *Counseling Psychologist*, 33, 479–500.

Carlson, E. B. (1997). *Trauma assessments: A clinician's guide*. New York, NY: Guilford Press.

Carter, R. T. (2007). Racism and psychological and emotional injury: Recognizing and assessing race-based traumatic stress. *The Counseling Psychologist*, 35, 13–105.

Carter, R. T., & Forsyth, J. M. (2009). A guide to the forensic assessment of race-based traumatic stress reactions. *The Journal of the American Academy of Psychiatry and the Law*, 37, 28–40.

Carter, R. T., & Sant-Barket, S. M. (2015). Assessment of impact of racial discrimination and racism: How to use the Race-Based Traumatic Stress Symptom Scale in practice. *Traumatology*, 21(1), 32–39.

Centers for Disease Control (2016). *Health United States, 2015*. Retrieved from http://www.cdc.gov/nchs/data/hus/hus15.pdf

Chae, D. H., Lincoln, K. D., & Jackson, J. S. (2011). Discrimination, attribution, and racial group identification: Implications for psychological distress among Black Americans in the National Survey of American Life (2001–2003). *American Journal of Orthopsychiatry*, 81(4), 498–506.

Charles, C. Z., Dinwiddie, G., & Massey, D. S. (2004). The continuing consequences of segregation: Family stress and college academic performance. *Social Science Quarterly*, 85(5), 1353–1373.

Charles, K. K., Hurst, E., & Stephens, M., Jr. (2006). Exploring racial differences in vehicle loan rates. Working Paper, NBER. April 2006.

Cheng, H. L., & Mallinckrodt, B. (2015). Racial/ethnic discrimination, posttraumatic stress symptoms, and alcohol problems in a longitudinal study of Hispanic/Latino college students. *Journal of Counseling Psychology*, 62(1), 38–49.

Cheng, H. L., Tran, A. G., Miyake, E. R., & Kim, H. Y. (2017). Disordered eating among Asian American college women: A racially expanded model of objectification theory. *Journal of Counseling psychology*, 64(2), 179.

Clark, R., Anderson, N. B., Clark, V. R., & Williams, D. R. (1999). Racism as a stressor for African Americans: A biopsychosocial model. *American Psychologist*, 54(10), 805–816.

Cooper, S. M., McLoyd, V. C., Wood, D., & Hardaway, C. R. (2008). Racial discrimination and the mental health of African American adolescents. In S. M. Quintana & C. McKown (Eds.), *Handbook of race, racism, and the developing child* (pp. 278–312). Hoboken, NJ: Wiley.

Dias, E., Eligon, J., & Oppell Jr., R. A. (2018). Philadelphia Starbucks arrests, outrageous to some, are everyday life for others. *The New York Times*. Retrieved from https://www.nytimes.com/2018/04/17/us/starbucks-arrest-philadelphia.html

Dovidio, J. F., & Gaertner, S. L. (2000). Aversive racism and selection decisions: 1989 and 1999. *Psychological Science*, 11(4), 315–319. doi:10.1111/1467-9280.00262

Earl, T. R., & Williams, D. R. (2009). Black Americans and mental health status. In H. A. Neville, B. M. Tynes, & S. O. Utsey (Eds.), *Handbook of African American Psychology* (p. 335). Thousand Oaks, CA: Sage.

Flores, E., Tschann, J. M., Dimas, J. M., Pasch, L. A., & de Groat, C. L. (2010). Perceived racial and ethnic discrimination, posttraumatic stress symptoms, and health risk behaviors among Mexican American adolescents. *Journal of Counseling Psychology, 57*(3), 264–273.

Gaston, S. (2016). The long-term effects of parental incarceration: Does parental incarceration in childhood or adolescence predict depressive symptoms in adulthood? *Criminal Justice and Behavior, 43*(8), 1056–1075.

Gee, G. C., Spencer, M., Chen, J., Yip, T., & Takeuchi, D. T. (2007). The association between self-reported racial discrimination and 12-month DSM-IV mental disorders among Asian Americans nationwide. *Social Science & Medicine, 64*(10), 1984–1996.

Gee, G. C., Walsemann, K. M., & Brondolo, E. (2012). A life course perspective on how racism may be related to health inequities. *American Journal of Public Health, 102*(5), 967–974.

Gerrard, M., Stock, M. L., Roberts, M. E., Gibbons, F. X., O'Hara, R. E., Weng, C. Y., & Wills, T. A. (2012). Coping with racial discrimination: The role of substance use. *Psychology of Addictive Behaviors, 26*(3), 550.

Gong, F., Xu, J., & Takeuchi, D. T. (2012). Beyond conventional socioeconomic status: Examining subjective and objective social status with self-reported health among Asian immigrants. *Journal of Behavioral Medicine, 35*(4), 407–419.

Graham, J. R., West, L. M., Martinez, J., & Roemer, L. (2016). The mediating role of internalized racism in the relationship between racist experiences and anxiety symptoms in a Black American sample. *Cultural Diversity and Ethnic Minority Psychology, 22*(3), 369.

Hall, W. J., Chapman, M. V., Lee, K. M., Merino, Y. M., Thomas, T. W., Payne, B. K., … & Coyne-Beasley, T. (2015). Implicit racial/ethnic bias among health care professionals and its influence on health care outcomes: A systematic review. *American Journal of Public Health, 105*(12), E60–E76.

Harrell, C. J. P. (1999). Manichean psychology: Racism and the minds of people of African descent. Washington, DC: Howard University Press.

Harrell, C. J. P., Burford, T. I., Cage, B. N., Nelson, T. M., Shearon, S., Thompson, A., & Green, S. (2011). Multiple pathways linking racism to health outcomes. *Du Bois Review: Social Science Research on Race, 8*(1), 143–157.

Harrell, S. P. (2000). A multidimensional conceptualization of racism-related stress: Implications for the well-being of people of color. *American Journal of Orthopsychiatry, 70*(1), 42–57. doi:10.1037/h0087722

Hicken, M. T., Lee, H., & Hing, A. K. (2018). The weight of racism: Vigilance and racial inequalities in weight-related measures. *Social Science & Medicine, 199*, 157–166.

Hollingsworth, D. W., Cole, A. B., O'Keefe, V. M., Tucker, R. P., Story, C. R., & Wingate, L. R. (2017). Experiencing racial microaggressions influences suicide ideation through perceived burdensomeness in African Americans. *Journal of Counseling Psychology, 64*(1), 104.

Holmes, S. C., Facemire, V. C., & DaFonseca, A. M. (2016). Expanding criterion A for posttraumatic stress disorder: Considering the deleterious impact of oppression. *Traumatology, 22*(4), 314-321. doi:10.1037/trm0000104

Hope, E. C., Hoggard, L. S., & Thomas, A. (2015). Emerging into adulthood in the face of racial discrimination: Physiological, psychological, and sociopolitical consequences for african american youth. *Translational Issues in Psychological Science, 1*(4), 342.

Hurd, N. M., Varner, F. A., Caldwell, C. H., & Zimmerman, M. A. (2014). Does perceived racial discrimination predict changes in psychological distress and substance use over time? An examination among Black emerging adults. *Developmental Psychology, 50*(7), 1910.

Inzlicht, M., & Kang, S. K. (2010). Stereotype threat spillover: How coping with threats to social identity affects aggression, eating, decision making, and attention. *Journal of Personality and Social Psychology*, 99(3), 467.

Jones, C. P. 2000. Levels of racism: A theoretic framework and a gardener's tale. *American Journal of Public Health*, 90(8): 1212–1215.

Jones, J. M. (1997). *Prejudice and racism* (2nd ed.). New York, NY: McGraw-Hill. Originally published in 1972.

Kaholokula, J. K. A., Antonio, M. C., Ing, C. K. T., Hermosura, A., Hall, K. E., Knight, R., & Wills, T. A. (2017). The effects of perceived racism on psychological distress mediated by venting and disengagement coping in Native Hawaiians. *BMC Psychology*, 5(1), 2.

Kessler, R. C., McGonagle, K. A., Zhao, S., Nelson, C. B., Hughes, M., Eshleman, S., … & Kendler, K. S. (1994). Lifetime and 12-month prevalence of DSM-III-R psychiatric disorders in the United States: Results from the National Comorbidity Survey. *Archives of General Psychiatry*, 51(1), 8–19.

Krieger, N. (2012). Methods for the scientific study of discrimination and health: an ecosocial approach. *American Journal of Public Health*, 102(5), 936–944.

Kwate, N. O. A., & Goodman, M. S. (2015). Cross-sectional and longitudinal effects of racism on mental health among residents of Black neighborhoods in New York City. *American Journal of Public Health*, 105(4), 711–718.

Leidenfrost, C. M., Calabrese, W., Schoelerman, R. M., Coggins, E., Ranney, M., Sinclair, S. J., & Antonius, D. (2016). Changes in psychological health and subjective well-being among incarcerated individuals with serious mental illness. *Journal of Correctional Health Care*, 22(1), 12–20.

Merritt, M. M., Bennett, G. G. J., Williams, R. B., Edwards, C. L., & Sollers, J. J. I., II. (2006). Perceived racism and cardiovascular reactivity and recovery to personally relevant stress. *Health Psychology*, 25(3), 364–369. doi:10.1037/0278-6133.25.3.364

Miller, R. R., Browning, S. L., & Spruance, L. M. (2001). An introduction and brief review of the impacts of incarceration on the African American family. *Journal of African American Men*, 6(1), 3–12.

Moody, M. (2016). From under-diagnoses to over-representation: Black children, ADHD, and the school-to-prison pipeline. *Journal of African American Studies*, 20(2), 152–163.

Mouzon, D. M., & McLean, J. S. (2017). Internalized racism and mental health among African-Americans, US-born Caribbean Blacks, and foreign-born Caribbean Blacks. *Ethnicity & Health*, 22(1), 36–48.

Mouzon, D. M., Taylor, R. J., Keith, V. M., Nicklett, E. J., & Chatters, L. M. (2017). Discrimination and psychiatric disorders among older African Americans. *International Journal of Geriatric Psychiatry*, 32(2), 175–182.

Murray, J., Farrington, D. P., & Sekol, I. (2012). Children's antisocial behavior, mental health, drug use, and educational performance after parental incarceration: a systematic review and meta-analysis. *Psychological Bulletin*, 138(2), 175.

Mutz, D. C., & Goldman, S. K. (2010). Mass media. In J. F. Dovidio, M. Hewstone, P. Glick, & V. M. Esses (Eds.), *The Sage Handbook of Prejudice, Stereotyping and Discrimination* (pp. 241–257). Thousand Oaks, CA: Sage.

National Public Radio (2017). You, me and them: Experiencing discrimination in America. Retrieved from https://www.npr.org/series/559149737/you-me-and-them-experiencing-discrimination-in-america

Neblett, E. W., Jr., Gaskin, A. L., Lee, D. B., & Carter, S. E. (2011). Racial and ethnic discrimination. In B. B. Brown & M. J. Prinstein (Eds.), *Encyclopedia of Adolescence* (vol. 2) (pp. 53–58). San Diego: Academic Press.

Nordberg, A., Twis, M. K., Stevens, M. A., & Hatcher, S. S. (2018). Precarity and structural racism in Black youth encounters with police. *Child and Adolescent Social Work Journal*, 35(5) 1–8.

Nunley, J. M., Pugh, A., Romero, N., & Seals, R. A. (2015). Racial discrimination in the labor market for recent college graduates: Evidence from a field experiment. *The BE Journal of Economic Analysis & Policy, 15*(3), 1093–1125.

O'Keefe, V. M., Wingate, L. R., Cole, A. B., Hollingsworth, D. W., & Tucker, R. P. (2015). Seemingly harmless racial communications are not so harmless: Racial microaggressions lead to suicidal ideation by way of depression symptoms. *Suicide and Life-Threatening Behavior, 45*(5), 567–576.

Oh, H., Yang, L. H., Anglin, D. M., & DeVylder, J. E. (2014). Perceived discrimination and psychotic experiences across multiple ethnic groups in the United States. *Schizophrenia Research, 157*(1–3), 259–265.

Paradies, Y. (2006). A systematic review of empirical research on self-reported racism and health. *International Journal of Epidemiology, 35*, 888–901.

Park, I. J., Du, H., Wang, L., Williams, D. R., & Alegría, M. (2018). Racial/ethnic discrimination and mental health in mexican-origin youths and their parents: Testing the "linked lives" hypothesis. *Journal of Adolescent Health, 62*(4), 480–487.

Pascoe, E. A., & Smart Richman, L. (2009). Perceived discrimination and health: A meta-analytic review. *Psychological Bulletin, 135*(4), 531–554. doi:10.1037/a0016059

Phillips, D., & Lauterbach, D. (2017). American Muslim immigrant mental health: The role of racism and mental health stigma. *Journal of Muslim Mental Health, 11*(1), 39–56.

Pierce, C. (1995). Stress analogs of racism and sexism: Terrorism, torture and disaster. In C. Willie, P. Rieker, B. Kramer, & B. Brown (Eds.), *Mental Health, Racism, and Sexism* (pp. 277–293). Pittsburgh, PA: University of Pittsburgh Press.

Pieterse, A. L., Todd, N. R., Neville, H. A., & Carter, R. T. (2012). Perceived racism and mental health among Black American adults: A meta-analytic review. *Journal of Counseling Psychology, 59*(1), 1–9. doi:10.1037/a0026208

Priest, N., Paradies, Y., Trenerry, B., Truong, M., Karlsen, S., & Kelly, Y. (2013). A systematic review of studies examining the relationship between reported racism and health and wellbeing for children and young people. *Social Science & Medicine, 95*, 115–127. doi:10.1016/j.socscimed.2012.11.031

Purdie-Vaughns, V., & Williams, D. R. (2015). Stand-your-ground is losing ground for racial minorities' health. *Social Science & Medicine, 147*, 341e343.

Robins, L. N., & Regier, D. A. (Eds.). (1991). *Psychiatric disorders in America: The Epidemiologic Catchment Area Study.* New York, NY: Free Press.

Rodriguez-Seijas, C., Stohl, M., Hasin, D. S., & Eaton, N. R. (2015). Transdiagnostic factors and mediation of the relationship between perceived racial discrimination and mental disorders. *JAMA Psychiatry, 72*(7), 706–713.

Rostain, A. L., Ramsay, J. R., & Waite, R. (2015). Cultural background and barriers to mental health care for African American adults. *The Journal of Clinical Psychiatry, 76*(3), 279–283.

Smedley, B. E., Stith, A. Y., & Nelson, A. R. (2003). *Unequal treatment: Confronting ethnic and racial disparities in health care.* Washington, DC: Institute of Medicine.

Soto, J. A., Dawson-Andoh, N. A., & BeLue, R. (2011). The relationship between perceived discrimination and generalized anxiety disorder among African Americans, Afro Caribbeans, and non-Hispanic Whites. *Journal of Anxiety Disorders, 25*(2), 258–265.

Steele, C. M. (1997). A threat in the air: How stereotypes shape intellectual identity and performance. *American Psychologist, 52*(6), 613.

Stewart, E. A., Baumer, E. P., Brunson, R. K., & Simons, R. L. (2009). Neighborhood racial context and perceptions of police-based racial discrimination among black youth. *Criminology, 47*(3), 847–887.

Suarez, L. M., Polo, A. J., Chen, C. N., & Alegría, M. (2009). Prevalence and correlates of childhood-onset anxiety disorders among Latinos and non-Latino Whites in the United States. *Psicologia Conductual, 17*(1), 89.

Sue, D. W., Capodilupo, C. M., Torino, G. C., Bucceri, J. M., Holder, A. M. B., Nadal, K. L., & Esquilin, M. (2007). Racial microaggressions in everyday life: Implications for clinical practice. *American Psychologist*, 62(4), 271–286. doi:10.1037/0003-066X.62.4.271

Syed, M., & Juan, M. J. D. (2012). Discrimination and psychological distress: Examining the moderat-
ing role of social context in a nationally representative sample of Asian American adults. *Asian
American Journal of Psychology*, 3(2), 104.

Taylor, J. (1990). Relationship between internalized racism and marital satisfaction. *Journal of Black
Psychology*, 16(2), 45–53.

Taylor, J., & Jackson, B. (1990). Factors affecting alcohol consumption in black women. Part II. *International Journal of the Addictions*, 25(12), 1415–1427.

Tobler, A. L., Maldonado-Molina, M. M., Staras, S. A., O'Mara, R. J., Livingston, M. D., & Komro,
K. A. (2013). Perceived racial/ethnic discrimination, problem behaviors, and mental health
among minority urban youth. *Ethnicity & Health*, 18(4), 337–349.

Torres, L., Driscoll, M. W., & Burrow, A. L. (2010). Racial microaggressions and psychological functioning among highly achieving African-Americans: A mixed-methods approach. *Journal of
Social and Clinical Psychology*, 29(10), 1074–1099.

Tynes, B. M., & Markoe, S. L. (2010). The role of color-blind racial attitudes in reactions to racial
discrimination on social network sites. *Journal of Diversity in Higher Education*, 3(1), 1–13.
doi:10.1037/a0018683

Umaña-Taylor, A. J., & Updegraff, K. A. (2007). Latino adolescents' mental health: Exploring the
interrelations among discrimination, ethnic identity, cultural orientation, self-esteem, and
depressive symptoms. *Journal of Adolescence*, 30(4), 549–567.

Underhill, M. R. (2018, July 20). Police calls for #LivingWhileBlack have gotten out of hand. Here's
what we can do about it. *Washington Post*. Retrieved from: https://www.washingtonpost.com
/news/post-nation/wp/2018/07/20/pothe-criminalization-of-blackness-and-what-we-can-do
-about-it/?utm_term=.2301fcfd4cdd

US Department of Health and Human Services. (2001). *Mental health: Culture, race, and ethnicity. A
supplement to mental health: A report of the Surgeon General*. Rockville, MD: Author.

van Ryn, M., Burgess, D. J., Dovidio, J. F., Phelan, S. M., Saha, S., Malat, J., … & Perry, S. (2011). The
impact of racism on clinician cognition, behavior, and clinical decision making. *Du Bois Review:
Social Science Research on Race*, 8(1), 199–218.

Verhaeghen, P., Aikman, S. N., & Van Gulick, A. E. (2011). Prime and prejudice: Co-occurrence in
the culture as a source of automatic stereotype priming. *British Journal of Social Psychology*, 50(3),
501–518.

Victor, D. (2018, May 11). When White people call the police on Black people. *New York Times*.
Retrieved from https://www.nytimes.com/2018/05/11/us/black-white-police.html

Vinkers, D. J., de Beurs, E., Barendregt, M., Rinne, T., & Hoek, H. W. (2011). The relationship between
mental disorders and different types of crime. *Criminal Behaviour and Mental Health*, 21(5),
307–320.

Walters, J. M. (2004). *Testing a biopsychosocial model of perceived racism among Latinos* (Doctoral dissertation, University of Illinois at Urbana-Champaign).

Wang, P. S., Demler, O., & Kessler, R. C. (2002). Adequacy of treatment for serious mental illness in
the United States. *American Journal of Public Health*, 92(1), 92–98.

Williams, D. R. (2012). Miles to go before we sleep: Racial inequities in health. *Journal of Health and
Social Behavior*, 53(3), 279–295.

Williams, D. R., Neighbors, H. W., & Jackson, J. S. (2003). Racial/ethnic discrimination and health:
Findings from community studies. *American Journal of Public Health*, 93(2), 200–208. doi:10.2105/
AJPH.93.2.200

Williams, D. R., & Mohammed, S. A. (2009). Discrimination and racial disparities in health: Evidence and needed research. *Journal of Behavioral Medicine, 32*(1), 20–47. doi:10.1007/s10865-008 -9185-0

Williams, D. R., & Mohammed, S. A. (2013a). Racism and health I: Pathways and scientific evidence. *American Behavioral Scientist, 57*(8): 1152–1173. doi:10.1177/0002764213487340

Williams, D. R., & Mohammed, S. A. (2013b). Racism and health II: A needed research agenda for effective interventions. *American Behavioral Scientist, 57*(8), 1200–1226.

Williams, D. R., Takeuchi, D. T., & Adair, R. K. (1992). Marital status and psychiatric disorders among blacks and whites. *Journal of Health and Social Behavior*, 140–157.

Williams, D. R., & Williams-Morris, R. (2000). Racism and mental health: The African American experience. *Ethnicity and Health, 5*(3–4), 243–268.

Williams, M. T., Gooden, A. M., & Davis, D. (2012). African Americans, European Americans, and Pathological stereotypes: An African-centered perspective. In G. R. Hayes & M. H. Bryant (Eds.), *Psychology of culture* (pp. 25–46). Hauppauge, NY: Nova Science Publishers.

Williams, M. T., Malcoun, E., Sawyer, B., Davis, D. M., Bahojb-Nouri, L. V., & Leavell Bruce, S. (2014). Cultural adaptations of prolonged exposure therapy for treatment and prevention of post-traumatic stress disorder in African Americans. *Behavioral Sciences, 4*(2), 102–124. doi:10.3390/bs4020102

Williams, M. T., Taylor, R. J., Mouzon, D. M., Oshin, L. A., Himle, J. A., & Chatters, L. M. (2017). Discrimination and symptoms of obsessive–compulsive disorder among African Americans. *American Journal of Orthopsychiatry, 87*(6), 636.

Zhang, A. Y., & Snowden, L. R. (1999). Ethnic characteristics of mental disorders in five US communities. *Cultural Diversity and Ethnic Minority Psychology, 5*(2), 134.

CHAPTER 6

Using Contextual Behavioral Science to Understand Racism and Bias

Jonathan W. Kanter,
University of Washington

Daniel C. Rosen,
Bastyr University

Katherine E. Manbeck,
University of Washington

Adam M. Kuczynski,
University of Washington

Mariah D. Corey,
University of Washington

Heather M. L. Branstetter,
Bastyr University

Introduction

What is racism? What defines a racist act? Traditional answers to these questions have focused on extreme acts of hatred committed by explicitly prejudiced individuals, allowing most White people to distance themselves from any associations with the terms. Contemporary racial dialogue, however, has upended this notion, leaving large numbers of White people, including mental health practitioners, disoriented and confused about what exactly constitutes racism and racist acts, whether they are personally culpable, and what to do to the extent that they are responsible. Terms with which White people may be unfamiliar are now emphasized as proxy indicators of racism, including "implicit bias," "color-blindness," "White privilege," and "microaggressions." This new language of racism—while acknowledging that explicit racism continues to be a major problem—focuses more sharply on the role and behavior of White people who explicitly claim anti-racist values and consider themselves to be "well intentioned."

In this chapter, we take a broad view of contemporary dialogue and intervention on racism and bias, offering a contextual behavioral science (CBS) view that clarifies the terms at issue as human actions–in–context and situates them in the known language and processes of CBS. We review the theoretical foundations and major research findings in support of the prevalent terms used, including "implicit bias," "color-blindness," "White privilege," and "microaggressions." Central to our chapter is the position that these terms are scientifically and experientially valuable, effectively pointing toward and clarifying important sources of oppression and discrimination experienced by people of color. However, as used in typical discourse and intervention efforts, these terms lack an integrative, conceptual framework or clear contextual behavioral basis to maximize intervention effectiveness. Furthermore, the psychological processes behind these terms that often render them aversive and produce avoidance need increased attention.

A key affective process discussed is intergroup anxiety (IGA), a regrettably normative, cross-situational anxiety response that in-group members have to out-group members (and vice versa) when anticipating or engaging in intergroup interactions (Stephan & Stephan, 1985). For many White individuals, during intergroup interactions, IGA is automatically elicited and—because our social context includes strong norms that it is unacceptable to display and even privately experience such feelings—results in experiential avoidance. We discuss how experiential avoidance, a key construct within CBS (e.g., Hayes, Wilson, Gifford, Follette, & Strosahl, 1996), may play a significant role in efforts to understand and intervene on contemporary racism. Our framework leads to a series of contextual behavioral intervention ideas, which are described in chapter 8 of this volume.

Our Current Context

Although a strong recent global resurgence of nationalism has legitimized explicit acts of racism and hatred in major subcultures of our society (Ulansky & Witenberg, 2017), powerful social norms place demands on most White people to distance themselves from such explicit racist ideas or practices (Sommers & Norton, 2006). Many White people denounce nationalism and racism explicitly and consider themselves to be non-racist and well intentioned in their interactions with people of color. Yet modern psychological science and critical theory has yanked out the safety net that has defined racism solely in these explicit terms.

The contemporary dialogue on racism, stimulated by developments in science and theory, and advanced by courageous activists and people of color who are willing to speak out and not stay silent about their experiences, is dominated by discussions of implicit racial biases that are exhibited by the vast majority of White Americans (Greenwald, Poehlman, Uhlmann, & Banaji, 2009). Likewise, contemporary dialogue emphasizes themes from social identity theory (Tajfel & Turner, 1986), which makes the bold but well-supported claim that for most of us, some level of racism is locked into identity development through the formation of self- and in-group-preferencing loyalties. Such dialogue confronts many White people with the choices that they make—in the service of protecting and advancing the interests of themselves, their families, and their communities—which are made in the context of being a member of an in the group that exerts power and privilege over others.

Dovidio introduced the term *aversive racism* specifically to describe the nature and myriad manifestations of implicit racial biases in White individuals who are often not aware of, and are defensive about, such processes (Dovidio & Gaertner, 2004). Consistent with aversive racism, current scholarship has focused on racial microaggressions—brief and commonplace daily verbal exchanges between White people and people of color, which are experienced by people of color as derogatory and racially biased. Microaggressions, presumably fueled by implicit biases, are likely to be justified by the White person as unintentional and sometimes followed by an accusation that the person of color has misinterpreted the White person's behavior or is being too sensitive (Sue et al., 2007). Such exchanges may be seen as microcosms of the larger national dialogue— an opportunity for change, growth, and connection that is transformed, instead, into a moment of resentment, confusion, and disconnection.

The investigation on racism now concerns itself with the degree or extremity of bias rather than its existence or absence; with everyday choices that serve one's self-interest that, at first glance, have nothing to do with race; and with subtle behaviors that indicate bias rather than explicitly hostile acts. Significant racial biases and subtle but chronically harmful choices and behaviors are well documented among health professionals who explicitly endorse egalitarian values and whose ethical guidelines are explicitly anti-racist, such as medical providers (Maina, Belton, Ginzberg, Singh, & Johnson, 2016), as well as psychologists and other mental health providers (Constantine, 2007).

An industry of diversity experts and trainers offering a host of antibias interventions for organizations and the public has grown over the past several decades in parallel with increased public discourse on normative social psychological processes that produce racial bias in most of us. Yet reviews of diversity training, broadly defined, conclude that there is very little evidence that typical diversity trainings are effective (Bezrukova & Spell, 2012) and even less evidence for *why* they produce positive changes if they do (Paluck & Green, 2009). Sue and colleagues (Sue, Torino, Capodilupo, Rivera, & Lin, 2009) have documented how White participants often react to participation in these interventions, including with shame, guilt, avoidance, defensiveness, hostility, and, at times, negative evaluations of the presenter (e.g., Boatright-Horowitz & Soeung, 2009). Such reactance is particularly the case for interventions that focus on microaggressions (e.g., Lilienfeld, 2017). Participants may be told not to microaggress, but are not given workable options for overriding automatic perceptual processes and stereotype activations that lead to microaggressions. It is not a surprise that so many diversity trainings are not effective and that White participants' anxieties are worse, rather than improved, by the end.

A Contextual Behavioral Lens

To frame this problem from a CBS perspective, a shift of focus is required. It is not easy to successfully intervene on psychological processes of which an individual has no awareness and for whom increasing awareness may be aversive (i.e., racial bias). Likewise, it is not easy to intervene on behaviors, presumably fueled by these processes, which the individual denies doing (i.e., microaggressions). Nor is it easy to ask White people who claim to be well-intentioned and non-racist to examine the conscious choices they make in the service of advancing themselves and their families. To people of color, these choices are often perceived as White people settling into the advantageous status quo rather than confronting it and engaging deeply with the social justice movements they claim to support.

The context seems promising for development within CBS (Hayes, Barnes-Holmes, & Wilson, 2012), the ultimate purpose of which, after all, "is to change the world in a positive and intentional way" (p. 1). The fit is not simply aspirational, in that the dominant intervention model within CBS (i.e., acceptance and commitment therapy [ACT]; Hayes, Strosahl, & Wilson, 1999) centers on normative psychological processes and on how to effectively help individuals willingly experience aversive private experiences such that behavior can be aligned more fully and meaningfully with one's values (e.g., being egalitarian and non-racist). However, a CBS understanding of racism with linked interventions has yet to be developed.

A first step to developing effective CBS interventions to address racism and existent health disparities is to define the key constructs in functional terms. This is not straightforward, as the terms employed in contemporary dialogues about racism, despite being highly valuable in describing problems, were not developed with contextual behavioral principles in mind. From a CBS perspective, prioritization is given to the development and scientific study of terms that are useful with respect to description (or prediction) and influence as a unified goal (Hayes et al., 2012). The current terms, while effective with respect to description or prediction (i.e., validation), are less effective with respect to influence. Stated differently, the current terms need to be adequately defined to clarify the functional, psychological processes that may most easily and effectively be intervened upon to decrease racism.

Thus, in the sections that follow, we review the theoretical foundations and major research findings in support of the prevalent terms used in contemporary discussions of racism. We then present a contextual behavioral framework that reformulates the prevalent terms as contextual behavioral processes, using known terms in CBS and, in particular, the language of ACT's hexaflex model of psychological flexibility (Hayes et al., 1999). We emphasize multiple hexaflex processes, including lack of contact with the present moment, self-as-content, fusion, and experiential avoidance, and suggest that they are key to understanding complications around discussing color-blindness, White privilege, and microaggressions. We assume the reader has a working knowledge of the hexaflex model. For useful introductions to the model, consider Luoma, Hayes, and Walser (2017) or Harris (2009).

A Review and Contextual Behavioral Understanding of Key Terms

In this section we define key terms from the psychological literature on race and racism, including a contextual behavioral perspective of each construct.

Implicit Bias

The construct of implicit bias—biases in feelings, thoughts, or actions toward others, presumably fueled by unconscious evaluative judgments and stereotypes—has proven to be useful and important to understanding racial bias (Greenwald et al., 2009), and serves as the starting point for our review. The term's scientific foundations lie in implicit social cognition, which seeks to explain widespread observations that many mental processes appear to function outside consciousness, and the term was rapidly applied to explain discrimination that could not be understood as resulting from explicitly expressed discriminatory attitudes. Although we make the case for shifting away from implicit bias in our intervention model, we do not question the significance of the construct for a description of the problem. Even small effects on implicit bias tests, when extrapolated to the large numbers of people for whom such effects are discernable, describe a significant societal problem (Greenwald, Banaji, & Nosek, 2015). The term orients public attention and public policy to the myriad, subtle, pervasive, and automatic expressions of implicit bias in White individuals' nonverbal and verbal behaviors and decision making that contribute to disparities in educational, criminal justice, health, housing, and other significant outcomes that, in turn, are major determinants of quality of life and life expectancy for people of color (for a recent review, see Staats, Capatosto, Tenney, & Mamo, 2017). Implicit bias also is important to consider for therapists, as a small but meaningful literature documents that psychologists demonstrate implicit biases against people of color (Abreu, 1999; Castillo, Brossart, Reyes, Conoley, & Phoummarath, 2007).

Despite the value of implicit bias in describing these problems, it is increasingly clear that most interventions that directly try to reduce implicit bias fail (Lai et al., 2014). Furthermore, the subset of interventions that have produced change show only small-to-moderate effects that are transient and not sustainable (Lai et al., 2016), and there is little evidence that changes in bias produce corresponding changes in behavior (Lai, Hoffman, & Nosek, 2013). The most popular measure of implicit bias (the Implicit Association Test [IAT]) has been fiercely criticized, in fact, as being a poor predictor of individual-level bias and discriminatory behavior (e.g., Oswald, Mitchell, Blanton, Jaccard, & Tetlock, 2013).

IMPLICIT BIAS IN CONTEXT

From a CBS lens, we question the utility of the dominant social cognitive and neuroscientific assumptions through which we view implicit bias, and suggest they have a downside. The concern is about how complex scientific findings on bias are filtered through these assumptions, translated into public discourse, and employed as the basis of interventions. Specifically, the process of translation may have reified the IAT into the *thing* that it purports to measure, located the *thing* as a discrete object inside the brain, and encouraged the illusion that intervening on the *thing* will be useful.

CBS questions such reification and instead prefers to focus on variables that can be situated as human actions–in–context, in line with the pragmatic position that a science of human actions–in–context will be more effective at solving society's significant problems (Hayes et al., 2012). Our view is that it is not helpful to view tests of implicit bias as referencing a core, underlying mental structure that can be rooted out, as there may be nothing there to grab hold of. Although we do not question that behavior is ultimately controlled by the brain, we are concerned that the scientific search for the "racist" part of the brain or the neurological basis of bias is overly simplistic and reductionistic, and we are skeptical that such a search will meaningfully inform the development of effective interventions. We are also concerned that the emphasis on implicit bias as the dominant driver of contemporary racism, and the assumption that it is an unconscious force influencing behavior largely outside of voluntary control, may in some ways make it harder for White people to take responsibility for their conscious choices and actions and engage in meaningful change efforts.

In our view, implicit bias is best viewed as an important quality of human actions–in–context—a label for the observation that our actions, from subtle performances on cognitive association tests to explicit and complex behavioral sequences extended over time, often systematically favor our in-groups and selves over out-groups and others—but implicit bias is not the *thing* that causes these actions. Thus, while implicit bias is an important construct—referencing a multitude of observed problems—it is not a useful construct to target for interventions and thus does not appear directly in the CBS model.

As we will discuss below, we suggest intergroup anxiety (IGA) as a central construct of interest. Importantly, IGA is not defined as a conscious process, and we know that, in general, anxiety often operates and biases behavior outside of awareness. We suggest that IGA does not account for all manifestations of bias, but in our view, it is a viable and more parsimonious explanation of many significant research findings related to implicit bias. Furthermore, emphasizing IGA suggests clear and obvious intervention approaches within CBS, particularly the notion of acceptance (rather than suppression or avoidance) of anxiety and other aversive bodily responses in intergroup interactions.

Color-blindness

There is much debate around the term *color-blindness* and what it means in a racial context. For many White individuals, racial color-blindness is proclaimed as a value, a fair-minded desire to ignore interracial divisions and view each person as an individual, in the service of the aspirational goal of a racially color-blind society in which, in the words of Martin Luther King Jr., individuals "will not be judged by the color of their skin, but by the content of their character" (King, 1964; Lilienfeld, 2017). The consensus among psychological practitioners, scientists, and scholars, however, is that color-blindness is, or at least leads to, a modern form of racism, involving denial of race, institutional racism, and White privilege.

Research on color-blindness, in fact, is unequivocal. The most well-used self-report measure of color-blindness is positively and robustly linked with multiple indicators of racism in White people (reviewed by Neville, Awad, Brooks, Flores, & Bluemel, 2013), including a higher likelihood of engaging in microaggressions (Kanter et al., 2017). While this measure has been criticized as being confounded with the other indicators of racism it predicts (Lilienfeld, 2017), multiple other unbiased and objective indicators of color-blindness tell the same story: Color-blindness backfires, producing not less racial prejudice but more (Apfelbaum, Norton, & Sommers, 2012). Color-blindness is associated with lower detection of overt racial discrimination by children, less intervention to correct clear social injustices by teachers (Apfelbaum, Pauker, Sommers, & Ambady, 2010), more errors by jurors in trials of Black defendants (Sommers & Norton, 2006), and less eye contact and friendliness in interracial interactions (Norton, Sommers, Apfelbaum, Pura, & Ariely, 2006). Color-blindness is also an issue for mental health professionals, with documented negative effects. Psychologists and trainees who report stronger color-blind attitudes show less empathy for and are more likely to blame clients of color for their problems (Burkard & Knox, 2004) and report less multicultural awareness and knowledge (Neville, Spanierman, & Doan, 2006).

Overall, it is clear that some White individuals and institutions, in particular legal and criminal justice institutions and organizations facing employment-discrimination issues, may be adopting color-blindness as a strategy to obfuscate and deny racist practices and defend in-group-favoring choices (Apfelbaum et al., 2012). On the other hand, evidence increasingly suggests that some degree of colorblindness is culturally normative for most White people as a strategy for appearing non-prejudiced, especially in mainstream social contexts that do not support expressions of prejudice. In fact, color-blindness emerges in US children around age ten without explicit training (Apfelbaum, Pauker, Ambady, Sommers, & Norton, 2008).

COLOR-BLINDNESS IN CONTEXT

Through our CBS lens, color-blindness is a value system, which may be thought of as a coherent verbal network of "if-then" rules (e.g., "If I do not notice race, then I cannot be a racist"). This value system is supported by mainstream social norms and adopted by many White people, who may then follow the rules of color-blindness as a way of adhering to social norms and appearing non-racist. In addition to being supported by social norms, it is a relatively low-effort choice (compared to other ways of demonstrating that one is not racist). Furthermore, the choice may be reinforcing in the short-term simply if one determines that one is complying with the rule and has successfully distanced oneself from any association with the category "racist" as per the social rule (i.e., "I clearly am not a racist, because I am trying to be color-blind"). Acts of color-blindness are also socially reinforced in the short-term by like-minded individuals who observe them (Apfelbaum, Sommers, & Norton, 2008). Further, color-blindness is negatively rein-forced by successful avoidance of aversive feelings that are elicited when a White person more directly confronts issues of privilege, advantage, and oppression in our society, as discussed below.

This social reinforcement and rule-compliance may be enough to sustain color-blind behavior even as other contingencies are not favorable and the behavior overall is dam-aging with respect to progress on anti-racist valued living in the long run. It is well-established, in fact, that in many cases, a reliance on rules to govern behavior renders the person less sensitive to the actual contingencies (Hayes, Brownstein, Zettle, Rosenfarb, & Korn, 1986). For example, a White individual, while interacting with a Black person, may perceive themselves to be acting in an unbiased manner and that the interaction is going well. The Black person in the interaction, however, is likely to perceive the White individual as biased and demonstrating subtle cues of unfriendliness, such as nervous laughter and poor eye contact (Norton et al., 2006). The Black person may be unlikely to feed these perceptions back to the White individual, reducing the White person's contact with the actual contingencies even further.

We predict that for some White people who developed in a context that provided local cultural and familial support for these values, the propensity to maintain a color-blind perspective may become quite strong. In some cultural contexts, such as evangeli-cal faith communities, color-blindness is explicitly, strongly cultivated and reinforced as an anti-racist value and an expression of God's will (Emerson & Smith, 2000). In such contexts, any race-based reaction to a person of color is a violation of color-blindness and essentially an act of racism (Apfelbaum et al., 2008), one of the most socially stigmatizing acts possible. The strength of conviction behind color-blindness in individuals who learned to be color-blind in these contexts—seemingly at odds with the insurmountable evidence that the task of color-blindness is unnatural, impossible, and self-defeating—may appear incomprehensible to scholars and activists, but our contextual behavioral view of such rigid adherence to ultimately unworkable rules is understandable in context.

White Privilege

White privilege—the notion that White people, regardless of their individual cir-cumstances, benefit from racism—has become a central premise of much contemporary discourse on racism. The term, which can be traced to the early writings of W. E. B. Du Bois (Roediger, 1991), was popularized for wider White audiences by Peggy McIntosh's (1989) influential essay "White Privilege: Unpacking the Invisible Backpack," which now is frequently cited as a classic and used by diversity trainers in their efforts to raise White people's awareness of their privilege (Case & Rios, 2017). It is not uncommon for the list of privileges in McIntosh's essay to form the basis of a *privilege walk*, a diversity workshop exercise in which White participants' advantages over participants of color are physically represented, step-by-step, as a head start in a walking race across the room.

White privilege is related to color-blindness in that having little awareness of, or explicitly denying, issues of White privilege makes it easier to maintain a color-blind stance (Neville et al., 2013).

While most psychologists believe that they are skilled at discussing cultural differences (Maxie, Arnold, & Stephenson, 2006), White privilege is a significant issue for mental health practitioners. Therapist trainees, especially those who are high in intergroup anxiety, are likely to have difficulties with willingness to confront privilege (Langrehr & Blackmon, 2016). These difficulties are pronounced for psychologists, who demonstrate less awareness of and willingness to address White privilege than do other mental health practitioners, such as social workers (Mindrup, Spray, & Lamberghini-West, 2011). In our opinion, it is important for White mental health practitioners to recognize that they are not immune from the cultural forces that produce these difficulties as normative processes for most White people.

Like color-blindness, some of the dialogue on privilege views White people as simply lacking awareness of the ways in which they have benefited from privilege, while other parts of the dialogue views White people as explicitly, selfishly motivated to deny obvious privileges of which they are aware. We believe that, like color-blindness, there is justification in being suspicious of some White individuals who fiercely deny privilege: the privileges seem blatantly obvious to most people of color, and the hostility expressed in the denial of privilege is noteworthy and easily experienced as microaggressive, if not explicitly racist (consider Fortgang, 2014).

Furthermore, it is hard to reconcile, at times, the life choices made by many seemingly privileged White people with their claimed intentions to dismantle racism and produce a more equitable society. Such choices include where to buy a home, where to send children to school, and how to invest savings. It is generally accepted that, from an evolutionary perspective, all people, regardless of race or social status, are vested with self-interest, and this interest will extend to the family and to the perceived in-group (Tajfel & Turner, 1986). In other words, people will make life choices to better themselves and their families. In the context of contemporary dialogue on racism, however, it is increasingly expected that White people take responsibility for understanding that the choices that they make, which favor themselves and their in-groups, occur in a context in which that in-group enjoys power and privilege over others. There are strong themes in the contemporary dialogue that White people who claim to be well intentioned and non-racist while making such life choices are inauthentic and insincere in these claims. From this perspective, there may be more courageous choices possible that would align the White person's behavior more closely with his or her own values.

Raising awareness of White privilege is difficult, especially when this more blaming view of privilege is emphasized. In fact, when presented with interventions designed to raise awareness of White privilege, White people are likely to claim personal hardships that allow them to deny personally benefiting from it, even if they recognize that other White people have benefited (Taylor Phillips & Lowery, 2015). Interventions to increase White awareness of privilege also routinely increase negative affect (Langrehr &

Blackmon, 2016) and guilt (Case & Rios, 2017), and result in negative evaluations of the trainer responsible for pointing this out (Boatright-Horowitz & Soeung, 2009). It also is likely the case that the trainer is preaching to the choir, at least relatively: White individuals who are most likely to deny White privilege also are most likely to score higher on other indicators of racism and avoid discussions of privilege altogether (e.g., nonmandatory diversity trainings) (Conway, Lipsey, Pogge, & Ratliff, 2017).

WHITE PRIVILEGE IN CONTEXT

White privilege can be understood in relation to identity development. From a CBS perspective, identity development partially involves developing a coherent way of talking about ourselves in terms of our attributes and qualities (e.g., Who am I? What kind of person am I?). This network of self-descriptions in CBS is known as *self-as-content* or the *conceptualized self* (see Hayes, 1995). Given the context in which many White people develop in this society, the conceptualized self that develops over time is problematic from a racial perspective. Specifically, while ideally we want to develop an experience of self that integrates individual, group, and universal aspects of identity, many White people do not have a meaningful, personal experience of their racial group and, instead, experience only individual-level aspects of identity (e.g., Sue & Sue, 2003). In our highly individualistic society, there is tremendous contextual support for defining oneself as an autonomous, self-determined individual in control of one's life outcomes (Ryan & Deci, 2002) and for acting to preserve and protect the interests of one's self and one's family; in fact, a lack of self-interest and self-determination is seen as a significant risk for psychological pathology (e.g., Rehm, 1977). This has been questioned by cross-cultural scholars, who note that collectivist societies, which cultivate stronger group and universal aspects of identity, demonstrate much lower rates of depression and other mental health problems than do individualistic societies (e.g., Chen, 1996).

One important by-product of such an individualistic emphasis in White people's conceptualized selves is difficulties with the notion of unearned White privilege. We expect variability in the degree to which White individuals define themselves and build coherent self-defining narratives of "who I am" as hard-working, self-efficacious, autonomous individuals. For some individuals, "I worked hard for and earned my achievements in life," or something similar, may be a central, defining feature of one's conceptualized self. Furthermore, a developmental context that reinforces such a strong, individual view of self likely provides little support for the development of a conceptualized self that includes a personally significant experience of Whiteness or membership in a privileged group defined by Whiteness.

While White identity development does not typically include a meaningful awareness of Whiteness or White group membership, very soon after birth, White people will start to demonstrate in-group favoritism toward other White people without awareness (Bar-Haim, Ziv, Lamy, & Hodes, 2006). In-group favoritism can be explicit and cognitively complex, but it does not need to be. Research demonstrates that humans will automatically, preconsciously favor their in-groups across a range of behavioral choices, from simple eye contact to friendship preferences, consumer choices, and voting behavior (Hammond & Axelrod, 2006). In other words, it is likely that a White person's behavior will favor and privilege other White people even as Whiteness and White privilege are denied. When these contradictions are observed by a person of color, a White person's claims around being well intentioned and non-racist likely will be experienced as insincere.

Like color-blindness, some contexts may produce extreme difficulties around White privilege and identity, specifically the context of White supremacy that pervades certain subcultures in the United States, both historically and currently. This context explicitly cultivates not a lack of but a very strong White group identity (e.g., Vance, 2016). Biased interpretations of out-group members as hostile and threatening are explicitly supported within the subculture, and there are limited meaningful experiences of non-stereotyped diversity to counteract such processes. Such a context predicts that an individual's con-ceptualized self may be rigidly individualistic, in-group preferencing may be explicitly and rigidly White, and significant difficulties with perspective taking toward people of color may result.

Microaggressions

As defined by Sue et al. (2007), microaggressions are "brief and commonplace daily verbal, behavioral, and environmental indignities, whether intentional or unintentional, that communicate hostile, derogatory or negative racial slights and insults to the target person or group" (p. 273). People of color, and, in particular, Black people, report experi-encing microaggressions regularly (Donovan, Galban, Grace, Bennett, & Felicié, 2013; Lewis, Chesler, & Forman, 2000; Smith, Allen, & Danley, 2007), as do members of other marginalized groups, including lesbian, gay, bisexual, transgender, and queer (LGBTQ) individuals; Asian Americans; Latinx; women; and other cultural groups (for reviews, see Sue, 2010; Wong, Derthick, David, Saw, & Okazaki, 2014).

The cumulative experience of microaggressions is associated with multiple negative health and mental health consequences, including increased serious psychological dis-tress (Chae, Lincoln, & Jackson, 2011), increased depression and decreased life satisfac-tion (Ayalon & Gum, 2011), increased risk for mood and substance use disorders (Clark, Salas-Wright, Vaughn, & Whitfield, 2015), increased anxiety (Liao, Weng, & West, 2016), and increased suicide risk (O'Keefe, Wingate, Cole, Hollingsworth, & Tucker, 2015). Similar to other public health concerns in which small doses of toxins, from sec-ond-hand smoke to fetal alcohol exposure, accumulate to produce measurable and sig-nificant negative health impacts, microaggressions appear to reflect this process at an interpersonal level.

It also is clear that microaggressive expressions are related to racism. Our research surveyed White people on how frequently they engage in expressions that are commonly interpreted as microaggressive, and found that White people's likelihood of engaging in microaggressions was significantly associated with higher scores on other well-validated measures of racism, including negative feelings toward Black people and explicit preju-dice (Kanter et al., 2017). Many White people, however, have difficulty understanding the impact of microaggressions. They may react defensively, claiming that the purported microaggression was unintentional, arguing that the expression should not be catego-rized as racist, and accusing the person of color reporting the microaggression as simply being too sensitive or "politically correct" (Lilienfeld, 2017).

MICROAGGRESSIONS IN CONTEXT

Microaggressions have entered the public discourse on racism and become a domi-nant theme in contemporary anti-racism workshops and seminars. Our experience sam-pling such workshops is that a typical strategy involves disseminating lists of different types of microaggressions, with examples, and cautioning participants against expressing these statements. While such lists as intervention efforts are well intended and likely function to validate the experiences of people of color who experience microaggressions, we are concerned that opportunities for more significant and sustainable behavior change are lost if intervention efforts emphasize such lists without a more in-depth func-tional analysis of the context in which microaggressions occur.

First, the lists do not consistently define microaggressive behaviors in terms of the psychological processes of the offender, which presumably would be helpful if the goal is to change the offender's behavior as well as validate the experiences of the victim. Similarly, the lists do little to help offenders overcome the obstacles to behavior change, such as potential threats to self and identity, that may become salient in the discussion. Third, the lists do not help individuals with alternate, improved behavior. In their sim-plest form, they simply identify the topography of problematic behavior and punish it by linking such behavior to racism.

We are not against punishment of racist behavior, but punishment should occur in the context of the goals of the intervention. In the case of presumably voluntary White workshop participants, and in the context of microaggressions that likely occur between individuals who are in meaningful ongoing relationships, the effectiveness of punishment to change the White person's behavior is questionable. CBS is clear that punishment only decreases behavior—it does not promote new behavior—and it produces counter-control in terms of aggressiveness and resistance, is only effective in the presence of the punisher, and renders the punisher as aversive and to be avoided (Sidman, 1989). In this context, the strong negative reactions and push-back against microaggression trainings is not surprising to the extent these trainings are experienced functionally as punishing. Our concern is not that racism should not be punished, it is that punishment will not produce the outcome we want, which is improved behavior from White people and resulting improved relationships between White people and people of color as experi-enced by people of color.

A Contextual Behavioral Framework

Our goal is to develop a framework that will facilitate predicting and influencing the behavior of White people who claim non-racist values and good intentions (e.g., therapists), and, in particular, we care about behavior in interracial interactions with consequences for the health and well-being of people of color and our communities. Our framework does not make assumptions regarding the veracity of the White person's claimed intentions. While many arguments can occur about if a White person "intended" to do something racist or not, our analysis largely renders irrelevant what the White person says in this regard. Typically, we have little awareness of the actual sources of contextual influence over our behavior, such that whatever is claimed as intended or unintended post hoc rarely maps on to the real influences on the behavior and is more likely a function of the context in which someone is asking for an explanation. Thus, our analysis aims to understand the problematic behavior in context, rather than as a function of internal motivation.

The value guiding our efforts is workability. The concern is that current intervention efforts lack a workable intervention model, given the psychological processes that are triggered in White participants during attempted interventions. We seek to design intervention efforts that produce not simply the reduction of problematic, biased behavior in White people (e.g., clinicians), but a closer alignment of actual behavior (rather than defensively claimed "intentions") with non-racist values, improved perspective taking, empathy, and the ability to form meaningful and healing relationships with, and as experienced by, people of color. We seek sustainable behavior change.

Figure 6.1 presents a visual depiction of our framework. It describes the sources of influence on a specific behavior of a specific person at a specific moment in context. Our framework emphasizes that all behavioral moments are embedded in context: the evolutionary, historical, and current context that collectively influences each person's behavior. This collective context is pervasively racist, and understanding this context helps us make sense of a person's actions. Within this context, the framework also locates the person's behavior as a function of their individual identity, including one's value systems (e.g., color-blindness), and beliefs about oneself and being White (e.g., White privilege). From this perspective, the person's automatic perceptual and attentional processes are considered: On what is the person's attention focused? What does he notice? And what is he not seeing or hearing? The center of the framework is presented next, examining the central role of intergroup anxiety (IGA), stereotyped beliefs and other cognitive processes, and one's avoidance of (or willingness to experience) these and other related internal processes. The final outcome of the model, one's overt behavior (e.g., microaggressions) is the collective outcome of these processes.

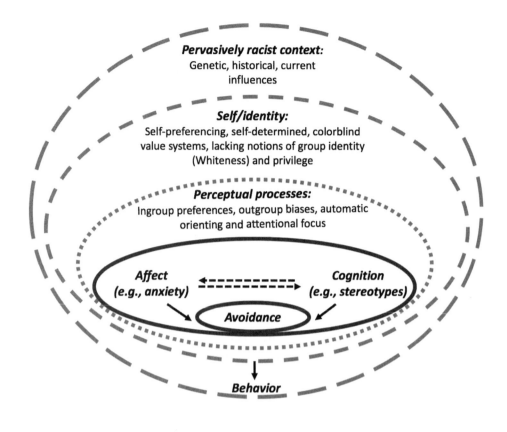

Figure 6.1.

A Pervasively Racist Context

Our framework starts with recognition of the overarching context in which biased actions occur, which is a major influence on the contextual behavioral psychological processes that give rise to these biased actions. Our view of context is very broad and inclusive of multiple sources of influence, including evolutionary or genetic influences, the person's history of learning and development, and current contextual influences on behavior.

Evolutionary influences and genetic predispositions must be acknowledged at the start, with a caution that genetic issues should not be overstated. Most scholars, to be clear, do not believe that we will ever find a gene for racism or that racist behavior is genetically predetermined. Much scholarship, in fact, has refuted the biological basis of race itself (e.g. Yudell, Roberts, DeSalle, Tishkoff, 2016). That said, there are some important considerations. First, humans appear to be genetically predisposed to identify with self-preferencing in-groups and feel threatened by out-groups (Tajfel & Turner, 1986). This is undoubtedly important for survival in a world in which groups band together to compete for scarce resources. However, who we define as in-group members and out-group members is not genetically predefined and is, instead, a function of our unique developmental context (Hammond & Axelrod, 2006). The assignment of content to in-group and out-group frames happens quickly: three-month-olds demonstrate a preference for same-race over other-race faces, but, crucially, only in homogeneous same-race facial environments (Bar-Haim et al. 2006). Once the in-group and out-group frame is filled in with specific content (e.g., White = in-group, Black = out-group), it influences perceptual processes and behavior automatically. Other genetically influenced traits, such as openness to experience, which negatively predicts generalized prejudice as well as right-wing and social dominance orientations (Ekehammar, Akrami, Gylje, & Zakrisson, 2004), are important to consider. Collectively, genetic influences can be seen as shifting risk for the shaping of racist behavior by environmental influences.

Regarding these environmental influences, our view is that the environment in which most White people develop is pervasively racist, and it is next to impossible to completely avoid social influences that cultivate negative stereotypes and biases against people of color. There is no denying the impact of these larger cultural forces in creating baseline levels of problematic psychological processes, which we describe next. Caregiver influences, other significant personal relationships, and the extent (or lack) of exposure to diversity during development undoubtedly play major roles. For example, most White people have few (if any) people of color in their social networks (Cox, Navarro-Rivera, & Jones, 2016), and their primary exposure to people of color is through biased media. For these individuals, it seems probable that this biased exposure sharpens in-group and out-group distinctions, decreases the likelihood of Whiteness becoming a meaningful aspect of identity, increases the likelihood of responding to people of color based on stereotypes, increases interracial anxiety, and increases the likelihood of microaggressions, due to misunderstandings and poor perspective taking. It is undoubtedly more difficult for an individual to develop clarity on racial issues, such as the extent of structural forces of racism that oppress people of color and the nuances of microaggressive behavior that are experienced as offensive by people of color, if one has no people of color with whom one is interacting and discussing these issues. Fortunately, most individuals have choices regarding their social context—where they spend time, recreate, and travel. Left unexamined, however, the default choices for most White people are proximate to other White people.

Identity Development: The Conceptualized Self

As reviewed earlier, color-blindness is one example of how White identity develops in this pervasively racist context. More broadly, from a CBS perspective, we consider identity development to be partially an issue of self-as-content, or the conceptualized self (Hayes, 1995; Hayes et al., 1999). The "content" of self-as-content refers to how one might respond when asked "who are you?" Our view is that many White peoples' conceptualized selves lack meaningful inclusion of a group identity around Whiteness. This, combined with strong community support for color-blindness as an anti-racist value system, produces conceptualized selves in which color-blindness is a rigidly held, defining value-system, tied to self-assessments that one is well-intentioned and non-racist. Furthermore, many White peoples' conceptualized selves include views that they are hard working, autonomous, and have earned what they have achieved as an individual. Collectively, all of this self-conceptualization makes it hard for White people to appreciate, at a deep and personal level, what it means to be White in a pervasively racist context, how privilege may operate and advantage White people in this context, and how out-group members may be at a serious disadvantage. It makes it harder for White people to accurately take the perspectives of and empathically attune to the lived experiences of out-group members.

We all typically hold our conceptualized selves tightly and feel threatened when the content is threatened. In CBS terms, we are fused with our content about ourselves. To the extent that a White person is rigidly fused to the notion that they are color-blind, and therefore not racist, this person may be quite closed to the possibility that someone could engage in racist behavior (e.g., microaggressions) without explicitly endorsing racist beliefs or racist intentions. Likewise, the degree to which one is fused with an identity as a self-efficacious individual likely predicts how threatening it will be to consider the notion of unearned White privilege. For some, a White privilege challenge to self-efficacy may be experienced as a fundamental attack on one's core self. The notion of incorporating such a view into one's self-conceptualization may be experienced as intolerable, and the self may be defended ferociously. All of this may occur without awareness of these processes and without a meaningful language system to describe them.

Perceptual Processes

The context also influences basic, automatic orienting and perceptual processes that are activated in interracial interactions, quickly biasing the White person from the start of an interaction and influencing the trajectory of the interaction (Richeson & Shelton, 2007). Based on in-group frames that are filled in by experience, racial categorizations are made in a tenth of a second (Ito & Urland, 2003), and other perceptual processes are hooked by racial features, all beyond voluntary control. Eye contact, in particular, demonstrates racial disparities. Specifically, White people are more likely to have attention drawn to the racially specific features of Black faces, such as the noses and mouths, and away from the eyes, in initial facial-recognition tasks (Kawakami et al., 2014). Such attentional hooks have important implications for normative interracial interactions. For example, eye contact is essential in recognizing, understanding the intentions of, and forming accurate impressions of others (e.g. Adams & Kleck, 2003), as well as in signaling affiliative intent and safety to conversational partners (Bourgeois & Hess, 2008), and even momentary lapses in synchrony between partners has consequences (Vicaria & Dickens, 2016).

Intergroup Anxiety and Cognitive Processes

The context in which the self develops, and which leads to biased perceptual processes, also supports the development of intergroup anxiety (IGA) (and other biased affective responses) and negative stereotypes (and other biased cognitive processes), which are elicited in interracial interactions. In our view, these affective and cognitive responses are contextually controlled and may be subtle or obvious. The individual who produces these responses may or may not have conscious awareness of them. Affect and cognition bidirectionally influence and augment each other, and interact with avoidance repertoires, as discussed below, to influence behavior.

IGA is defined as an overarching, cross-situational anxiety response to an out-group that is experienced when anticipating or engaging in intergroup interactions (Stephan & Stephan, 1985). In our pervasively racist historical and cultural context, IGA is regrettably normative. The basic in-group and out-group processes, described above, that establish people of color as an out-group and orient perceptual processes to racially specific stimuli, are likely enough to establish some normative level of intergroup anxiety for White people unless their developmental histories include significant exposure to people of color (Mindrup et al., 2011). However, in a cultural milieu infused with negative stereotypes of people of color, specifically related to being different, inferior, and dangerous, these basic processes are massively augmented. Negative stereotypes related to people of color are continuously primed and automatically activated in this environment (Devine, 1989; Dixon & Maddox, 2005), with corresponding hyper-activations of the amygdala (e.g., whenever a darker or Black person's face is present) (Chekroud, Everett, Bridge, & Hewstone, 2014). In this context, IGA is seemingly inevitable, normative, and expected, varying in severity depending on a person's unique history, exposure, and genetic predispositions (i.e., with respect to openness to experience and anxiety sensitivity). White IGA responses, when elicited in interactions with people of color, are well-documented (Britt, Bonieci, Vescio, Biernat, & Brown, 1996).

Avoidance

To summarize our model thus far, we started by emphasizing the pervasively racist historical and social context into which White people are born and in which White people are raised. This context accounts for the pervasiveness, for many White people, of automatically activated perceptual biases, rigidly held identities that emphasize color-blindness, and the feeling of being threatened by notions of privilege, negative stereotypes, and IGA. Yet, even as the context makes these problems highly likely and largely unavoidable for many White people, the context also supports the emergence of strong, aversive responses to these responses. Being labeled a racist in our society, at least in most quarters, carries a heavy functional load, located in a relational network with closed-mindedness, hatred, ignorance, and violence (Sommers & Norton, 2006), eliciting disgust when applied to others and shame when applied to the self, and significant social and legal punishment contingencies are in place. The problem is that the word "racist," in our current context, is applied as a label for highly likely and largely unavoidable behavior.

The situation seems perfectly poised to generate experiential avoidance (EA). Specifically, EA involves when "a person is unwilling to remain in contact with particular private experiences (e.g., bodily sensations, emotions, thoughts, memories, behavioral predispositions) and takes steps to alter the form or frequency of these events and the contexts that occasion them" (Hayes et al., 1996, p. 1154). Fundamental to the construct of EA is that it develops through normative social-psychological processes, particularly societal rules and language systems that encourage EA as a logical belief system and recipe for life success (Hayes et al., 1999). The clinical theory of EA is that it persists because EA is negatively reinforcing in the short term (i.e., aversive experiences are temporarily reduced or avoided), even though it is damaging with respect to living a value-driven life in the long term, which requires, at times, openness to aversive experiences. Research indicates that EA sits on a continuum, with some individuals on the open and accepting end and others on the avoidant end, who are likely to be quite rigidly avoidant, explicit about avoidance as a life value (e.g., "My goal is to feel happy at all times"), and resistant to change (Bond et al., 2011).

It may be useful to construe the context of contemporary racism for White individuals similarly. From this perspective, our context supports race-based EA: an unwillingness to contact private experiences stimulated by racial differences, such as perceptual biases, negative stereotypes, and IGA, even though these experiences appear to be involuntarily and automatically activated by the context. Likewise, race-based EA may be seen in an unwillingness to consider larger life choices as relevant to racism and privilege and a preference for defining racism as either explicit hatred or a function of involuntary, subtle processes. Color-blindness can be seen as an explicit articulation of rules for race-based EA. Thus, some White individuals may be avoidant of any contexts that trigger private experiences stimulated by racial differences and may try to avoid awareness of (e.g., suppress) these private experiences themselves (Plant & Butz, 2006). They may avoid dialogues on race or racism or spaces in which interactions with people of color are likely. White individuals may be avoidant of any suggestions that they may be, or appear to be, racist and may offer their attempts to follow the rules of color-blindness as a defense against these suggestions.

Furthermore, like EA, which ranges from relatively low, culturally normative levels to pathologically pervasive and rigid levels, we expect race-based EA to sit on a continuum. Some—presumably those for whom diversity has been a larger part of their life experience—will demonstrate less automatic activation of stereotypes and IGA, endorse lower levels of color-blindness, express more openness to people of color and multicultural orientations, and engage in more choices that favor people of color. Others, in contrast, will be high in IGA, rigidly color-blind, explicit about color-blindness as a life value, fiercely defensive against notions of privilege, and resistant to change. For individuals on the more rigid or extreme end of the race-based EA continuum, the characterization of "White fragility" (DiAngelo, 2011) may be appropriate, though inadequate to functionally explain this behavior in a contextually useful (or accurate) way.

Microaggressions

Microaggressions, in particular, may be understood as resulting from these functional contextual processes. For example, a White individual, hooked by automatic attentional processes that bias them to notice out-group features, may comment on a Black woman's hair, ask an Asian man where he is from, try speaking in Spanish to a Latinx waiter, or ask a mixed ethnicity woman if she is Black or White. Any of these comments may be experienced as microaggressive by the person of color, who may be aware that the functional influence behind the comment is biased attention to their racial features, even if the White person is not aware.

Likewise, the White person may get hooked by a stereotype and express it, either directly or indirectly, such as asking a Black law student if they received a minority fellowship or referring to a Black doctor as a nurse or assistant instead of as a doctor, or starting talking with a Mexican man about soccer without knowing if he is personally interested in the sport. All of this may be experienced as microaggressive by the person of color, even as the White person is not aware that they are acting from stereotypes. Similarly, the White person may get hooked by IGA and express it nonverbally, such as through nervous laughter or poor eye contact. Alternately, the White person's behavior may be dominated by avoidance, including physical distancing, attempting to change the topic to avoid sensitive issues, carefully choosing words that have no association with race or racism, or prematurely ending a conversation. All of this may happen without much conscious intentionality from the White person but may be noticed and reacted to negatively by the person of color.

Microaggressions around color-blindness, privilege, and avoidance may be particularly likely when the conversational context emphasizes racial inequities or racial differences, including when life choices made by White people are more likely to be examined in the context of differences in power, privilege, and structural advantages. In such a context, a White person would benefit from a more developed sense of Whiteness and privilege as aspects of identity, more comfort with and willingness to engage in racial dialogue, and—ultimately—a willingness to examine and reconsider life choices in the context of one's stated anti-racist values. When these characteristics are lacking, the person of color may find a racially themed discussion to be invalidating of their experiences of the reality of racism, such as when a White person demonstrates a lack of awareness of the depth of structural issues, expresses color-blindness (e.g., "all lives matter"), or is unable to acknowledge the potential benefits and privileges of being White and the ways in which power and privilege have impacted their choices.

Conclusion

In this chapter, we reviewed research and theory on implicit bias, color-blindness, White privilege, and microaggressions. Overall, research on these terms clearly shows that they describe important and valid facets of racism, racist behavior, and obstacles to progress toward a more equitable, non-racist society. Bias exists in policies and individual behavior across all of our society's institutions and structures: education, criminal justice, health, housing, and employment. Color-blindness, a value system adopted by many White people, functions as an obstacle to progress in this biased context. The ways in which many White people are raised and socialized to define themselves as individuals, without meaningful awareness of how Whiteness, at the group level, confers advantages and privileges, and how White people will fiercely defend themselves against notions of Whiteness and privilege, are additional obstacles. In this biased context, self-interested choices that "well-intentioned" White people make often go unexamined, and microaggressions occur frequently. Despite White people's arguments that microaggressions are unintentional and harmless, the extant research is straightforward. Day-to-day microaggressive experiences result in stress, confusion, hypervigilance, and other significant responses for people of color, which accumulate to represent a public health hazard, significantly contributing to physical and mental health disparities over time.

It is clear why diversity trainers and advocates focus their efforts on increasing awareness of bias, pointing out the problems associated with color-blindness, pushing White people to acknowledge and own their privileges, cautioning White people about microaggressive expressions, and trying to educate them when microaggressions occur. Yet, as reviewed above, these efforts typically produce little behavior change, and White resistance is strong.

We believe that both researchers and mental health professionals can and need to do better in dismantling racial health disparities and addressing racial bias within our field. In this chapter, we described, in contextual behavioral terms, the behavior of White people that is characterized as demonstrating or denying bias, color-blindness, White privilege, and microaggressions, in the service of behavior change strategies that are more effective and sustainable than simply encouraging people to suppress behavior. In our description, we moved away from implicit bias and toward the construct of IGA, which may function as a more effective intervention target. We describe how IGA may develop in a normative US cultural context, as White people come to experience people of color as threatening out-group members due to White people's lack of exposure to diversity during development, as pervasive negative stereotypes that people of color are dangerous augment this threatening out-group status, and as White individuals learn that interactions with people of color are fraught with peril due to the possibility that the White person will be perceived as racist in some way. Race-based experiential avoidance (EA) can easily develop in this context, and color-blindness can be seen as an explicit articulation of race-based EA, which comes to function as a rule for how to be non-racist in this context. This rule has the unfortunate effect of rendering White people who rigidly follow it even less sensitive to the actual contingencies, including their own biased behavior and the structural racism all around them.

For many White individuals, identity development occurs within a narrow band that emphasizes individuality and rarely results in the experience of Whiteness or privilege as a personally or emotionally significant aspect of the conceptualized self. This narrow band of identity development makes it even harder to engage in perspective taking toward people of color, and makes it harder to make life choices most consistent with anti-racist values. In other words, all of these developmental and contextual factors inter-act to produce a White individual who is highly likely to demonstrate hypocrisy in life choices and engage in microaggressions on a fairly regular basis, if he is not avoiding interactions with people of color altogether.

We hope that the analysis we offered in this chapter inspires readers who are familiar with CBS into action. Much research is needed, and we hope our analysis is a fertile ground for the development of hypotheses that would explore contemporary racism in terms of contextual behavioral processes. We also hope that our analysis will inspire intervention development, especially to the degree that our analysis maps on to the six core processes of ACT's model of psychological flexibility: defusion, acceptance, contact with the present moment, self-as-context, values, and committed action. For example, we suggest that—until the pervasively racist cultural context that White individuals are born and raised in can be changed—it is regrettably normative for most White individu-als to experience some degree of IGA and negative stereotypes as active psychological processes. These private experiences are unwelcome and unbidden, and largely out of voluntary control. Acceptance and defusion interventions, targeting IGA and negative stereotypes respectively, may reduce reliance on rule-governed experiential avoidance and color-blindness strategies that make the situation worse, not better, and may reduce the impact of IGA and negative stereotypes on behavior.

In chapter 8 of this volume we offer some specific intervention ideas that we have developed and evaluated in line with these suggestions. However, we see the field of pos-sibility as wide open and believe there is great promise for CBS to produce progress on one of society's greatest problems. Wholesale systemic and structural changes are needed to address the larger issues that produce the pervasively racist context in which the psy-chological processes we have described in this chapter unfold. We believe that CBS-informed interventions have the potential not only to reduce bias in White individuals and improve interracial behavior and relationships, whether therapeutic or otherwise, but also to strengthen values-based life choices and actions in line with courageously confronting the status quo, collective community building, political action, and other forms of activism that are undoubtedly necessary to influence these larger forces.

KEY POINTS FOR CLINICIANS

• A new language of racism, including implicit bias, awareness of White privilege, color-blindness, and microaggressions, emphasizes normative processes that occur in most White individuals.

• These processes can be understood in contextual behavioral terms, clarifying their nature and possible intervention strategies.

• Implicit bias may be seen as an umbrella term for various biased behaviors that often occur without awareness.

• Many White individuals have difficulty with awareness of White privilege because normative identity development does not emphasize group identity or Whiteness and instead prioritizes individuality.

• Color-blindness can be seen as rule-governed behavior ("If I do not notice race, then I cannot be racist") that typically backfires, producing more racist behavior, not less.

• Microaggressions are the behavioral manifestations of these and other processes.

• A broad emphasis on race-based experiential avoidance may help us develop more effective interventions targeting the modern language of racism.

References

Abreu, J. M. (1999). Conscious and nonconscious African American stereotypes: Impact on first impression and diagnostic ratings by therapists. *Journal of Consulting and Clinical Psychology, 67,* 387–393. https://doi.org/10.1037//0022-006X.67.3.387

Adams, R. B., & Kleck, R. E. (2003). Perceived gaze direction and the processing of facial displays of emotion. *Psychological Science, 14,* 644–647. https://doi.org/10.1046/j.0956-7976.2003.psci_1479.x

Apfelbaum, E. P., Norton, M. I., & Sommers, S. R. (2012). Racial color blindness: Emergence, practice, and implications. *Current Directions in Psychological Science, 21*(3), 205–209. https://doi.org/10.1177/0963721411434980

Apfelbaum, E. P., Pauker, K., Ambady, N., Sommers, S. R., & Norton, M. I. (2008). Learning (not) to talk about race: When older children underperform in social categorization. *Developmental Psychology, 44*(5), 1513–1518. https://doi.org/10.1037/a0012835

Apfelbaum, E. P., Pauker, K., Sommers, S. R., & Ambady, N. (2010). In blind pursuit of racial equality? *Psychological Science, 21*(11), 1587–1592. https://doi.org/10.1177/0956797610384741

Apfelbaum, E. P., Sommers, S. R., & Norton, M. I. (2008). Seeing race and seeming racist? Evaluating strategic colorblindness in social interaction. *Journal of Personality and Social Psychology, 95*(4), 918–932. https://doi.org/10.1037/a0011990

Ayalon, L., & Gum, A. M. (2011). The relationships between major lifetime discrimination, everyday discrimination, and mental health in three racial and ethnic groups of older adults. *Aging & Mental Health, 15*(5), 587–594. https://doi.org/10.1080/13607863.2010.543664

Bar-Haim, Y., Ziv, T., Lamy, D., & Hodes, R. M. (2006). Nature and nurture in own-race face processing. *Psychological Science, 17*(2), 159–163. https://doi.org/10.1111/j.1467-9280.2006.01679.x

Bezrukova, K., & Spell, C. S. (2012). Reviewing diversity training: Where we have been and where we should go. *Academy of Management Learning & Education, 11*(2), 207–227. https://doi.org/10.5465/amle.2008.0090

Boatright-Horowitz, S. L., & Soeung, S. (2009). Teaching White privilege to White students can mean saying good-bye to positive student evaluations. *American Psychologist, 64*(6), 574–575. https://doi.org/10.1037/a0016593

Bond, F. W., Hayes, S. C., Baer, R. A., Carpenter, K. M., Guenole, N., Orcutt, H. K., … & Zettle, R. D. (2011). Preliminary psychometric properties of the acceptance and action questionnaire-II: A revised measure of psychological inflexibility and experiential avoidance. *Behavior Therapy, 42*(4), 676–688. https://doi.org/10.1016/j.beth.2011.03.007

Bourgeois, P., & Hess, U. (2008). The impact of social context on mimicry. *Biological Psychology, 77,* 343–352.

Britt, T. W., Bonieci, K. A., Vescio, T. K., Biernat, M., & Brown, L. M. (1996). Intergroup anxiety: A person x situation approach. *Personality and Social Psychology Bulletin, 22*(11), 1177–1188.

Burkard, A. W., & Knox, S. (2004). Effect of therapist color-blindness on empathy and attributions in cross-cultural counseling. *Journal of Counseling Psychology, 51*(4), 387–397. http://doi.org/10.1037/0022-0167.51.4.387.

Capodilupo, C. M., Nadal, K. L., Corman, L., Hamit, S., Lyons, O. B., & Weinberg, A. (2010). The manifestation of gender microaggressions. In D. W. Sue (Ed.), *Microaggressions and marginality: Manifestation, dynamics, and impact* (pp. 193–216). Hoboken, NJ: John Wiley.

Case, K. A., & Rios, D. (2017). Educational interventions to raise awareness of White privilege. *Journal on Excellence in College Teaching, 28*(1), 137–156.

Castillo, L. G., Brossart, D. F., Reyes, C. J., Conoley, C. W., & Phoummarath, M. J. (2007). The influence of multicultural training on perceived multicultural counseling competencies and implicit racial prejudice. *Journal of Multicultural Counseling and Development, 35*(4), 243–255. https://doi.org/10.1002/j.2161-1912.2007.tb00064.x

Chae, D. H., Lincoln, K. D., & Jackson, J. S. (2011). Discrimination, attribution, and racial group identification: Implications for psychological distress among Black Americans in the National Survey of American Life (2001–2003). *American Journal of Orthopsychiatry, 81*(4), 498–506. https://doi.org/10.1111/j.1939-0025.2011.01122.x

Chekroud, A. M., Everett, J. A. C., Bridge, H., & Hewstone, M. (2014). A review of neuroimaging studies of race-related prejudice: Does amygdala response reflect threat? *Frontiers in Human Neuroscience, 8*(179). https://doi.org/10.3389/fnhum.2014.00179

Chen, C. N. (1996). Anxiety and depression: East and West. *International Medical Journal, 3,* 3–5.

Clark, T. T., Salas-Wright, C. P., Vaughn, M. G., & Whitfield, K. E. (2015). Everyday discrimination and mood and substance use disorders: A latent profile analysis with African Americans and Caribbean Blacks. *Addictive Behaviors, 40,* 119–125. https://doi.org/10.1016/j.addbeh.2014.08.006

Constantine, M. G. (2007). Racial microaggressions against African American clients in cross-racial counseling relationships. *Journal of Counseling Psychology, 54*(1), 1–16. https://doi.org/10.1037/0022-0167.54.1.1

Conway, J. G., Lipsey, N. P., Pogge, G., & Ratliff, K. A. (2017). Racial prejudice predicts less desire to learn about white privilege. *Social Psychology, 48*(5), 310–319. https://doi.org/10.1027/1864-9335/a000314

Cox, D., Navarro-Rivera, J., & Jones, R. P. (2016). Race, religion, and political affiliation of Americans' core social networks. *Public Religion Research Institute*. Retrieved from: https://www.prri.org /research/poll-race-religion-politics-americans-social-networks/

Devine, P. G. (1989). Stereotypes and prejudice: Their automatic and controlled components. *Journal of Personality and Social Psychology*, 56(1), 5–18. http://doi.org/10.1037/0022-3514.56.1.5

DiAngelo, R. (2011). White fragility. *International Journal of Critical Pedagogy*, 3(3), 54–70. https://doi .org/10.1177/0278364910382803

Dixon, T. L., & Maddox, K. B. (2005). Skin tone, crime news, and social reality judgments: Priming the stereotype of the dark and dangerous black criminal. *Journal of Applied Social Psychology*, 35(8), 1555–1570. https://doi.org/10.1111/j.1559-1816.2005.tb02184.x

Donovan, R. A., Galban, D. J., Grace, R. K., Bennett, J. K., & Felicié, S. Z. (2013). Impact of racial macro- and microaggressions in Black women's lives: A preliminary analysis. *Journal of Black Psychology*, 39(2), 185–196. https://doi.org/10.1177/0095798412443259.

Dovidio, J. F., & Gaertner, S. L. (2004). Aversive racism. *Advances in Experimental Social Psychology*, 36, 1–52. https://doi.org/10.1016/S0065-2601(04)36001-6

Ekehammar, B., Akrami, N., Gylje, M., & Zakrisson, I. (2004). What matters most to prejudice: Big five personality, social dominance orientation, or right-wing authoritarianism? *European Journal of Personality*, 18(6), 463–482. https://doi.org/10.1002/per.526

Emerson, M. O., & Smith, C. (2000). Divided by faith: Evangelical religion and the problem of race in America. New York, NY: Oxford University Press.

Fortgang, T. (2014). Why I'll never apologize for my white male privilege. *Time: Education*. Retrieved from http://time.com/85933/why-ill-never-apologize-for-my-white-male-privilege/

Greenwald, A. G., Banaji, M. R., & Nosek, B. A. (2015). Statistically small effects of the Implicit Association Test can have societally large effects. *Journal of Personality and Social Psychology*, 108(4), 553–561. https://doi.org/10.1037/pspa0000016.

Greenwald, A. G., & Krieger, L. H. (2006). Implicit bias: Scientific foundations. *California Law Review*, 94(4), 945–968. https://doi.org/10.15779/Z38GH7F.

Greenwald, A. G., Poehlman, T. A., Uhlmann, E. L., & Banaji, M. R. (2009). Understanding and using the Implicit Association Test: III. Meta-analysis of predictive validity. *Journal of Personality and Social Psychology*, 97(1), 17–41. https://doi.org/10.1037/a0015575.

Hammond, R. A., & Axelrod, R. (2006). The evolution of ethnocentrism. *Source: The Journal of Conflict Resolution*, 50(6), 926–936. Retrieved from http://www.jstor.org/stable/27638531

Harris, R. (2009). *ACT Made Simple*. Oakland, CA: New Harbinger.

Hayes, S. C. (1995). Knowing selves. *The Behavior Therapist*, 18, 94–96.

Hayes, S. C., Barnes-Holmes, D., & Wilson, K. G. (2012). Contextual behavioral science: Creating a science more adequate to the challenge of the human condition. *Journal of Contextual Behavioral Science*, 1(1–2), 1–16. https://doi.org/10.1016/j.jcbs.2012.09.004.

Hayes, S. C., Brownstein, A. J., Zettle, R. D., Rosenfarb, I., & Korn, Z. (1986). Rule-governed behavior and sensitivity to changing consequences of responding. *Journal of the Experimental Analysis of Behavior*, 45(3), 237–256. https://doi.org/10.1901/jeab.1986.45-237.

Hayes, S. C., Strosahl, K. D., & Wilson, K. G. (1999). *Acceptance and commitment therapy: An experiential approach to behavior change*. New York, NY: Guilford Press.

Hayes, S. C., Wilson, K. G., Gifford, E. V, Follette, V. M., & Strosahl, K. (1996). Experimental avoidance and behavioral disorders: A functional dimensional approach to diagnosis and treatment. *Journal of Consulting and Clinical Psychology*, 64(6), 1152–1168. https://doi.org/10.1037/0022 -006X.64.6.1152

Ito, T. A., & Urland, G. R. (2003). Race and gender on the brain: Electrocortical measures of attention to the race and gender of multiply categorizable individuals. *Journal of Personality and Social Psychology*, 85(4), 616–626. https://doi.org/10.1037/0022-3514.85.4.616

Kanter, J. W., Williams, M. T., Kuczynski, A. M., Manbeck, K. E., Debreaux, M., & Rosen, D. C. (2017). A preliminary report on the relationship between microaggressions against Black people and racism among White college students. *Race and Social Problems*, *9*(4), 291–299. https://doi .org/10.1007/s12552-017-9214-0

Kawakami, K., Williams, A., Sidhu, D., Choma, B. L., Rodriguez-Bailón, R., Cañadas, E., ... & Hugenberg, K. (2014). An eye for the I: Preferential attention to the eyes of ingroup members. *Journal of Personality and Social Psychology*, *107*(1), 1–20. https://doi.org/10.1037/a0036838

King, M. L., Jr. (1964, June). Wesleyan Baccalaureate. Hartford, Connecticut.

Lai, C. K., Hoffman, K. M., & Nosek, B. A. (2013). Reducing implicit prejudice. *Social and Personality Psychology Compass*, *7*(5), 315–330. https://doi.org/10.1111/spc3.12023

Lai, C. K., Marini, M., Lehr, S. A., Cerruti, C., Shin, J. E. L., Joy-Gaba, J. A., ... & Nosek, B. A. (2014). Reducing implicit racial preferences: I. A comparative investigation of 17 interventions. *Journal of Experimental Psychology: General*, *143*(4), 1765–1785. https://doi.org/10.1037/a0036260

Lai, C. K., Skinner, A. L., Cooley, E., Murrar, S., Brauer, M., Devos, T., ... & Nosek, B. A. (2016). Reducing implicit racial preferences: II. Intervention effectiveness across time. *Journal of Experimental Psychology: General*, *145*(8). https://doi.org/10.1037/xge0000179

Langrehr, K. J., & Blackmon, S. M. (2016). The impact of trainees' interracial anxiety on white privilege remorse: Motivation to control bias as a moderator. *Training and Education in Professional Psychology*, *10*(3), 157–164. https://doi.org/10.1037/tep0000118

Lewis, A. E., Chesler, M., & Forman, T. A. (2000). The impact of "colorblind" ideologies on students of color: Intergroup relations at a predominantly White university. *Journal of Negro Education*, *69*(1–2), 74–91.

Liao, K. Y. H., Weng, C. Y., & West, L. M. (2016). Social connectedness and intolerance of uncertainty as moderators between racial microaggressions and anxiety among Black individuals. *Journal of Counseling Psychology*, *63*(2), 240. https://doi.org/10.1037/cou0000123

Lilienfeld, S. O. (2017). Microaggressions: Strong claims, inadequate evidence. *Perspectives on Psychological Science*, *12*(1), 138–169. https://doi.org/10.1177/1745691616659391

Lin, A. I. (2010). Racial microaggressions directed at Asian Americans. In D. W. Sue (Ed.), *Microaggressions and marginality: Manifestation, dynamics, and impact* (pp. 85–102) Hoboken, NJ: John Wiley & Sons.

Luoma, J. B., Hayes, S. C., & Walser, R. D. (2017). *Learning ACT: An acceptance and commitment therapy skills training manual for therapists.* (2nd Ed.). Oakland, CA: New Harbinger.

Maina, I. W., Belton, T. D., Ginzberg, S., Singh, A., & Johnson, T. J. (2016). A decade of studying implicit racial/ethnic bias in healthcare providers using the implicit association test. *Social Science and Medicine*, *199*, 219–29. https://doi.org/10.1016/j.socscimed.2017.05.009

Maxie, A. C., Arnold, D. H., & Stephenson, M. (2006). Do therapists address ethnic and racial differences in cross-cultural psychotherapy? *Psychotherapy: Theory, Research, Practice, Training*, *43*(1), 85. https://doi.org/10.1037/0033-3204.43.1.85

McIntosh, P. (1989). White privilege: Unpacking the invisible backpack. *Peace and Freedom Magazine*, *July/August*, 10–12. Retrieved from http://code.ucsd.edu/pcosman/Backpack.pdf

Mindrup, R. M., Spray, B. J., & Lamberghini-West, A. (2011). White privilege and multicultural counseling competence: The influence of field of study, sex, and racial/ethnic exposure. *Journal of Ethnic & Cultural Diversity in Social Work*, *20*(1), 20–38. https://doi.org/10.1080/15313204.2011 .545942.

Mooney, C., & Viskontas, I. (2014). The science of your racist brain. *Mother Jones.* Retrieved from https://www.motherjones.com/politics/2014/05/inquiring-minds-david-amodio-your-brain -on-racism/

Neville, H. A., Awad, G. H., Brooks, J. E., Flores, M. P., & Bluemel, J. (2013). Color-blind racial ideology theory, training, and measurement implications in psychology. *American Psychologist*, *68*(6), 455–466. https://doi.org/10.1037/a0033282.

Neville, H., Spanierman, L., & Doan, B. T. (2006). Exploring the association between color-blind racial ideology and multicultural counseling competencies. *Cultural Diversity and Ethnic Minority Psychology, 12*(2), 275. http://doi.org/10.1037/1099-9809.12.2.275

Norton. M. I., Sommers, S. R., Apfelbaum, E. P., Pura, N., Ariely, D. (2006). Color blindness and inter-racial interaction. *Psychological Science, 17*(11), 949–953. https://doi.org/10.1111/j.1467-9280.2006.01810.x

O'Keefe, V. M., Wingate, L. R., Cole, A. B., Hollingsworth, D. W., & Tucker, R. P. (2015). Seemingly harmless racial communications are not so harmless: Racial microaggressions lead to suicidal ideation by way of depression symptoms. *Suicide and Life-Threatening Behavior, 45*(5), 567–576. https://doi.org/10.1111/sltb.12150

Oswald, F. L., Mitchell, G., Blanton, H., Jaccard, J., & Tetlock, P. E. (2013). Predicting ethnic and racial discrimination: A meta-analysis of IAT criterion studies. *Journal of Personality and Social Psychology, 105*(2), 171–192. https://doi.org/10.1037/a0032734

Paluck, E. L., & Green, D. P. (2009). Prejudice reduction: What works? A review and assessment of research and practice. *Annual Review of Psychology, 60*(1), 339–367. https://doi.org/10.1146/annurev.psych.60.110707.163607.

Plant, E. A., & Butz, D. A. (2006). The causes and consequences of an avoidance-focus for interracial interactions. *Personality and Social Psychology Bulletin, 32*(6), 833–846. https://doi.org/10.1177/0146167206287182.

Rehm, L. P. (1977). A self-control model of depression. *Behavior Therapy, 8*(5), 787–804. https://doi.org/10.1016/S0005-7894(77)80150-0

Richeson, J. A., & Shelton, J. N. (2007). Negotiating interracial interactions: Costs, consequences, and possibilities. *Current Directions in Psychological Science, 16*(6), 316–320. https://doi.org/10.1111/j.1467-8721.2007.00528.x.

Roediger, D. R. (1991). *The wages of whiteness: Race and the making of the American working class.* New York, NY: Verso.

Ryan, R. M., & Deci, E. L. (Eds.), (2002). Self-determination theory and the facilitation of intrinsic motivation, social development, and well-being. *American Psychologist, 55*, 68–78. https://doi.org/10.1037/0003-066X.55.1.68.

Sidman, M. (1989). *Coercion and its fallout.* Boston, MA: Authors Cooperative.

Smith, W. A., Allen, W. R., & Danley, L. L. (2007). "Assume the position … You fit the description": Psychosocial experiences and racial battle fatigue among African American male college students. *American Behavioral Scientist, 51*(4), 551–578. http://doi.org/10.1177/0002764207307742

Sommers, S. R., & Norton, M. I. (2006). Lay theories about White racists: What constitutes racism (and what doesn't). *Group Processes & Intergroup Relations, 9*(1), 117–138. https://doi.org/10.1177/1368430206059881

Staats, C., Capatosto, K., Tenney, L., & Mamo, S. (2017). *Implicit Bias Review.* Kirwan Institute for the Study of Race and Ethnicity. Retrieved from http://kirwaninstitute.osu.edu/wp-content/uploads/2017/11/2017-SOTS-final-draft-02.pdf

Stephan, W. G., & Stephan, C. W. (1985). Intergroup anxiety. *Journal of Social Issues, 41*(3), 157–175. https://doi.org/10.1111/j.1540-4560.1985.tb01134.x

Sue, D. W. (2010). *Microaggressions in everyday life: Race, gender, and sexual orientation.* Hoboken, NJ: John Wiley & Sons.

Sue, D. W., Capodilupo, C. M., Torino, G. C., Bucceri, J. M., Holder, A. M. B., Nadal, K. L., & Esquilin, M. (2007). Racial microaggressions in everyday life: Implications for clinical practice. *American Psychologist, 62*(4), 271–286. https://doi.org/10.1037/0003-066X.62.4.271

Sue, D. W., & Sue, D. (2003). *Counselling the culturally diverse: Theory and practice.* New York, NY: Wiley.

Sue, D. W., Torino, G. C., Capodilupo, C. M., Rivera, D. P., & Lin, A. I. (2009). How White faculty perceive and react to difficult dialogues on race: Implications for education and training. *The Counseling Psychologist, 37*(8), 1090–1115. https://doi.org/10.1177/0011000009340443

Tajfel, H., & Turner, J. C. (1986). The social identity theory of intergroup behavior. In S. Worchel & W. G. Austin (Eds.), *Psychology of intergroup relations* (pp. 7–24). Chicago: Nelson Hall.

Takaki, R. (2008). A different mirror: A history of multicultural America. New York, NY: Back Bay Books.

Taylor Phillips, L., & Lowery, B. S. (2015). The hard-knock life? Whites claim hardships in response to racial inequity. *Journal of Experimental Social Psychology, 61*, 12–18. https://doi.org/10.1016/j.jesp.2015.06.008

Ulansky, E., & Witenberg, W. (2017). Is nationalism on the rise globally? *Huffington Post.* Retrieved from https://www.huffingtonpost.com/elena-ulansky/is-nationalism-on-the-ris_b_10224712.html

Vance, J. D. (2016). *Hillbilly elegy: A memoir of a family and culture in crisis.* New York, NY: Harper-Collins Publishers.

Vicaria, I. M., & Dickens, L. (2016). Meta-analyses of the intra- and interpersonal outcomes of inter-personal coordination. *Journal of Nonverbal Behavior, 40*(4), 335–361. doi:10.1007/s10919-016-0238-8.

Williams, M. T., Kanter, J. W., & Ching, T. H. W. (2017). Anxiety, stress, and trauma symptoms in African Americans: Negative affectivity does not explain the relationship between microaggres-sions and psychopathology. *Journal of Racial and Ethnic Health Disparities, 5*(5), 1–9. https://doi.org/10.1007/s40615-017-0440-3

Wong, G., Derthick, A. O., David, E. J. R., Saw, A., & Okazaki, S. (2014). The what, the why, and the how: A review of racial microaggressions research in psychology. *Race and Social Problems, 6*(2), 181–200. https://doi.org/10.1007/s12552-013-9107-9

Yudell, M., Roberts, D., DeSalle, R., & Tishkoff, S. (2016). Taking race out of human genetics. *Science, 351*(6273), 564–565. https://doi.org/10.1126/science.aac4951

PART 2

Best Practices in Training and Psychotherapy

Cultural Competence 101

TEACHING ABOUT RACE AND RACISM

Monnica T. Williams,
University of Connecticut

Introduction

Perhaps there is no subject more challenging than the intricacies of race and racism in American culture. It has become clear that simply teaching facts about cultural differences between racial and ethnic groups is not adequate to achieve cultural competence in learners, as less visible constructs are far more potent drivers of behaviors and attitudes. These constructs include implicit bias, stereotypes, White privilege, intersectionality, microaggressions, and other topics that require a critical appraisal of one's self and one's role as a participant in a structurally racist society (Case, 2007). Because students may be hindered by a lifetime of deeply ingrained stereotypes and prejudices, traditional lectures and readings are often not sufficient to bring about a multicultural shift in perspective, even for students who consider themselves to be open-minded and progressive.

Classroom discussion is an important component to training, but it takes practice and skill to successfully engage potentially resistant students, with White students typically more resistant to the realities of racism than students of color. In fact, as noted in chapter 6, attempts to raise awareness of bias in White students can actually increase interracial anxiety, helplessness, guilt, and fear of being misunderstood, leading to avoidance and defensiveness (Case, 2007; Perry, Dovidio, Murphy, & Van Ryn, 2015; Sue, Rivera, Capodilupo, Lin, & Torino, 2010). Contact has long been recognized as an effective tool for reducing racism, and it appears to work through decreasing anxiety and increasing empathy toward the out-group (Pettigrew, Tropp, Wagner, & Christ, 2011). To that end, in addition to presenting accurate information, trainings should include meaningful discussion and experiential components with a focus on mutually reciprocal conversations across race (Lai et al., 2014).

This training approach evolved from years of experience as a diversity researcher and educator, having trained a wide range of students, clinicians, faculty, and allied professionals. One key approach to training is rooted in principles derived from the therapeutic technique known as functional analytic psychotherapy (FAP; Tsai et al., 2009), where student behavior is shaped through the use of interpersonal reinforcers such as empathy, statements of caring, and self-disclosure. FAP has been described as a modality that can help improve therapeutic relationships across racial differences (Miller, Williams, Wetterneck, Kanter, & Tsai, 2015) and also as a technique for teaching therapists (e.g., Schoendorff & Steinwachs, 2012). The training approach described here is for educators who are looking for guidance in navigating this challenging terrain. Because comprehensive diversity education in clinical training programs is a relatively recent requirement, faculty may have never received cultural training of any sort, and so this information may be new to faculty as well.

The training outlined in this chapter was used as part of a day-long training entitled the Racial Harmony Workshop, and it covers the didactic elements that were included in that workshop. The focus is on Black-White racism, but many of the topics discussed apply to other marginalized ethnic and racial groups as well, and the material is suitable for learners at every stage of professional development, including clinical trainees. This chapter provides a step-by-step description of the techniques that were used to effectively engage participants and will be particularly beneficial to readers who are interested in conducting diversity trainings. Presentation slides are provided as supplemental material, and it may be helpful to reference these while reading this chapter.

Delivering the Workshop

Overview

INTRODUCTIONS

It is recommended that trainings for mixed audiences be conducted by a diverse pair, whenever possible, to facilitate engagement across racial groups (for example, a Black female and a White male). This is also a good way to model a mutually respectful, equitable interracial relationship, and it provides opportunities to model allyship. At the start of the workshop, each facilitator provides a brief personal introduction. In addition to academic credentials, some personal information should be included to help humanize the instructors (e.g., background, family information, hobbies, and so forth). To prepare participants for the discussions and experiential parts to come, we note the importance of connecting with others as a way to understand each other and to overcome bias and racism. We also acknowledge that this is often challenging when others are from different racial and ethnic backgrounds.

To facilitate openness, safety and confidentiality are important. We ask participants to be open and to pledge to keep everything learned about others confidential. That being said, we cannot guarantee that others will adhere to this pledge, and so participants should consider this before sharing. We also note that the workshop will be uncomfortable at times, and so people can go at their own pace, while at the same time, we will be encouraging openness, sharing, and taking interpersonal risks as a means to facilitate connection.

Often students enter these trainings with anxieties that if they speak up, they may appear racist or prejudiced in some way. Given that all audiences (public, undergraduates, graduates, medical students, and even professionals in psychology and medicine) have reported this topic matter to be difficult at times, we let participants know early that we are making some assumptions about them—all good assumptions. We explain, "If you experience discomfort during this workshop, it is because you are one or more of the following groups: (1) caring, empathetic people, the least likely to offend others, and who want to avoid harming others; (2) people exposed to racism either personally or in your environment; and (3) people who want to grow as a person and do even better."

After the introductions are complete, we start with an ice-breaker exercise to help people start the process of interacting. This could be something like going around the room and asking everyone to introduce themselves, while sharing a fun fact about who they are.

Didactics

CULTURE AND RACE

The training begins with defining key concepts, which can be confusing and are often misused. The following terms should be defined as follows (Shiraev & Levy, 2016):

- *Culture*
    - *Attitudes* include beliefs (e.g., political, ideological, religious, moral), values, general knowledge (empirical and theoretical), opinions, superstitions, and stereotypes.
    - *Behaviors* include a wide variety of norms, roles, customs, traditions, habits, practices, and fashions.
    - *Symbols* represent things or ideas, the meaning of which is bestowed on them by people; a symbol may have the form of a material object, a color, a sound, a slogan, a building, or anything else.

- *Ethnicity:* Cultural heritage shared by group of people, typically with a common ancestral origin, language, traditions, and often religion and geographic territory.

- *Nationality:* Shared by people who are citizens of the same country; a political and legal designation.

- *Religious affiliation:* An individual's acceptance of knowledge, beliefs, and practices related to a particular faith.

- *Race:* Group of people classified by specific, similar physical characteristics and assumed ancestry.

Race is the most problematic of these terms—it is basically a "box people put you in based on how you look." It is important to emphasize that the term "race" includes biological, cultural, and social components. Thus, we prefer the term "ethnoracial" to "racial" in most cases. We then review US racial and ethnic categories as per the census definition. Explaining how these categories have changed over the years illustrates how such groupings are more of a social construction than biological fact. We also discuss the difficulties of redefining Hispanic as an ethnic group rather than a racial group, as the newest US Census procedures force Hispanics to choose either White, Black, Native American, or Asian as their race. As a result, on the last census, over 40 percent of Hispanics did not identify with any race at all, selecting "Other" (Ríos, Romero, & Ramírez, 2014).

Finally, we discuss the changing demographics of our country. The newest census projections put White Americans as a minority at 2042, underscoring the importance of understanding and appreciating our nation's growing people groups of color. We note that some people are anxious about this shift and what it might mean for White people.

COLOR-BLINDNESS VERSUS MULTICULTURALISM

No discussion of race and racism would be complete without addressing the topic of color-blindness (Terwilliger, Bach, Bryan, & Williams, 2013). Color-blindness is the racial ideology that posits the best way to end discrimination is by treating individuals as equally as possible, without regard to race, culture, or ethnicity. At its face value, color-blindness seems like a good thing. It focuses on commonalities between people, such as their shared humanity. However, color-blind ideology is actually a form of racism. As the most prevalent approach to racial differences in this country, many students will initially have difficulty comprehending this. We explain that the reason color-blindness is a form of racism is because it acts as if racial, ethnic, and cultural differences don't exist, maintains the status quo by not seeing inequities, and fails to embrace positive qualities in each cultural group. As the person of color leading the workshop, I say, "As a person of color, I like who I am, and I don't want any aspect of that to be unseen or invisible. The need for color-blindness implies there is something shameful about the way God made me and the culture I was born into that we shouldn't talk about. Thus, color-blindness has helped make race into a taboo topic that polite people cannot openly discuss. And if you can't talk about it, you can't understand it, much less address the racial problems that afflict our society. In fact, being unwilling to acknowledge racial differences makes it appear as if you do not understand how to interact properly with people from other groups."

If color-blindness is the wrong approach, we ask, how did it happen that so many embrace it? Color-blindness is something we learn from an early age. Our parents teach it to us through their words and actions, though perhaps not intentionally. For example, what do you say when you are at the playground, and your child says, "Mommy, look at that Black girl!" A typical parent might say, "Hush!" or "That's not polite!" or you just turn red and give the child an angry look or even a smack. Any of those communicate to the child that race is not an okay thing to talk about. What could the parent have said instead?

Identity can be thought of at three levels: (1) individual: we are all unique snow-flakes; (2) group: we are all members of certain groups that we identify with; and (3) universal: we are all human beings (Sue & Sue, 2012). Focusing only on the universal and ignoring the other two levels can be hurtful, especially to people who have suffered because of their individual characteristics or group identities. Instead, we introduce *multiculturalism*, which means we appreciate people's group identities based on their heritage. Race is a group that people belong to, and we want to recognize and appreciate it rather than ignore it. Even though it is a problematic social construction, it has very real consequences for group members, who may have suffered due to their group membership and who may have pride in their group and its accomplishments. To do multiculturalism right, we have to create a new version of the Golden Rule: "Don't treat people the way *you* want to be treated. Treat them the way *they* want to be treated."

RACIAL AND ETHNIC IDENTITY

Racial and ethnic identity development is a process that can be challenging for people of all races, White and non-White alike. People often start at a stage where they don't think much about their race and ethnicity. Over time, and when faced with challenges connected to their race and ethnicity, they decide what this aspect of their identity means to them (Sue & Sue, 2012). A stronger, positive ethnic identity protects people of color from some of the harms of racism (Williams, Chapman, Wong, & Turkheimer, 2012; Williams et al., 2018). It can be said that Black and White people live in two different Americas due to differential experiences arising from race. Black families tend to teach their children about the realities of discrimination from an early age to prepare and protect them through a process called "racial socialization" (Hughes et al., 2006). This may include teaching children about the accomplishments of Black people throughout history and also teaching children how to recognize and prepare for racism. Immigrant families may be less likely to engage in racial socialization if they came from countries where they didn't experience racial stigma or oppression.

White people have an ethnoracial identity as well. Most White people do not think about their own Whiteness, do not define themselves by skin color, and consequently experience themselves as *non-racialized*. They also do not see how their Whiteness has given them *power and privilege* compared to people of color, especially if their own experience of their lives has been of hard work and struggle. This can make developing a positive and prosocial White racial identity challenging. However, without deconstructing Whiteness as *race*, *privilege*, and *social construction*, we cannot begin to think in ways that are explicitly anti-racist (Dlamini, 2002; Neville, Worthington, & Spanierman, 2001). There are invisible systems of dominance built into every structure in our society. The racism that puts non-Whites at an unfair disadvantage confers unfair advantages to White people, including those who have worked hard and struggled. This system is a reflection of *dysfunction* at societal level, which we call our *social psychopathology*.

DiAngelo (2011) notes that White people in our society live in a social environment that protects and insulates them from racial stress. This perpetuates the non-racialized view of self and decreases the ability of White people to tolerate racial stress. Discussions about race induce discomfort and may trigger a range of defensive moves—for example, a display of emotions such as anger, fear, and guilt, and behaviors such as arguing, silence, and leaving the stress-inducing situation (avoidance). These behaviors function to reinstate White racial equilibrium and can make productive discussions about race challenging.

PATHOLOGICAL STEREOTYPES

Stereotypes are beliefs that all people within a particular group possess the same traits or characteristics. As instructors, we may use our own experiences to discuss this issue. For example, "When I first moved to Kentucky I held some stereotypes about the sort of people who lived there.... I thought that people were walking around barefoot and in overalls, with missing teeth and shotguns. But when I went to the mall, everyone looked normal, just like me, and I had to acknowledge that my stereotypes were wrong."

Stereotypes are often false or incorrect ideas attributed to particular members of a group, based on illogical reasoning, and represent unfair generalizations that do not change when presented with accurate information. *Pathological stereotypes* about people are a means of explaining and justifying differences between groups and using these differences to oppress the out-group (Williams, Gooden, & Davis, 2012). We prompt people to consider stereotypes they may have about certain groups, for example, about women, Hispanic people, Black men, Black teens, Asian Americans, and so forth. It is critical to understand that social status or group position determines the stereotype content, not the actual personal characteristics of group members (Jost & Banaji, 1994). Groups that have fewer social and economic advantages will be stereotyped in a way that helps explain disparities, such as lower employment rates or greater incarceration.

To illustrate the pervasiveness of stereotypes, I show a "Successful Black Man (psychologist) Meme." At the top, it says "I hated the projects" and at the bottom it continues, "that I had to do for my doctoral dissertation, but I confess it made me a better psychologist." Why is this meme funny? Because we all know the stereotypes about Black men being poor, and so the word "projects" evokes images of run-down public housing, which is not meant at all in this counter-stereotypical example. If you found the meme funny, it illustrates how we are all impacted by stereotypes, even if we do not agree with them.

It is very important to emphasize that stereotypes are not true, otherwise a discussion about negative stereotypes can be really unpleasant for people of color, who worry that they are being judged based on these stereotypes. African Americans are described with primarily derogatory stereotypes that include qualities such as lazy, ignorant, unintelligent, criminal, poor, loud, angry, and hostile. Current stereotypes include some seemingly "positive" terms as well, such as athletic, religious, and musical. Because we all have knowledge of the pathological stereotypes, very often we make wrong assumptions about others, and stereotypes about African Americans are not reality. There are four examples we like to share, one historical and three current.

Historical example:

- Jim Crow laws assumed that Black people were contaminated or unclean to justify segregation, yet Black women typically worked as maids, nannies, and cooks for White people, which does not make sense if Black people are, in fact, contaminated (i.e., the movie *The Help* is a good example).

We then move on to current examples. Students are often surprised by these:

- Fewer Black youth abuse drugs than White or Hispanic youth (Centers for Disease Control [CDC], 2000).

- Black fathers are more involved with their children than White fathers (Jones & Mosher, 2013).

- Although Blacks, on average, earn less than Whites, most Black people are not poor (Fontenot, Semega, Kollar, 2018).

The persistence of these negative stereotypes maintains our dysfunctional class system, and both negative and seemingly positive stereotypes continue to keep African Americans in a disadvantaged status. Negative stereotypes suggest that Blacks are intellectually deficient and lazy, which justifies the denial of educational and employment opportunities, while positive stereotypes, such as athleticism and musical talents, push African American youth away from college in favor of efforts to become sports stars or entertainers, which are professions in which the vast majority will fail (Williams, Gooden & Davis, 2012).

RACISM AND MICROAGGRESSIONS

Although many students will readily accept that racism exists, they often lack an understanding of how pervasive and harmful it can be for people of color. Although it is less acceptable to be openly racist than in past decades, racism continues to be widespread, because we are all drenched in negative social messages about minorities (pathological stereotypes). All of us absorb these messages and are influenced to some degree, and this affects how we think and act. This can be illustrated by advertisements with racist themes. For example, a Dove soap ad from 2011 showed three women in front of a before-and-after image of cracked and smooth skin; with a Black woman on the "before" side, a White woman on the "after" side, and a Hispanic woman in the middle.

The news and social media also perpetuate racism. A lynching postcard from the turn of the century is compared to a picture of an unarmed Black man being killed by police on national news, while the helicopter pilot makes derogatory remarks about the victim. Because of the long history of unfettered police violence against African Americans, these images can be oppressive and traumatizing to African Americans (Bor, Venkataramani, Williams, & Tsai, 2018). These widespread images communicate that Black people are disposable and not worthy of human dignity.

We end this segment with a discussion by presenting a list of examples of various types of racism. White students tend to underestimate the frequency and impact that racism has on people of color, and Black students tend to keep these experiences to themselves to avoid being invalidated, which perpetuates the lack of understanding. It is quite powerful for White students to hear the first-hand accounts of racism that have taken place right on their own campuses and the painful events experienced by a person of color in the very same classroom. Some examples we provide of racism include:

- being followed in stores ("shopping while Black"),

- insensitive remarks by coworkers and friends (microaggressions),

- profiling by law enforcement ("driving while Black"),

- racial slurs,

- Confederate monuments (environmental microaggressions),

- threats,

- #AllLivesMatter, and

- others?

We share our own experiences of encountering and committing racist acts to help students feel more comfortable divulging their own experiences. We provide lots of positive reinforcement for these disclosures and commend students for their honesty and bravery in sharing. In terms of who perpetrates and suffers from racism, we note that people of any group can perpetrate racism and discrimination, including other ethnoracial minorities, women, sexual minorities (LGBT), and disabled persons. Anyone of any race can suffer as a result of racism and discrimination. However, to discriminate the perpetrator must have some degree of power over the victim—for example, White over Black, men over women, boss over employee, police officer over citizen. The power differential can be social or formal.

Here we point out that most people have some bias, even if they don't want to. Data from the Implicit Associations Test (IAT) shows that when given a test where people are supposed to pair positive versus negative words with Black versus White faces, people tend to have more trouble pairing the Black faces with the positive words. If we look at the test results on a scale where positive numbers indicate a preference for European Americans, 0 indicates no preference for either group, and negative numbers indicate a preference for African Americans, we find that males are a bit more biased than females (0.36 versus 0.30), non-Hispanics are a bit more biased than Hispanics (0.34 versus 0.31), and Whites are a lot more biased than Blacks (0.40 versus 0.04) (Iyengar, Hahn, Dial, & Banaji, 2009; Mooney, 2014). This is on a scale where >0.15 is little or no bias, 0.15–0.35 is slight bias, and 0.35–0.65 is moderate bias. So on average White people have a moderate pro-White and anti-Black bias, whereas on average Blacks are unbiased. Now we have arrived at the heart of the problem. Even though people may recognize that racism is wrong and illogical, most people will still have racist thoughts and engage in racist behaviors.

Racism we define as the routine, institutionalized mistreatment of a person based on membership in a disempowered racial group. In the United States, African Americans experience the most racial discrimination, followed by Hispanic Americans and Asian Americans (Chao, Mallinckrodt, & Wei, 2012), although discrimination against other groups, such as women and sexual minorities, is common as well. There are many types of racism (i.e., "old-fashioned racism," symbolic racism, aversive racism). Here we take a moment to discuss what is probably the most common manifestation of racism—microaggressions (Pierce, 1970). Microaggressions are small racist acts that are not clearly racially motivated and, as such, create uncertainty and anxiety in people of color, because it is hard to determine if the experience was actually a discriminatory act (Sue et al., 2007). This causes uncertainty as to whether or not the negative interaction was caused by personal factors or racism. It is especially stressful because, unlike overt discriminatory acts, which provide a clear explanation for the cause of the negative behavior, microaggressions are easily deniable by the perpetrator. Thus, it can be hard for a person of color to figure out what really just happened in a given situation, and asking the perpetrator is unlikely to be helpful.

Microaggressions can be actions too. Here we show a picture of a White man and Black man walking down the street. The White man inexplicably crosses the street and keeps walking on the other side. We urge students to think about the Black man in this picture. "Put yourself in his shoes. What might he be thinking and feeling? What if this happened to you every day?" The purpose of this exercise is to help promote empathy for the experience of being ostracized. Often participants believe the person of color is feeling angry, which is to be expected, based on stereotypes of angry Black people, but this is a great place to discuss how the person of color may be feeling other things as well—confused, sad, lonely, or even suicidal as a result of ongoing ostracization (e.g., O'Keefe, Wingate, Cole, Hollingsworth, & Tucker, 2015).

We then share several examples from real counseling sessions in which a therapist a therapist committed a microaggresion against a client. Examples provided include:

- "I don't see you as Black. I just see you as a regular person."

- "If Black people just worked harder, they could be successful like other people."

- "Let's hope you weren't treated that way due to racism."

- "Don't be too sensitive about the racial stuff. I didn't mean anything bad or offensive."

- "I'm not racist, because some of my best friends are Black."

(Constantine, 2007; DeLapp & Williams, 2015)

We invite student responses as to why each one is a microaggression and what message the client might receive from the communication. We also point out some common examples of microaggressive experiences on campus, such as White people asking Blacks if they can touch their hair. This is actually a common request made of Black students with very curly hair and is generally unwelcome (Kanter et al., 2017). Another example might be a White professor telling Black students specifically that they should all sign up for tutoring since his class is difficult. Although the professor means well, such a comment is still insulting and hurtful to Black students, whom he implies are unintelligent with this "helpful" suggestion.

In fact, racism in all of its forms hurts. Research shows that not only is racism interpersonally painful, but it is also connected to a host of mental health problems, including stress (Clark, Anderson, Clark, & Williams, 1999), PTSD symptoms (Pieterse, Todd, Neville, & Carter, 2012), serious psychological distress (Chae, Lincoln, & Jackson, 2011; Chao et al., 2012), depression (Banks & Kohn-Wood, 2007), binge drinking (Blume, Lovato, Thyken, & Denny, 2012), suicidality (O'Keefe et al., 2015), and even psychosis and schizophrenia (Berger & Sarnyai, 2015).

Racism can be traumatic, and the trauma is cumulative, as shown in figure 7.1 (Williams, Metzger, Leins, & DeLapp, 2018). Many people of color already have traumatic cultural histories (e.g., for African Americans, this would include kidnapping from Africa, slavery, segregation, discrimination, community trauma), and this history alone is a source of ongoing low levels of stress (Kira, 2010). On top of that is overt and covert ongoing racism experienced on a regular basis. On top of that is a stressor that could be large or small, but that pushes a person over the line from feeling stressed to traumatized. Atop of that is the invalidation that the person encounters when trying to get social support. The last layer is the institutional barriers that make it harder for people of color to find professional help, such as low income or the lack of available culturally competent clinicians. Thus, racism is often an accumulation of insults for people of color, resulting in ongoing, unresolved traumatization.

CLINICAL IMPLICATIONS

For all the reasons described above, people of color tend underutilize health care services; they worry about mistreatment, being hospitalized involuntarily, or being used as guinea pigs (Ayalon & Alvidrez, 2007). People of color have greater distrust of the medical establishment and mental health care and may believe medical institutions hold racist attitudes (Whaley, 2001). This may be due in part to past medical abuses in communities of color, such as the US government-funded Tuskegee Syphilis Study, Guatemala STD experiments, Johns Hopkins University Baltimore Lead Paint Study, experimental Native American infant vaccination programs, and many others, some of which are ongoing today (Suite, La Bril, Primm, & Harrison-Ross, 2007). As a result, people of color may not seek care until problems are severe and thus end up in the emergency room or, worse yet, incarcerated.

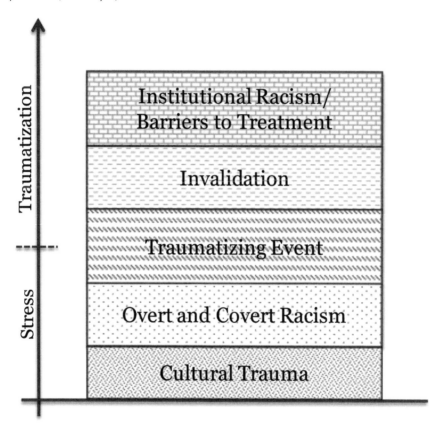

Figure 7.1.

Additionally, most people of color have already encountered discrimination in other medical contexts, and so they may be cautious in a new situation, especially if they are expected to be vulnerable and bear their emotions. This understandable caution may be misinterpreted as paranoia by mental health clinicians, contributing to overdiagnosis of psychosis in people of color (Whaley, 2001). Indeed, African Americans are consistently over diagnosed with schizophrenia and are more likely to be admitted as inpatients, even after controlling for severity of illness and other demographic variables (OR=2.52; Snowden, Hastings, & Alviderez, 2009). However, as noted above, discrimination and racism can also increase risk for psychotic disorders (Berger & Sarnyai, 2015).

In sum, there are several causes of mental health disparities. Persistent experiences of discrimination lead to psychological and physiological distress and also avoidance of health care providers who are primarily White. Concurrently, clinician bias leads to disparities (errors) in clinician decision making and poor (microaggressive) communication with clients. This leads to negative client reactions, making it less likely they will comply with provider recommendations or return for care (e.g., Penner, Blair, Albrecht, & Dovidio, 2014). In sum, racial bias may be invisible to perpetrators (clinicians), but is often very visible to those affected by it (clients of color).

RESPONDING TO RACISM

Well-intentioned White people who care about Black people may feel helpless and overwhelmed in the face of the pervasive reality of racism. Kanter and Rosen (2016) offer some practical strategies for making a difference.

- *Learn:* Our understanding of "racism" today is very different from "racism" of the past. Learn the new language.

- *Accept:* Get better at accepting, rather than avoiding, difficult feelings surrounding race.

- *Explore:* Get curious about your own stereotypes and biases, and learn how to deal with them.

- *Commit:* Get active and be part of the solution.

- *Connect:* Take risks to forge real relationships with others who are different from you.

Most importantly, when someone opens up about racial issues, *don't question* experiences of discrimination and racism (Hays, 2009). We underscore this as follows: "This is not the time to question whether or not it was really a racial event. Don't look for alternative explanations. You weren't there, so there is no need for you to suggest anything different happened. Victims need to feel heard, believed, and understood. Don't minimize the experience—that person is in the best position to know what happened and how it made them feel. Instead, deeply validate that person's experiences and feelings."

How can people of color navigate racism? Having a clinician who is a racial match may be helpful, but it does not guarantee a cultural match and may be complicated by the ethnic identity development of the client (for more on this, see chapter 9, "Culturally Responsive Assessment and Diagnosis for Clients of Color"). We also recommend the following steps for people color (DeLapp & Williams, 2016):

- Place the blame where it belongs (recognize our cultural dysfunction).

- Seek social support within one's community (e.g., close friends, family).

- Limit exposure to cues of racism, as needed, while recovering (e.g., signing off social media).

- Utilize religious or spiritual practices for comfort (e.g., prayer, meditation).

- Participate in restful and relaxing activities (e.g., enjoyable activities, self-care).

- Engage in peaceful activism (making meaning from pain).

- Educate others—and be patient! (facilitate mutual understanding).

Racism can be hurtful, and it's not fair. But it can also be an opportunity to educate others and improve relationships. For example, if a person has microaggressed against someone else, and they are able to talk about it and solve the problem, the person who committed the microaggression is much less likely to do it again, and through that conversation, the world has been made a little bit better for everyone.

EXPERIENTIAL EXERCISES

Experiential exercises can help to reduce interracial anxieties through disconfirmation of cognitive distortions (e.g., pathological stereotypes) and habituation to feared stimuli (e.g., talking about race, worries about being perceived as a racist). Positive intergroup interactions will reduce stressful intergroup interactions, and success depends on the ability of each person to listen well and demonstrate appropriate empathy and understanding (Davies, Tropp, Aron, Pettigrew, & Wright, 2011; Holoien, Bergsieker, Shelton, & Alegre, 2015; Shelton, Trail, West, & Bergsieker, 2010). When cross-racial participants exchange personally vulnerable details of their lives with each other, interracial anxiety decreases and intimacy and friendship increases (Page-Gould, Mendoza-Denton, & Tropp, 2008). Thus, White participants are encouraged to listen with empathy to the narratives of Black participants and then reciprocally disclose vulnerable details from their own lives, and vice versa.

One example of an effective experiential exercise we use in such workshops is called the "interracial therapeutic dyad." Participants are instructed to break into interracial groups of two people. One person plays the role of the therapist (White person), and one takes the role of the client of color. The client is to share a real experience of racism that happened to them. The therapist then practices responding with caring and sensitivity. After ten minutes, the two people switch roles, and the person of color takes on the role of the therapist and the White person takes the client role. The White person will share a real stereotype they held or a racially insensitive act they committed. The therapist will practice responding to this disclosure with caring and sensitivity. After this exercise, time is provided for participants to discuss how it went to the larger group; people usually report feeling anxious at the start of the exercise but more relaxed and emotionally closer afterward. This is a good place to emphasize the importance of practicing interracial dialogues and nurturing cross-racial friendships.

Conclusion

Practical Implementations

As noted, the bulk of this training was used as part of a day-long workshop, titled the Racial Harmony Workshop, that integrated the didactics above with additional experiential exercises focused on mutually reciprocal conversations across race (described in Kanter, Williams, & Rosen, 2018). This integrated approach was tested in a randomized trial with Black and White undergraduate students (Williams et al., 2018). As described in Kanter et al., the four specific experiential exercises of the Racial Harmony Workshop involved students breaking into small groups or pairs and included (1) one that involved noticing each other with eye contact, (2) another that focused on exploring discomfort through personal narratives, (3) a racial identity exploration exercise, and (4) an ending exercise with the large group expressing appreciations and a plan for future new behaviors. Results indicated positive benefits for both Black and White participants, including increased mood and positive feelings toward Black people for the White students and increased racial identity for the Black students.

Components of this approach have also been integrated with other experiential exercises targeting bias in medical students to improve clinician emotional rapport in interracial encounters, with an emphasis on improved interactions with patients in racially challenging moments. Twenty-five medical students and recent graduates were randomized to the intervention or a waitlist. Coders assessed video recordings of clinician rapport and responsiveness during simulated interracial patient encounters with standardized Black patients (actors) who presented specific racial challenges to clinicians. Improvements in emotional rapport and responsiveness, attitudes toward minorities, and working alliance with the Black standardized patients were observed by raters and reported by the clinicians who received the intervention (Kanter et al., citation forthcoming). Thus, research supports the usefulness of this approach as a potentially important and effective component of interventions to reduce racism and bias and improve outcomes for people of color in domains of public health significance.

Summary

This chapter is intended as a roadmap for interactive classroom discussions that teach students about race and racism, the first leg on their journey toward cultural competence. These are challenging concepts to teach, so do not attempt this training without having done your own personal anti-racism work first. Practice having difficult discussions and anticipate in advance how you will respond to hard questions. It is useful to have data handy to help respond to common racial misconceptions. Those who have not conducted diversity trainings before are encouraged to read the references provided to learn more about the information presented here. Finally, keep in mind that maintaining an atmosphere of safety, mutual respect, and caring in the room is critical for success.

Remember, that cultural competence is a lifelong process, so simply mastering the material described here will not make one competent. It may not be possible for a person to become competent in a culture they are not part of, but it is possible for instructors and clinicians to learn the skills needed to help others across racial and ethnic divides. Cultural humility is perhaps the key concept (Foronda, Baptiste, Reinholdt, & Ousman, 2016), as the more we learn, the more we realize we need to learn.

KEY POINTS FOR CLINICIANS

- Teaching students about race and racism in America is possibly the most difficult aspect of helping learners achieve cultural competence.

- Racism is embedded into nearly all social structures, institutions, and policies, and thus can be challenging to recognize.

- People may commit racist acts without realizing it, causing distress in targets.

- The use of interpersonal reinforcers such as empathy, statements of caring, and self-disclosure can facilitate learning about challenging material.

- This approach has been included in interventions shown to reduce racism among students and improve rapport with clients.

References

Ayalon, L., & Alvidrez, J. (2007). The experience of black consumers in the mental health system: Identifying barriers to and facilitators of mental health treatment using the consumers' perspective. *Issues in Mental Health Nursing, 28*, 1323–1340. doi:10.1080/01612840701651454

Banks, K., & Kohn-Wood, L. P. (2007). The influence of racial identity profiles on the relationship between racial discrimination and depressive symptoms. *Journal of Black Psychology, 33*(3), 331–354.

Berger, M., & Sarnyai, Z. (2015). "More than skin deep": Stress neurobiology and mental health consequences of racial discrimination. *The International Journal on the Biology of Stress, 18*(1), 1–10. doi:10.3109/10253890.2014.989204

Blume, A. W., Lovato, L. V., Thyken, B. N., & Denny, N. (2012). The relationship of microaggressions with alcohol use and anxiety among ethnic minority college students in a historically White institution. *Cultural Diversity and Ethnic Minority Psychology, 18*(1), 45–54.

Bor, J, Venkataramani, A. S., Williams, D. R., & Tsai, A. C. (2018). Police killings and their spillover effects on the mental health of black Americans: A population-based, quasi-experimental study. *The Lancet, 392*(10144), 302–310. doi:10.1016/S0140-6736(18)31130-9

Case, K. A. (2007). Raising white privilege awareness and reducing racial prejudice: Assessing diversity course effectiveness. *Teaching of Psychology, 34*(4), 231–235.

Centers for Disease Control (CDC). (2000). Youth Risk Behavior Surveillance, United States, 1999. *Mortality and Morbidity Weekly Report: Surveillance Summaries, 49*(SS05), 1–96.

Chae, D. H., Lincoln, K. D., & Jackson, J. S. (2011). Discrimination, attribution, and racial group identification: Implications for psychological distress among Black Americans in the National Survey of American Life (2001–2003). *American Journal of Orthopsychiatry, 81*(4), 498–506.

Chao, R. C., Mallinckrodt, B., & Wei, M. (2012). Co-occurring presenting problems in African American college clients reporting racial discrimination distress. *Professional Psychology: Research and Practice, 43*(3), 199–207. doi:10.1037/a0027861

Clark, R., Anderson, N. B., Clark, V. R., & Williams, D. R. (1999). Racism as a stressor for African Americans: A biopsychosocial model. *American Psychologist, 54*(10), 805–816.

Constantine, M. G. (2007). Racial microaggressions against African American clients in cross-racial counseling relationships. *Journal of Counseling Psychology, 54*(1), 1–16.

Davies K. R., Tropp L. R., Aron A., Pettigrew T. F., & Wright S. C. (2011). Cross-group friendships and intergroup attitudes: A meta-analytic review. *Personality and Social Psychology Review, 15*, 332–351. doi: 10.1177/1088868311411103

DeLapp, R. C. T., & Williams, M. (2016, July 18). Proactively coping with racism. *Psychology Today* [blog]. Retrieved from: https://www.psychologytoday.com/blog/culturally-speaking/201607/proactively-coping-racism

DeLapp, R. C. T., & Williams, M. T. (2015). Professional challenges facing African American psychologists: The presence and impact of racial microaggressions. *The Behavior Therapist, 38*(4), 101–105.

Devine, P. G., Forscher, P. S., Austin, A. J., & Cox, W. L. (2012). Long-term reduction in implicit race bias: A prejudice habit-breaking intervention. *Journal of Experimental Social Psychology, 48*(6), 1267–1278. doi:10.1016/j.jesp.2012.06.003

DiAngelo, R. (2011). White fragility. *The International Journal of Critical Pedagogy, 3*(3), 54–70.

Dlamini, S. N. (2002). From the other side of the desk: Notes on teaching about race when racialised. *Race, Ethnicity & Education, 5*(1), pp. 51–56.

Fontenot, K., Semega, J., & Kollar, M. (2018, September). *Income and Poverty in the United States: 2017, Current Population Reports.* Washington D. C; US Census Bureau (pp. 60–63). Retrieved from https://www.census.gov/content/dam/Census/library/publications/2018/demo/p60-263.pdf

Foronda, C., Baptiste, D., Reinholdt, M. M., & Ousman, K. (2016). Cultural humility: A concept analysis. *Journal of Transcultural Nursing, 27*(3), 210–217. doi:10.1177/1043659615592677

Hays, P. A. (2009). Integrating evidence-based practice, cognitive–behavior therapy, and multicultural therapy: Ten steps for culturally competent practice. *Professional Psychology: Research and Practice, 40*(4), 354–360. http://dx.doi.org/10.1037/a0016250

Holoien, D. S., Bergsieker, H. B., Shelton, J. M., & Alegre, J. M. (2015). Do you really understand? Achieving accuracy in interracial relationships. *Journal of Personality and Social Psychology, 108*, 76–92.

Hughes, D., Rodriguez, J., Smith, E., Johnson, D., Stevenson, H., & Spicer, P. (2006). Parents' ethnic-racial socialization practices: A review of research and directions for future study. *Developmental Psychology, 42*(5) 747–770.

Iyengar, S., Hahn, K., Dial, C., & Banaji, M. (2009). Understanding explicit and implicit attitudes: A comparison of racial group and candidate preferences in the 2008 election. Conference proceedings from the American Political Science Association. Retrieved from http://pcl.stanford.edu/research/2010/iyengar-understanding.pdf

Jones, J., & Mosher, W. D. (2013, December 20). *Fathers' involvement with their children: united states, 2006–2010.* Division of Vital Statistics, Centers for Disease Control. National Health Statistics Reports, 71. Retrieved from http://www.cdc.gov/nchs/data/nhsr/nhsr071.pdf

Jost, J. T., & Banaji, M. B. (1994). The role of stereotyping in system-justification and the production of false consciousness. *British Journal of Social Psychology, 33*, 1–27.

Kanter, J., & Rosen, D. (2016). What well-intentioned White people can do about racism. *Psychology Today* [blog]. Retrieved from https://www.psychologytoday.com/blog/culturally-speaking/201608 /what-well-intentioned-white-people-can-do-about-racism

Kanter, J. W., Rosen, D. C., Manbeck, K., Branstetter, H., Kuczynski, A., Corey, M., Maitland, D., & Williams, M. T. (under review). Improving provider responsiveness and emotional rapport in racially charged interactions: A preliminary randomized trial.

Kanter, J. W., Williams, M. T., Kuczynski, A. M., Manbeck, K., Debreaux, M., & Rosen, D. (2017). A preliminary report on the relationship between microaggressions against Blacks and racism among White college students. *Race and Social Problems*, 9(4), 291–299. doi:10.1007/s12552-017 -9214-0

Kanter, J. W., Williams, M. T., & Rosen, D. (2018). *Manual for experiential exercises in Racial Harmony Workshop* (Unpublished manuscript). University of Washington, Seattle, WA.

Kira, I. A. (2010). Etiology and treatment of post-cumulative traumatic stress disorders in different cultures. *Traumatology*, 16(4), 128–141. doi:10.1177/1534765610365914

Lai, C. K., Marini, M., Lehr, S. A., Cerruti, C., Shin, J. L., Joy-Gaba, J. A., … & Nosek, B. A. (2014). Reducing implicit racial preferences: I. A comparative investigation of 17 interventions. *Journal of Experimental Psychology: General*, 143(4), 1765–1785. doi:10.1037/a0036260

Miller, A., Williams, M. T., Wetterneck, C. T., Kanter, J., & Tsai, M. (2015). Using functional analytic psychotherapy to improve awareness and connection in racially diverse client-therapist dyads. *The Behavior Therapist*, 38(6), 150–156.

Mooney, C. (2014, December 1). The science of why cops shoot young black men. And how to reform our bigoted brains. *Mother Jones*. Retrieved from http://www.motherjones.com/politics/2014/12 /science-of-racism-prejudice/

Neville, H., Worthington, R., & Spanierman, L. (2001). Race, power, and multicultural counseling psychology: Understanding white privilege and color blind racial attitudes. In J. Ponterotto, M. Casas, L. Suzuki, & C. Alexander (Eds.) *Handbook of Multicultural Counseling* (pp. 257–288). Thousand Oaks, CA: Sage.

O'Keefe, V. M., Wingate, L. R., Cole, A. B., Hollingsworth, D. W., & Tucker, R. P. (2015). Seemingly harmless racial communications are not so harmless: Racial microaggressions lead to suicidal ideation by way of depression symptoms. *Suicide and Life-Threatening Behavior*, 45(5), 567–576. doi:10.1111/sltb.12150

Page-Gould, E., Mendoza-Denton, R., & Tropp, L. R. (2008). With a little help from my cross-group friend: Reducing anxiety in intergroup contexts through cross-group friendship. *Journal of Personality and Social Psychology*, 95(5), 1080–94.

Penner, L. A., Blair, I. V., Albrecht, T. L., & Dovidio, J. F. (2014). Reducing racial health care disparities: A social psychological analysis. *Health and Well-Being*, 1(1) 204–212.

Perry, S. P., Dovidio, J. F., Murphy, M. C., & van Ryn, M. (2015). The joint effect of bias awareness and self-reported prejudice on intergroup anxiety and intentions for intergroup contact. *Cultural Diversity and Ethnic Minority Psychology*, 21(1), 89–96. doi:10.1037/a0037147

Pettigrew, T. F., Tropp, L. R., Wagner, U., & Christ, O. (2011). Recent advances in intergroup contact theory. *International Journal of Intercultural Relations*, 35(3), 271–280. doi:10.1016/j.ijintrel.2011 .03.001

Pierce, C. (1970). Offensive mechanisms. In F. Barbour (Ed.), *In the Black seventies* (pp. 265–282). Boston, MA: Porter Sargent.

Pieterse, A. L., Todd, N. R., Neville, H. A., & Carter, R. T. (2012). Perceived racism and mental health among Black American adults: A meta-analytic review. *Journal of Counseling Psychology*, 59(1), 1–9.

Ríos, M., Romero, F., & Ramírez, R. (2014, March). *Race reporting among Hispanics: 2010. working paper No. 102*. Population Division. Washington, DC: US Census Bureau. Retrieved from https://www

.census.gov/content/dam/Census/library/working-papers/2014/demo/shedding-light-on-race
-reporting-among-hispanics/POP-twps0102.pdf

Schoendorff, B., & Steinwachs, J. (2012). Using Functional Analytic Therapy to train therapists in Acceptance and Commitment Therapy, a conceptual and practical framework. *International Journal of Behavioral Consultation and Therapy, 7*(2–3), 135–137. doi:10.1037/h0100948

Shelton, J. N., Trail, T. E., West, T. V., & Bergsieker, H. B. (2010). From strangers to friends: The interpersonal process model of intimacy in developing interracial friendships. *Journal of Social and Personal Relationships, 27,* 71–90. doi:10.1177/0265407509346422

Shiraev, E. B., & Levy, D. A. (2016). *Cross-cultural psychology: Critical thinking and contemporary applications,* 6th ed. London: Routledge.

Snowden, L . R., Hastings, J. F., & Alviderez, J. (2009) Overrepresentation of Black Americans in psychiatric inpatient care. *Psychiatric Services, 60*(6), 779–785.

Sue, D. W., Capodilupo, C. M., Torino, G. C., Bucceri, J. M., Holder, A., Nadal, K. L., & Esquilin, M. (2007). Racial microaggressions in everyday life: Implications for clinical practice. *American Psychologist, 62*(4), 271–286.

Sue, D. W., Rivera, D. P., Capodilupo, C. M., Lin, A. I., & Torino, G. C. (2010). Racial dialogues and White trainee fears: Implications for education and training. *Cultural Diversity and Ethnic Minority Psychology, 16*(2), 206–214. doi:10.1037/a0016112

Sue, D. W., & Sue, D. (2012). *Counseling the culturally diverse: Theory and practice.,* 6th ed. Hoboken, NJ: John Wiley & Sons.

Suite, D. H., La Bril, R., Primm, A., & Harrison-Ross, P. (2007). Beyond misdiagnosis, misunderstanding and mistrust: relevance of the historical perspective in the medical and mental health treatment of people of color. *Journal of the National Medical Association, 99*(8), 879–885.

Terwilliger, J. M., Bach, N., Bryan, C., & Williams, M. T. (2013). Multicultural versus colorblind ideology: Implications for mental health and counseling. In A. Di Fabio (Ed.), *Psychology of counseling* (pp. 111–122). Hauppauge, NY: Nova Science Publishers.

Tsai, M., Kohlenberg, R. J., Kanter, J. W., Kohlenberg, B., Follette, W. C., & Callaghan, G. M. (2009). *A guide to functional analytic psychotherapy: Awareness, courage, love, and behaviorism.* New York, NY: Springer.

Whaley, A. L. (2001). Cultural mistrust and mental health services for African Americans: A review an meta-analysis. *Counseling Psychology, 29*(4), 513–531.

Williams, M. (2011, December). Colorblind ideology and racism. *Psychology Today* [blog]. Retrieved from http://www.psychologytoday.com/blog/colorblind/201112/colorblind-ideology-is-form-racism

Williams, M. T., Chapman, L. K., Wong, J., & Turkheimer, E. (2012). The role of ethnic identity in symptoms of anxiety and depression in African Americans. *Psychiatry Research, 199*(1), 31–36. doi:10.1016/j.psychres.2012.03.049

Williams, M. T., Duque, G., Chapman, L. K., Wetterneck, C. T., & DeLapp, R. C. T. (2018). Ethnic identity and regional differences in mental health in a national sample of African American young adults. *Journal of Racial and Ethnic Health Disparities, 5*(2), 312–321. doi:10.1007/s40615-017-0372-y

Williams, M. T., Gooden, A. M., & Davis, D. (2012). African Americans, European Americans, and pathological stereotypes: An African-centered perspective. In G. R. Hayes & M. H. Bryant (Eds.), *Psychology of Culture* (pp. 25–46). Hauppauge, NY: Nova Science Publishers.

Williams, M. T., Kanter, J. K., Oshin, L., Pena, A, Ching, T. H. W., Kuczynski, A., & Printz, D. (2018, February). Reducing microaggressions and promoting interracial connection: The racial harmony workshop. Faculty poster session for CLAS at the University of Connecticut, Storrs, CT.

Williams, M. T., Metzger, I., Leins, C., & DeLapp, C. (2018). Assessing racial trauma within a DSM-5 framework: The UConn Racial/Ethnic Stress & Trauma Survey. *Practice Innovations, 3*(4), 242–260. doi:10.1037/pri0000076

CHAPTER 8

Becoming an Antiracist White Clinician

Daniel C. Rosen,
Bastyr University

Jonathan W. Kanter,
University of Washington

Matthieu Villatte,
Bastyr University

Matthew D. Skinta,
Roosevelt University

Mary Plummer Loudon,
The Seattle Clinic

A new civil rights movement is happening, with racial justice at its core. Within a mental health context, this movement has increasingly focused on the elimination of racial disparities in the access, quality, and outcomes of clinical services (Rosen, Nakash, & Alegría, 2014). To address the current inequitable mental health delivery system, we must intervene at multiple levels, extending from policy decisions to the clinical behavior of providers. Though the field of multicultural psychology has called on mental health clinicians to adopt culturally responsive practices for decades (American Psychological Association, 2003, 2017; Arredondo et al., 1996), the current sociopolitical landscape has called many White clinicians to attention with an increased sense of urgency, including a recognition of the ways each of us may be led astray by biases outside our awareness. Taking action to address these biases, however, remains a challenge; there is a paucity of evidenced-based recommendations to inform clinical practice.

Whereas efforts to inform the practices of mental health providers are most often focused on specific interventions (e.g., topographical behavior), in this chapter, we shift the frame to first consider how our psychological science informs the more subtle process-level behaviors and clinical choices we make in the context of interracial care delivery. Our attention therein is focused on White providers working with clients of color.

Just as those of us who aspire to be antiracist White clinicians must actively commit to dismantling the external structures of racial health disparities, we must also actively engage in transforming our relationship to intrapersonal processes that may obstruct our capacity to deliver culturally responsive care. As psychologists who have spent years working in this area with different people in multiple contexts, we believe there is a critical role for applied psychological science in this effort, specifically, contextual behavioral science (CBS).

In chapter 6, we reviewed four major terms related to the new language of racism and racial bias essential to position this work within our current science and the sociopolitical zeitgeist. These terms included "implicit bias," "color-blindness," "White privilege," and "microaggressions." We described how each of these terms may be understood in terms of CBS processes—that is, human actions–in–context—and then we described a framework (see figure 6.1) that situated each of them as a sequence of intrapersonal psychological processes that may influence behavior in interracial interactions and that may be targeted by interventions from within acceptance and commitment therapy's (ACT) hexaflex model (Hayes, Strosahl, & Wilson, 2012). This framework emphasized (1) perceptual processes that lead to objectification of people of color, targeted with present moment awareness interventions; (2) elicited race-based anxiety and negative stereotypes, leading to experiential avoidance, targeted with defusion and acceptance interventions; and (3) rigidly held conceptualized selves, leading to color-blindness and lack of awareness of White privilege, targeted with self-as-context and acceptance interventions.

In the current chapter, we follow chapter 6 by describing each of these intervention pathways in detail. We then add a fourth intervention pathway that focuses on increasing clarity around antiracist values and engaging in committed actions that function to increase interracial connections. While the earlier intrapersonal processes were targeted with interventions from ACT, this final interpersonal pathway introduces interventions that we have been developing derived from functional analytic psychotherapy (FAP; Tsai et al., 2009).

Overall, the interventions presented in this chapter do not focus on the illusive elimination of racial anxieties and thoughts directly. Instead, we view such strategies as race-based experiential avoidance (EA)—an unwillingness to contact private experiences stimulated by racial differences, such as negative racial stereotypes and anxieties— and see it as a major obstacle to change. Our aim is to increase willingness to experience these private events, not as an act of passive acceptance or tolerance of racist processes, but in the service of opening up flexibility around how one responds to these reactions in moments that matter and in direct service to our clients' needs. The aim is to experience private reactions with mindful awareness such that their functional control over behavior is diminished and, instead, to locate and act on culturally responsive clinical behaviors. Said differently, the aim is to show up for our clients as the clinicians we want to be. With an assumed set of a priori values (e.g., social justice, equity), and consistent with a CBS lens, we have set out to identify the processes that strengthen the clinician's focus on the guiding question, "What would the clinician I want to *be* choose to *do* in this clinical moment?"

The overall goal of this chapter, therefore, is to help clinicians strengthen their culturally responsive practices and counter their own racial biases. We acknowledge that all of us (the authors) are in the process of *becoming* anti-racist clinicians ourselves, and have attempted to write from a place of aspiration and humility rather than one of any falsely achieved authority. Though we hope the chapter will be useful to many readers, the chapter is addressed to White clinicians.

Clinician Challenges and CBS-Informed Interventions

In this section, we present four problematic psychogical processes at the root of biased or racist clinical behavior and our suggested interventions and strategies for working through them. The interventions, largely drawn from the ACT and FAP therapeutic traditions, are offered in service of orienting clinicians to making choices consistent with antiracist values.

Clinician Challenge: Objectification

A starting point for any clinical interaction is the providers' attention, their focus. It stands to reason that if we are not focusing on our clients' central concerns and behaviors, delivering effective care becomes impossible. The myriad ways that humans are distracted by internal (e.g., private thoughts and sensations) and external (e.g., screens, sounds) stimuli are obstacles to this central task. Moreover, as humans categorize information based on our in-group and out-group differences (Tajfel & Turner, 1986), our attention is often immediately hooked by the features of others that are different from our own. This happens automatically and quickly. For example, we notice racial features in as little as a tenth of a second (Ito & Urland, 2003). This "noticing" has significant consequences, as demonstrated by a Yale Child Center Study (Gilliam, Maupin, Reyes, Accavitti, & Shic, 2016) that observed how teachers' differential attention (measured via eye-tracking) led to inequitable suspensions and expulsions of Black boys. As clinicians, we clearly need to be aware of ways our attention may be outside of our conscious control, including ways in which we automatically seek to confirm preconceived ideas or make perceived differences salient beyond their clinical relevance.

Functionally, we have found utility in describing this process and its related class of behaviors in the context of interracial interactions as *objectifying*, defined as moments when a White person's attention is drawn to racially distinct features of a person of color, and their responding is dominated by these cues. Simple examples of objectifying questions that occur in a clinical context include "Where are you from?" (e.g., to an Asian person), "Do you play any sports?" (e.g., to a Black man), or the self-disclosure "I love Bibimbap!" to a Korean client. Note that these examples are not framed for present purposes as good or bad or right or wrong, but rather as verbal behavior likely controlled by one's attention being hooked by noticeable differences rather than by clinical relevance. Paradoxically, while these efforts may be appraised by White clinicians as attempts to relate to their clients, they often leave clients of color feeling stereotyped, confused, and disconnected, as they make salient and objectify differences in power and privilege between them.

To further concretize this concept, consider the initial clinical intake. Imagine walking into a waiting room and meeting your client for the very first time. What do we know about the White clinician's attention in these moments? As noted, we know that White people are more likely to have their attention automatically drawn to the racially specific features of a Black person's face and away from the eyes (Kawakami et al., 2014). We also know that humans in many cultures, and in this case, many clients, rely on this eye contact to determine the providers' intent and to feel safe (Bourgeois & Hess, 2008; Adams & Kleck, 2003). Herein lies the relevance of attending to our attention.

Proposed CBS Intervention: Present Moment Awareness and Flexibility

A variety of contact techniques focused on actively attending to internal experiences (e.g., thoughts, feelings, sensations) in the present moment are likely well known to CBS practitioners, and they can be adapted and implemented in supporting culturally responsive practice. Generally consistent with well-used mindfulness techniques that encourage practitioners to pay attention, on purpose, in an open and non-judgmental way (Kabat-Zinn, 1994), we suggest that these techniques function to support complementary ACT processes that follow this section (e.g., acceptance, defusion). In other words, first, with mindful attention to the present moment, we notice our attentional hooks and then increase flexibility by unhooking.

Our first recommendation is to bring awareness into the clinical encounter such that one's attention stays focused "on purpose" on one's client and, more specifically, on their eyes. We presume this is especially relevant in the first moments of the first visit, when we are most at risk of objectifying and stereotyping one another. From an ACT point of view, this requires both an initial awareness of this attentional or perceptual bias and the ability to engage in committed action (e.g., culturally appropriate levels of eye contact).

Other examples of being accountable for our attention include the recognition that phone calls from Black clients are returned at lower rates than White clients (Kugelmass, 2016; Shin, Smith, Welch, & Ezeofor, 2016) and that biases often drive the questions we ask (or don't ask) our clients during the clinical intake, as well as the diagnosis we assign (Alegría et. al, 2008). Once these behaviors are understood as often operating outside of awareness, clinicians may choose to direct their attention through preventive means. We suggest, for example, setting up equitable practices in how phone calls are returned (e.g., in the order they were received), which intake questions are asked (e.g., defined by a structured protocol consistent with the questions you determine are essential to the intake session), and diagnostic decision making (Nakash, Rosen & Alegría, 2009; Rosen, Nakash, Kwong, & Branstetter, 2017).

At the moment-to-moment level of clinical practice, however, such preventive strategies are much more challenging to access. The multitude of factors that demand our attention in the clinical interaction renders any simple formula quite useless. Here, we are back to the very hard work of mindfulness, of staying attentive to ourselves to accurately experience the here and now, to contact the present moment.

Simple mindfulness exercises may help us better notice our attentional hooks and the resulting negative racial thoughts and anxieties that might occur outside of awareness when interacting with clients of color. In the context of a workshop developing these skills, participants are led through a traditional eyes-closed mindfulness meditation that facilitates non-judgmental contact with the present moment (e.g., notice the sound of the facilitator's voice, the feel of one's body in one's clothes, one's breathing, heartbeat, any thoughts and feelings that arise) without a focus on racial themes. Then, maintaining gentle, mindful contact with the present moment, racial themes are introduced. Participants are asked to open their eyes and view a series of photos of people of color, potential clients, in different settings (e.g., in a law office, on a street corner in front of a corner grocery, at a police station) and arriving at their clinical appointment. The facilitator encourages participants to slow down and notice, with more exquisite attention and openness than is typical, where one's attention is drawn and any negative stereotypical thoughts (to the extent one is able to recognize them) and emotions that may be elicited by the pictures.

After the exercise, participants discuss how this process might apply to specific clients, and how such an exercise, if practiced over time, could produce new contact-with-the-present-moment skills that could be brought to bear in clinical interactions that matter. The goal in this type of exercise is for White clinicians to improve their non-judgmental, mindful awareness of how and where they pay attention, and of the resulting thoughts, anxieties, and other feelings that show up. Combined with defusion and acceptance exercises that follow, we believe this work facilitates access to value-consistent, culturally responsive practice with greater ease and flexibility.

Clinician Challenge: Avoidance of Internal Experiences

One by-product of growing up in a racist society is that racist thoughts will be learned, internalized, and cued by contextual features, such as a Black person's face, without our intent (e.g., Greenwald & Krieger, 2006). Likewise, our history and context also make interracial anxiety almost inevitable and cued instantly in interracial interactions. We know, for example, that most White people demonstrate instantaneous hyperactivations of the amygdala (a key index of the body's threat-response system) when presented with stimuli of a Black person's face (Chekroud, Everett, Bridge, & Hewstone, 2014).

From our perspective, a fundamental piece of the puzzle is that, in addition to growing up in a society that wires us to automatically have these negative private experiences, society also taught us that it is wrong to have them. Worse, society gave us no tools to manage them successfully. Thus, we often resort to ineffective strategies: avoidance, denial, and suppression. We may leave the room during a conversation about race, stay quiet in an interaction with a person of color to avoid saying something offensive, avoid spaces in which interactions with people of color are likely, or steer clear of people of color altogether. More specific to clinical work, the provider may set up their practice in a predominantly White neighborhood (without giving it a second thought), set fees accessible only to upper-income (and mostly White) clients, or, without awareness, be slower to return phone calls from clients of color or ignore those calls entirely.

We also avoid the psychological experiences themselves (i.e, interracial anxieties and negative stereotypes), dismissing, denying, and pushing them out of awareness. Social norms produce shame around admitting to others, and even recognizing in ourselves, that such private reactions occur. We pretend the reactions are not there, get defensive, and sometimes lie, both to ourselves and to others, to avoid looking bad. In combating racist thoughts that arise unbidden, the most common reaction we might have is to attempt to suppress those thoughts (e.g., Condor, Figgou, Abell, Gibson, & Stevenson, 2006). Thought suppression, however, is known to be a generally unsuccessful tactic and may even increase the frequency with which we experience the very thoughts we are trying to avoid (e.g., Wegner, 1992).

As previously noted, we see such efforts as race-based experiential avoidance (EA). Similar to how EA is generally defined (Hayes, Wilson, Gifford, Follette, & Strosahl, 1996, p. 1154), race-based EA may be defined as an unwillingness to contact private experiences stimulated by racial differences, such as negative racial stereotypes (i.e., cognitions) and anxieties (i.e., affect), and taking steps to avoid these experiences and the contexts that occasion them. The most pernicious aspect of race-based EA is that, even though it may be motivated by a desire not to be racist (and treat all people well), it results in avoidance of the very contexts and learning opportunities required for engaging in culturally responsive behavior. Avoidance is not a growth strategy.

The extreme end of the continuum of race-based EA may be thought of as what DiAngelo (2011) has described as "White fragility," in which White people experience even small amounts of racial stress as intolerable, triggering a range of defensive moves such as anger, fear, guilt, and behaviors such as argumentation, silence, and leaving the stress-inducing situation. Functionally defined, White fragility is the outcome of a history of avoided cognitions and emotions related to racism and privilege, such that even small exposures are experienced as overwhelmingly aversive, leading to increasingly restrictive behaviors.

Proposed CBS Interventions: Defusion and Acceptance

Rather than trying to change, avoid, or suppress race-based thoughts and anxieties, the aim is to experience them gently, with openness, and with less functional impact on behavior, thereby increasingly one's psychological flexibility to access values-based, culturally responsive actions. A host of defusion and acceptance techniques are available as ACT interventions that can readily be modified for these targets. Such techniques help the clinician explore racial biases and anxiety in an accepting and non-judgmental fashion (e.g., "leaves on a stream," the "physicalizing" exercise), relate to negative racial thoughts and feelings in ways that disrupt normative contexts that support tight relations between thoughts, feelings, and behavior, and extinguish the behavioral avoidance functions that co-occur with racially biased thoughts and anxieties. Here we present several examples.

DEFUSING FROM DIFFICULT THOUGHTS

It may be helpful for clinicians to willingly call to mind and explore, with defusion exercises, some of the more difficult and threatening race- and racism-related thoughts that occur. Consider the following thought: *I am a racist.* Your mind likely will immediately fight with this thought, bringing forth all of the examples and facts that disprove such an accusation or perhaps logically questioning the basis of the statement itself (e.g., *Perhaps I have at times engaged in racist behavior, but that does not make me a racist person!*). Defusion asks you to notice this fight and not get hooked by it. In this moment, it does not matter if the thought is true or false. In this moment, *I am a racist* is just a thought. Instead of fighting with it, notice, with curiosity, the emotional reactions the thought elicits. Perhaps employ the word repetition task, in which you rapidly repeat the thought or phrase aloud for thirty seconds, as an exploration of defusion (Masuda, Hayes, Sackett, & Twohig, 2004). Notice what happens to your emotions as you do this.

To be clear, the goal of such work, using this particular example, is not to help White clinicians accept that they are racist. Nor is it a strategy to dismiss the thought, such that it becomes trivialized or functionally meaningless. The goal is to increase flexibility around that thought or variations on it (such as feedback that one has behaved insensitively, microaggressed, or displayed a lack of awareness of privilege), such that the thought, feedback, or accusation is not automatically pushed away, denied, fought against, or avoided, all of which, paradoxically, may make it more likely that one will act in racist ways in response to the accusation. Instead, with defusion, there may be increased flexibility in response to the thought or accusation, allowing for a deeper consideration of the context in which the feedback or accusation occurs and responding in ways that are more likely to be curious and in service of our clients.

EXPLORING EMOTIONS

Defusion and acceptance often go hand in hand. Earlier, we discussed practicing mindful awareness of attentional hooks in the presence of racial cues. Here, we expand that suggestion, to practicing acceptance of any private reactions that arise when faced with racism more broadly defined (e.g., news coverage of disproportionate rates of arrest or shooting of Black people by police, content presented in workplace diversity trainings), including when one is accused of racist or insensitive behavior oneself.

The basic stance of willingness is to approach, with curiosity, whatever emotions are experienced, even those feelings or sensations that cannot easily be named. Explore the physical aspects of those emotions, such as tightness or constriction in your chest, or a fluttering sensation in the belly. In difficult moments, it might be easier to notice your body's physical response to discomfort rather than to parse the complex mix of co-occurring emotions. Depending on individual degrees of EA related to these feelings, behaviors to block or disengage with the uncomfortable content may be elicited by this physical, affective response prior to any intentional decision making. It may be helpful, if you desire to raise your awareness, to find opportunities for intentional practice. The following is a sample meditation script that you might record for yourself and listen to as a personal practice.

MEDITATION ON DISCOMFORT WITH RACISM AND PRIVILEGE

Seat yourself in a comfortable position. Begin with closed eyes or a soft downward gaze, and bring your awareness gently to your breath. Silently note "in" or "out" with each breath, without controlling or forcing your breath in a particular way. After a few moments, bring to mind a specific, uncomfortable interaction dealing with race and racism. This may be an argument with family or colleagues about privilege, a caring colleague of color pointing out racial bias in your work, or an article or event in the news that evoked discomfort. Perhaps a student or supervisee labeled you as "racist," and it felt awful. If possible, bring a clear, specific image to mind in that very moment. It might be the face of a person you interacted with, or the image on the news. Allow a single comment or expression from that discussion to come to mind. Without attempting to argue or think through better responses, use these cues as an opportunity to sink into the discomfort of the moment. Notice what happens to your breathing. Scan your body for any points of tension, noticing if any muscles tighten up as you reexperience this moment. Bring your awareness into the core of your body, observing any sensations you may feel. As you begin to gain a sense of your emotional and bodily reaction to the discomfort in the moment, imagine that each breath you take in brings some spaciousness into the experience. Without attempting to make the experience go away, allow yourself to sink deeper into your body's reaction. As you practice this, a number of experiences might arise. You might have earlier memories of this feeling come to mind, related to other discussions or interactions related to racism. You might feel a variety of secondary emotions, such as sadness, regret, or anger (at yourself, others, society). Notice these and the corresponding effect on your body. When you are ready, allow the image to fade, and come back to noticing your breath. The sensation of breathing in, and the sensation of breathing out. You might take the opportunity to write in a journal after this practice, to aid in remembering your observations.

The aim of acceptance exercises like this meditation is for clinicians to practice a willingness to fully feel difficult or unwanted emotions related to the realities of racism to increase in-session behavioral flexibility, connecting with our values, and engaging in culturally responsive practice.

Clinician Challenge: Rigid and Unexamined Self-Identity, or Fusion with Self-as-Content

As examined in chapter 6, self-as-content, or conceptualized self, refers to our at-times rigid identification with certain concepts, such as man, woman, Black, Latinx, straight, gay, hard working, smart, Christian, Jewish, Muslim, and so on. In other words, self-as-content refers to what many refer to as our identity, or how we answer the question, "Who are you?" People typically define and relate to themselves primarily through such concepts, and our interactions with the world become shaped by these concepts and their wide-ranging relational networks. For example, a White person raised in the United States who strongly identifies as a *man* might interact with other people through the socially derived concept of being a man and a range of associated beliefs. Specifically, he might think that as a man, he needs to take responsibility for the successes and failures in his life independently of others, always work hard to take care of his partner and children without complaint, never show any weaknesses or vulnerability, and expect or demand to be taken seriously to advance his point of view.

Our conceptualized selves are, of course, a function of how we developed and were influenced by our immediate familial, local, and larger social contexts. And in addition to recognizing what is included in one's self-as-content, we also need to understand what is *not* included. Specifically, many White people in the United States are raised without incorporation of Whiteness into their self-as-content. This is predictable: as a majority group member, the social context in which many White people are raised and operate does not distinguish Whiteness as a salient characteristic that matters to interactions and outcomes, as is the case for minoritized group members operating in a majority-White context. While it is common for many people of color to discuss around the family dinner table what it is like to be a person of color in this society, it is relatively rare for discussions of Whiteness to occur in White families. Thus, Whiteness does not get elaborated as an emotionally meaningful aspect of one's conceptualized self.

From a CBS perspective, conceptualized selves per se are not necessarily problematic, so long as they do not reduce our ability to interact flexibly with the world, according to multiple and, at times, co-occuring values. The degree to which such self-concepts are held rigidly may cause difficulty in certain contexts. For example, the White male person above, with a strongly held identity as a man but without a clear and conscious identity as a White person, may not exhibit much flexibility around the notion that White male privilege has conferred him unfair advantages and been partially responsible for his success in life. He may experience such a notion as a threat to his identity and self-worth and react defensively. While this is a problematic reaction from our perspective as educators and researchers committed to social justice and equity, it is also a problematic reaction from his own perspective to the degree that he also claims values related to humility, fairness, and not being racist in his actions.

Operating from a self-as-content perspective can interfere with the work of White clinicians serving clients of color in several ways. First, White clinicians might not be able to look at their own biases and missteps because they are too attached to their identity as "non-racist" (i.e, *If I am non-racist, I can't be doing racists things*), even less so if they are attached to their identities as "clinicians" (i.e., *As a clinician, I can't be racist because I am a compassionate person who helps others*). As in the example above, it may be hard for some White clinicians to fully embrace notions of White privilege and respond with humility in moments that matter, and this, likewise, makes it harder for them to fully embrace the perspectives and life experiences of their clients of color.

Second, a lack of appreciation of racial aspects of identity may produce a retreat to color-blindness, which may result in ignoring or avoiding clients' self-concepts relevant to therapeutic work. Specifically, a White clinician who conceptualizes their client's identity without including their racial and ethnic identity will likely miss any clinical issues linked to racism, as well as a host of potential cultural strengths. Third, alternately, for those White clinicians capable of acknowledging their own racial identity as White people and their client's identity as a person of color, they might still struggle to recognize their commonalities, concluding that these identities prevent them from serving their client (i.e., *As a White clinician, I have no way of relating to a person of color*).

Proposed CBS Intervention: Self-as-Context

To counteract the problematic effects of rigidly held identities that produce gaps in understanding and experiencing race-related issues, contextual behavioral psychologists have developed the concept of self-as-context, or the observer self, which corresponds to a more transcendent and inclusive approach to one's identity (McHugh & Stewart, 2012). At the core of self-as-context lies the distinction between our experiences and our perspective on these experiences. While these experiences are constantly changing across times and places, the observer within us, who is conscious of these changing experiences as they unfold, is consistently there, noticing, across time. In addition, while self-concepts are constructed based on experiences (e.g., *I have a clinical license—I am a psychologist*), our perspective on these experiences is not bound to any particular experience. Therefore, identifying with the perspective we have on our experiences allows us to include all experiences, even those that seem incompatible when we operate from a self-as-content point of view (e.g., *If I am humanistic therapist, I can't also have racist beliefs, let alone engage in microaggressions*).

Contextual behavioral psychologists have developed numerous techniques to facilitate a more expansive and flexibly held self, such as meditation exercises, imagery, and perspective-taking questions. For example, Hayes, Strosahl, and Wilson (2012) described an exercise inviting the listeners to remember a time when they were five years old and to picture the moment as if they were reliving it (a shift of perspective in time). The listeners are invited to repeat the process with episodes from the more recent past (e.g., five years ago, last summer) and to progressively become aware that, beyond changes in physical appearances and psychological experiences, their noticing activity is stable over time. This exercise is thus meant to help the listeners get in touch with the continuous perspective taking on all experiences described earlier, which provides stability as experiences and self-concepts change. (For a comprehensive description of self-as-context techniques, we encourage the reader to consult McHugh, Stewart, & Almada, 2019). Although a number of these techniques were developed for therapeutic interventions, they are generally suitable for self-development.

Cultivating a self-as-context point of view may help White clinicians recognize and deal with their biases toward people of color, recognize privileges associated with being White, and reduce the risk of engaging in harmful microaggressions in clinical practice.

For example, consider a client of color saying to a White clinician, "You don't get it," when discussing an issue of racism. A more expansive sense of self (as a perspective rather than a set of concepts) may decrease the risk of self-defensiveness in this moment because, from this perspective, there is no identity to defend. Actions, beliefs, and feelings can be explored and questioned safely because they do not alone define the person. For example, the clinician may be less likely to reject this feedback if they are not attached to beliefs such as *I am not racist* or *I am a compassionate therapist*. They may recognize that racist actions can coexist with compassionate actions and that racist and anti-racist beliefs may coexist within the same person. With such a stance, they may be better able to listen to the feedback and consider the perspective of their client rather than defending against a rigidly held view of self. Ultimately, with practice cultivating self-as-context, one may become curious and open to information that contradicts self-related concepts and beliefs, more likely to notice one's own biases, and more likely to listen to feedback from others about these biases.

A clinician interacting with their client with a more loosely held and expansive sense of self may be able to connect more deeply regardless of particular features of identity (e.g., race, gender, age), because a sense of commonality is established through their respective stable perspectives on their experiences. In other words, the clinician recognizes that, beyond their differences at the level of self-concepts, they have in common a capacity to observe and integrate a variety of experiences and identities. One might simply say they are both human. This, however, is different from color-blindness, because commonality found at the level of self-as-context does not require denial of coexisting

individual and group differences. In other words, one can simultaneously seek commonalities and appreciate and validate group differences. Here, self-as-context is consistent
with the principle of equity.

Finally, with improving one's access to self-as-context may come improved perspective taking. Consistent with a perspective-taking exercise developed by Vilardaga and
Hayes (2009), we want clinicians' experiences of common humanity to facilitate deep
connection with the journey that each client has taken to arrive, ultimately, in one's
office. What are the client's hopes, dreams, struggles, and yearnings? How has life shaped,
punished, and changed them? What is the client hiding because it is too painful to share?
How does the client long to be seen? This effort is often particularly important for clients
of color, whose lifetime experiences of racial slights and oppressions may result in feelings
of not being seen by White people as a person of worth or, worse yet, not being seen at
all, and feeling invisible (Franklin & Boyd-Franklin, 2000).

Clinician Challenge: Social Distance and Disconnection

Thus far, this section has focused largely on intrapersonal processes. We have
emphasized the private experiences of the White clinician (i.e., perceptual, cognitive,
and affective processes, and issues of self and identity), and the ways these processes may
manifest as microaggressions with clients of color. In fact, clients of color frequently report
experiencing microaggressions from White mental health clinicians, the most frequent
being minimizing or avoiding discussions of race and race-related issues altogether
(Constantine, 2007). Several studies have documented that experiences of microaggressions in therapy negatively impact the therapeutic alliance, treatment satisfaction, and
treatment length for clients of color (Owen, Tao, Imel, Wampold, & Rodolfa, 2014).

We have also presented how we might harness interventions to disrupt the functional impact of these processes on behavior when interacting with clients of color. For
example, a clinician may, through continued work with the ideas of this chapter, become
less controlled by race-based anxieties and stereotypes, less fused with a narrow band of
identity that constrains awareness of Whiteness and privilege, and more able to experience and embrace the lived reality of clients of color, even if doing so elicits anxiety, guilt,
and other aversive reactions.

This commitment assumes a set of a priori values held by the White clinician, typically related to equity, inclusion, and social justice. We have found that the desire for
deep and authentic relationships also stands as a particularly powerful value for White
clinicians engaged in antiracist work—both with one's clients and in one's life outside the
office. The distance between these declared values and the lived experience, for many
White people, however, often feels vast, as most of us live in cities still structured by
segregation and systemic racism.

The work of the antiracist White clinician, therefore, necessarily extends beyond altering intrapersonal processes. Specifically, we know from decades of research on contact theory that it is not enough to engage in private work alone to overcome racism. To support deep and meaningful connection with other people, we must, of course, develop relationships and social connections (Pettigrew & Tropp, 2006).

There are many ways for two people to be in relationship with one another, and not all are equally effective at reducing prejudice. Specifically, according to contact theory, the interpersonal exchanges that form the basis of interracial contact must be experienced as equitable by both groups (Pettigrew & Tropp, 2006). However, much naturally occurring contact between people of color and White people is not equitable. For example, White police officers who patrol Black communities achieve frequent contact, but the White officer is almost always in a position of power in relation to the Black community member, and thus, contact does not predictably reduce police prejudice. Many other examples of inequitable contact exist across employment, legal, educational, and even volunteer settings. In all of these settings, frequent contact occurs, but the White person in the interaction is often in a position of power while the Black person is in a position of vulnerability, and such contact does not reliably reduce prejudice and discrimination. Likewise, White clinicians may have frequent contact with Black clients, but since the contact is not equitable, it is not surprising that clinicians consistently display biases against Black patients that do not decrease over time (Maina, Belton, Ginzberg, Singh, & Johnson, 2016).

A key insight into this problem is provided by the dominant psychological science model on how close and trusting relationships form—the Interpersonal Process Model (IPM; Reis & Shaver, 1988). According to the IPM, equity in close and trusting relationships involves *reciprocity*: *both* members of the dyad must experience and express vulnerability (Sprecher, Treger, Wondra, Hilaire, & Wallpe, 2013) and *both* must respond well to each other's vulnerability (Reis & Clark, 2013). When this full process occurs, closeness and trust develop. This is found across multiple relationship types, including interracial relationships (Davies, Tropp, Aron, Pettigrew, & Wright, 2011; Page-Gould, Mendoza-Denton, & Tropp, 2008; Shelton, Trail, West, & Bergsieker, 2010).

Thus, the IPM makes an important prediction: for both individuals to benefit from interracial contact, they must both experience vulnerability. This also applies to clinical encounters. For White clinicians, efforts to engage in reciprocally vulnerable contact with clients of color will improve their empathy and perspective taking in relation to their client. For a client of color, a White clinician who is reciprocally vulnerable and authentic may help the client feel more trust and safety to move into a deeper, more authentic, and healing relationship with their clinician. Conversely, the absence of connection and trust in the therapeutic relationship often leads to the discontinued care, lack of adherence to treatment recommendations, and poor treatment outcomes that are at the root of racial mental health disparities.

Proposed CBS Interventions: Values, Committed Action, and Connection

What might this look like in terms of interventions for White clinicians? To facilitate reciprocal and equitable vulnerable exchanges in our training interventions, we have modified exercises used to train therapists in Functional Analytic Psychotherapy (FAP). FAP is a CBS-consistent treatment approach that optimizes client repertoires via therapist authentic, contingent responding to in-session behavioral targets, including applications for racially diverse client-therapist dyads (Miller, Williams, Wetterneck, Kanter, & Tsai, 2015). FAP therapist trainings utilize structured experiential exercises intended to strengthen clinicians' abilities to engage in mutually and reciprocally vulnerable interactions often evoke relevant behavioral targets (Kanter, Tsai, Holman, & Koerner, 2013). The specific experiential exercises used in standard FAP trainings can be adapted for purposes of evoking reciprocal and equitably vulnerable exchanges within racially diverse dyads. For example, in one training exercise, participants form small interracial groups (e.g., four to six individuals) and take turns briefly (e.g., 6 minutes) sharing their personal life histories, while the others in the group listen and respond with genuine empathy and emotion. Participants, when telling their life histories, are encouraged to share not simply autobiographical facts, but more vulnerable events that have shaped who they are, in the service of connecting. Other possible exercises include sharing stories of grief, betrayal, discrimination, and positive memories.

Consistent with the learning that occurs in these exercises, White clinicians are encouraged to intentionally expand their social circles and create opportunities for meaningful contact and connections on their own. How one does this depends on one's context, but the goal is not tokenism or superficial relating. Said simply, it may be time to make some friends. The key, from our perspective, is that these exchanges are characterized by mutual sharing and vulnerability, not self-interest or one-sided sharing. Such efforts could include committing to small acts of connection, such as deliberately sitting next to a person of color on the bus and greeting them, attending diversity dialogues that are publically available, choosing restaurants, events, and hobbies that require stepping outside one's comfort zone and usual social circles, and leaning into these opportunities with social engagement. Efforts to build and deepen ongoing relationships are key, such as talking to coworkers to whom one does not usually talk and inviting people of color to coffee or family dinners. The value brought to all of these experiences is not observational but, instead, to participate with vulnerability in service of meaningful connection.

Such exchanges are unlikely to succeed without previous work that creates flexibility around the private experiences that are likely to show up in these interactions. Thus, all of the ACT processes described above come into play. Engage with others, paying exquisite attention, with defusion and acceptance, to any distracting thoughts (e.g., objectifying) and emotions (e.g., anxiety) that might arise, while either sharing or listening. Notice urges for race-based EA, lean in to those urges, and build real, genuine moments of connection with people of color—relationships characterized by equal status and power within the relationship and by mutual vulnerability and caring for one another (Okech & Champe, 2008).

Through building such relationships, over time, deeper empathy and perspective taking for the lived experiences of people of color can develop. While such relationships are valuable in and of themselves, such learning also facilitates the ability of White clinicians to truly connect with and understand their clients of color.

How might such work improve clinical interactions between White clinicians and clients of color? As previously documented, a common racial microaggression in clinical care is the White provider's tendency to ignore, reject, or dismiss race-related content in session. Consider the following example: You, a White clinician, are having a first session with James, a Black male client. At the beginning of the session, James thanks you for scheduling his session and then shares how hard it was to get an appointment. "I had to call twenty therapists," he explains. "Most of them didn't even call me back. The ones who did said they couldn't take me. One said she could take me but only at nine in the morning, but I can't be late to work! I bet a White man would have gotten more call-backs and would have been offered a better time!"

How might you respond to James in this moment? In our sampling of White clinicians' responses to this prompt, we find that many have an automatic defensive reaction and an impulse to defend the other White clinicians. For example, you may want to explain to James that clinicians have busy schedules, and there are many reasons why clients do not get called back, and it is not necessarily racism that is fueling the problem. You may want to explain that you have many White colleagues and that you do not experience them as racist, that managing a clinical schedule is hard.

We hope, if a White clinician has been doing the work suggested in this chapter, that the clinician may gently notice urges to respond in this way, without fusion, and not get hooked by them. For James, it is likely these responses would be experienced as invalidating and disruptive to trust and the building of a strong therapeutic alliance. It is the case, in fact, that James's experience is common for Black clients and is documented by empirical evidence: in an experimental study, Kugelmass (2016) found that an insured, working-class Black man had, on average, to make sixteen calls to get a preferred-time therapy appointment with a new therapist for every one call a middle-class White woman had to make.

Although we do not contend that there is a perfect response to offer James in this moment, we hope that the work of this chapter facilitates a full appreciation of the vulnerability inherent in James's choice to share the experience with the clinician. James has likely shared previous experiences of racism with White individuals in the past, and he has probably learned to expect to be misunderstood and responded to poorly, with more prejudice and microaggressions (Shelton, Douglass, Garcia, Yip, & Trail, 2014; Shelton, Richeson, & Salvatore, 2005), as the average White person typically underestimates the severity of ongoing discrimination and disparities experienced by people of color (Kraus, Rucker, & Richeson, 2017).

While we would need to understand James's individual challenges, values, and goals to arrive at an actual case conceptualization, James's choice to share may be an indicator that he is willing to trust and to try again, and it may be a key moment for the clinician. To help the clinician with how to respond, we would like to suggest two important domains: Providing safety and providing validation. Recognizing the vulnerability in James's disclosure, rather than getting hooked by defensiveness, clarifies that the first thing James likely needs is to feel safe, to know that his disclosure will not get punished, and to know that it will not lead to further harm.

How might you express such safety to James? The foundations for trust and safety may have been established in previous sessions, such that you are not starting from scratch. In the moment, however, it may be useful to amplify these themes. How would it feel to respond with something along the lines of the following?

I want you to know that I'll do my best to create a safe space for you to talk about your experiences with me. And I'm going to be conscious about needing to earn your trust, in part, by listening carefully when you tell me what you've been dealing with as a Black man.

Validation contributes to a sense of safety and connection. Can you, fully and without a hint of ambivalence or defensiveness, open up to the reality and depth of racism in his life, such that his experience—and his interpretation of it as an indicator of racism in the mental health profession—is fully, unequivocally validated and heard? Consider the following:

I believe you 100 percent. You're absolutely right about Black clients getting called back less often than White clients by providers—I actually came across a study that demonstrated just how extreme that imbalance is. I know this is just one of countless examples of this kind of bias that you have to deal with. And I want to do better by you.

Safety and validation are experienced both verbally and nonverbally. For example, one person suppressing facial expressiveness in an interaction has documented effects on their counterpart, including raising blood pressure, disrupting rapport, and decreasing motivation to pursue a relationship with the suppressor (Butler, Egloff, Wilhelm, Smith, Erickson, & Gross, 2003). How are your eye contact and facial expressiveness during this interaction? Can you allow yourself to fully express your reaction with your whole body and face?

The examples above are not intended as a script that can be applied to clients. Rather, we hope sharing these more concrete responses will inspire clinicians as to how we might step out of our own comfort zones and explicitly orient to the client's needs in our own voices. We also note that for clinicians who are less familiar with responding in a vulnerable way during moments like these, the work feels risky. We suggest that this vulnerability is a good thing and an asset in our attempt to connect in real and meaningful ways in service of our clients' needs.

Participating with vulnerability in clinical work, regardless of the client, may seem odd to some clinicians. To be clear, the encouragement is not to disregard important therapeutic boundaries or to over-share autobiographical details of one's own life with clients. The encouragement, rather, is toward authenticity and humility with clients of color, which is likely a vulnerable move for many White clinicians. Specifically, the interracial anxieties that may be present when interacting with clients of color may push clinicians to adopt a more neutral or professional stance with clients as a defense against this anxiety. We encourage gentle attention to these feelings and a willingness to fully, vulnerably connect with the client. This may mean letting your feelings fully show, and verbally disclosing them when a client is retelling experiences of racism or trauma, sharing with a client that you are nervous when you start a new relationship, including relationships with clients of color, because you really want to get it right, or sharing difficulties that you are experiencing in your own life, as appropriate, to join your client in vulnerability and promote a more egalitarian and humble therapeutic relationship.

Research Findings

Several converging lines of evidence provide empirical support for the ideas in this chapter. First, many of the ACT component processes discussed herein have received empirical support in lab-based, experimental studies (Levin, Hildebrandt, Lillis, & Hayes, 2012), and we expect that these processes are broadly relevant and that the generalization to racist content is reasonable. That said, some research has explored ACT components as interventions targeting prejudice directly and has shown that flexibility around prejudical thoughts can be increased by engaging hexaflex processes (Hayes et al., 2004; Lillis & Hayes, 2007). We specifically recently evaluated these specific techniques in several studies. These included a six-hour workshop to increase connectedness among Black and White undergraduate students (Kanter & Williams, 2018), a six-hour workshop to improve White medical student provider empathy in interactions with Black patients (Rosen et al., 2018), and a five-hour workshop to decrease political polarization and improve connectedness between conservative and liberal college students (Manbeck et al., 2018). In all cases, improved connectedness between workshop participants was found immediately after the interventions and one month later (when measured), and, when measured, we found a decreased likelihood of microaggressing among White participants after the interventions.

Conclusion

There is no doubt that, across therapeutic orientations and client presentations, it is crucial for the clinician to create a strong therapeutic alliance and relationship with the client, characterized by empathy, positive regard, genuineness, a collaborative process, and an ability to successfully address and repair ruptures that may occur (Norcross, 2011).

It also is clear that when White clinicians interact with clients of color, many of these abilities are diminished by the harmful processes discussed above. It is likely that race-based EA plays a central role. In this chapter, employing the theoretical model described in chapter 6 of this volume, we have attempted to articulate how the psychological processes grounded in ACT and FAP can be harnessed and applied in this setting to strengthen culturally responsive practices and to counter racial bias.

We hope this chapter inspires additional research. To date, race-based EA has not been adequately studied as an intervention target, and many lab-based experimental component processes could be designed to clarify and evaluate the interventions discussed in this chapter. For example, researchers may explore the effects of different defusion and acceptance, self-as-context, perspective-taking, and values and committed action interventions on the functional control of race-based thoughts and feelings. Workshop interventions that combine component processes may be evaluated with larger samples, in different contexts, and against different comparison conditions.

For White clinicians hoping for help now, we make the obvious point that reading this chapter is not enough to produce sustainable behavior change and that growth comes from committed action. We hope, however, that this chapter inspires such action in White clinicians, as well as those who aim to help them change. There will be many challenges. The psychological obstacles described throughout this chapter arise frequently and unexpectedly. Skill, humility, self-awareness, and sensitivity are always needed. This requires a continuous reorienting to the value of leaning into these challenges and being prepared to engage present-moment, defusion, acceptance, self-as-context, values, and committed-action processes as an ongoing stream, applied to both the self and others.

We find this work to be challenging, innovative, and personally meaningful. It is challenging and innovative in that the basic CBS frame, to not try to get rid of negative racial thoughts and feelings, may be misinterpreted as an acceptance of racism itself. That is antithetical to our aim. A societal sea-change may be required for the mainstream to appreciate that acceptance of private events is required in the service of long term-behavioral, and even societal, change. Our hope, and the meaning in the work, is that this CBS approach may improve culturally responsive care and decrease harmful racist behaviors in clinical interactions between White clinicians and clients of color. We hope this will improve clinical outcomes and quality of life for our clients. Racism is one of humanity's greatest challenges, and the clinical encounter is a key moment of vulnerability for clients of color, who come seeking help and may ultimately be harmed. CBS, from its philosophical roots, scientific methods, and community values, is in a strong position to address this problem and make important contributions. The work, however, is up to each of us.

KEY POINTS FOR CLINICIANS

- A contemporary understanding of racism emphasizes not only explicit racism but subtle processes, including microaggressions, color-blindness, White privilege, and implicit biases that affect clinical choices and behaviors of White clinicians and outcomes for clients of color.

- Contextual behavioral processes and interventions may be brought to improve the capacity of White clinicians to deliver antiracist, culturally responsive care to clients of color.

- Interventions that improve contact with the present moment may decrease objectifying behaviors.

- Interventions that facilitate defusion and acceptance processes may increase culturally responsive behavior in the presence of inaccurate negative stereotypes, interracial anxieties, and other aversive feelings that typically lead to avoidance and other disconnecting responses.

- Interventions that target self-as-context may increase flexibility around rigidly held identities and facilitate increased openness to issues of White privilege and color-blindness.

- Interventions that target values and committed action may help White clinicians engage in deeper and more meaningful relationships with people of color that improve empathy and perspective taking.

References

Adams, R. B., & Kleck, R. E. (2003). Perceived gaze direction and the processing of facial displays of emotion. *Psychological Science, 14,* 644–647. https://doi.org/10.1046/j.0956-7976.2003.psci_1479.x

Alegría, M., Nakash, O., Lapatin, S., Oddo, V., Gao, S., Lin, J., & Normand, S. L. (2008). How missing information in diagnosis can lead to disparities in the clinical encounter. *Journal of Public Health Management and Practice, 14* (Suppl), S26–35. doi:10.1097/01.PHH.0000338384.82436.0d

American Psychological Association. (2003). Guidelines on multicultural education, training, research, practice, and organizational change for psychologist. *American Psychologist, 58,* 377–402.

American Psychological Association. (2017). *Multicultural guidelines: An ecological approach to context, identity, and intersectionality.* Retrieved from http://www.apa.org/about/policy/multicultural-guidelines.pdf

Arredondo, P., Toporek, R., Brown, S. P., Jones, L., Locke, D. C., Sanchez, J., & Stadler, H. (1996). Operationalization of the multicultural counseling competencies. *Journal of Multicultural Counseling and Development, 24,* 42–78.

Bourgeois, P., & Hess, U. (2008). The impact of social context on mimicry. *Biological Psychology, 77,* 343–352.

Burkard, A. W., & Knox, S. (2004). Effect of therapist color-blindness on empathy and attributions in cross-cultural counseling. *Journal of Counseling Psychology, 51*(4), 387–397. http://doi.org/10.1037/0022-0167.51.4.387

Butler, E. A., Egloff, B., Wilhelm, F. H., Smith, N. C., Erickson, E. A., & Gross, J. J. (2003). The social consequences of expressive suppression. *Emotion, 3*, 48–67. http://doi.org/10.1037/1528-3542.3.1.48

Chekroud, A. M., Everett, J. A. C., Bridge, H., & Hewstone, M. (2014). A review of neuroimaging studies of race-related prejudice: Does amygdala response reflect threat? *Frontiers in Human Neuroscience, 8*(179). https://doi.org/10.3389/fnhum.2014.00179

Condor, S., Figgou, L., Abell, J., Gibson, S., & Stevenson, C. (2006). "They're not racist…": Prejudice denial, mitigation and suppression in dialogue. *British Journal of Social Psychology, 45*(3), 441–462.

Constantine, M. G. (2007). Racial microaggressions against African American clients in cross-racial counseling relationships. *Journal of Counseling Psychology, 54*(1), 1–16.

Cooper, L. A., Roter, D. L., Carson, K. A., Beach, M. C., Sabin, J. A., Greenwald, A. G., & Inui, T. S. (2012). The associations of clinicians' implicit attitudes about race with medical visit communication and patient ratings of interpersonal care. *American Journal of Public Health, 102*(5), 979–987. https://doi.org/10.2105/AJPH.2011.300558

Cooper, L. A., Roter, D. L., Johnson, R. L., Ford, D. E., Steinwachs, D. M., & Powe, N. R. (2003). Patient-centered communication, ratings of care, and concordance of patient and physician race. *Annals of Internal Medicine, 139*(11), 907. https://doi.org/10.7326/0003-4819-139-11-200312020-00009

Davies, K., Tropp, A., Aron, A. Pettigrew, & Wright, (2011). Cross-group friendships and intergroup attitudes. *Personality and Social Psychology Review, 15*(4), 332–351. doi:10.1177/1088868311411103

DiAngelo, R. (2011). White fragility. *The International Journal of Critical Pedagogy, 3*(3), 54–70.

Franklin, A. J., & Boyd-Franklin, N. (2000). Invisibility syndrome: A clinical model of the effects of racism on African-American males. *Journal of Orthopsychiatry, 70*, 33–41.

Gilliam, W. S., Maupin, A. N., Reyes, C. R., Accavitti, M., & Shic, F. (2016). *Do early educators' implicit biases regarding sex and race relate to behavior expectations and recommendations of preschool expulsions and suspensions? A research study brief.* New Haven: Yale University Child Study Center.

Greenwald, A. G., & Krieger, L. H. (2006). Implicit bias: Scientific foundations. *California Law Review, 94*(4), 945–967.

Hayes. S. C., Bissett, R., Roget, N., Padilla, M., Kohlenberg, B. S., Fisher, G., et al. (2004). The impact of acceptance and commitment training and multicultural training on the stigmatizing attitudes and professional burnout of substance abuse counselors. *Behavior Therapy, 35*, 821–835. http://dx.doi.org/10.1016/S0005-7894(04)80022-4

Hayes, S. C., Wilson, K. G., Gifford, E. V, Follette, V. M., & Strosahl, K. (1996). Experimental avoidance and behavioral disorders: A functional dimensional approach to diagnosis and treatment. *Journal of Consulting and Clinical Psychology, 64*(6), 1152–1168. https://doi.org/10.1037/0022-006X.64.6.1152

Hayes, S. C., Strosahl, K., & Wilson, K. G. (2012). *Acceptance and commitment therapy: The process and practice of mindful change* (2nd ed.). New York, NY: Guilford Press.

Ito, T. A., & Urland, G. R. (2003). Race and gender on the brain: Electrocortical measures of attention to the race and gender of multiply categorizable individuals. *Journal of Personality and Social Psychology, 85*(4), 616–626. https://doi.org/10.1037/0022-3514.85.4.616

Kabat-Zinn, J. (1994). *Wherever you go, there you are: Mindfulness meditation in everyday life.* New York, NY: Hyperion.

Kanter, J. W., Tsai, M., Holman, G., & Koerner, K. (2013). Preliminary data from a randomized pilot study of web-based functional analytic psychotherapy therapist training. *Psychotherapy, 50*(2). doi:10.1037/a0029814

Kanter, J. W., & Williams, M. T. (2018, July). Facilitating racial harmony on college campuses: A randomized trial. In M. Corey (Chair), *It is time to discuss race and politics: Applying CBS to address social divisions.* Symposium presented at the Association for Contextual Behavioral Science 16th Annual World Conference, Montréal, Canada.

Kawakami, K., Williams, A., Sidhu, D., Choma, B. L., Rodriguez-Bailón, R., Cañadas, E., … & Hugenberg, K. (2014). An eye for the I: Preferential attention to the eyes of ingroup members. *Journal of Personality and Social Psychology, 107*(1), 1–20. https://doi.org/10.1037/a0036838

Keng, S.-L., Waddington, E., Lin, B. X. T., Tan, M. S. Q., Henn-Haase, C., & Kanter, J. W. (2016). Effects of functional analytic psychotherapy on therapist trainees in Singapore: A randomized controlled trial. *Clinical Psychology & Psychotherapy, 24,* 1014–1027. https://doi.org/10.1002/cpp.2064

Kraus, M. W., Rucker, J. M., & Richeson, J. A. (2017). Americans misperceive racial economic equality. *Proceedings of the National Academy of Sciences, 114*(39), 10324–10331.

Kugelmass, H. (2016). "Sorry, I'm not accepting new patients": An audit study of access to mental health care. *Journal of Health and Social Behavior, 57*(2), 168–183. https://doi.org/10.1177/0022146516647098

Langrehr, K. J., & Blackmon, S. M. (2016). The impact of trainees' interracial anxiety on White privilege remorse: Motivation to control bias as a moderator. *Training and Education in Professional Psychology, 10*(3), 157–164. https://doi.org/10.1037/tep0000118

Levin, M. E., Hildebrandt, M. J., Lillis, J., & Hayes, S. C. (2012). A meta-analysis of laboratory-based component studies suggested by the psychological flexibility model. *Behavior Therapy, 43*(4), 741–756. doi:10.1016/j.beth.2012.05.003

Lillis, J., & Hayes, S. C. (2007). Applying acceptance, mindfulness, and values to the reduction of prejudice: A pilot study. *Behavior modification, 31*(4), 389–411.

Maina, I. W., Belton, T. D., Ginzberg, S., Singh, A., & Johnson, T. J. (2016). A decade of studying implicit racial/ethnic bias in healthcare providers using the implicit association test. *Social Science and Medicine,* 1–11. https://doi.org/10.1016/j.socscimed.2017.05.009

Maitland, W. M., Kanter, J. W., Tsai, M., Kuczynski, A. M., Manbeck, K. M., & Kohlenberg, R. J. (2016). Preliminary findings on the effects of online Functional Analytic Psychotherapy training on therapist competency. *Psychological Record, 66*(4), 627–637. https://doi.org/10.1007/s40732-016-0198-8

Manbeck, K. E., Kanter, J. W., Kuczynski, A. M., Fine, L., Corey, M. D., & Maitland, D. W. M. (2018). Improving relations among conservatives and liberals on a college campus: A preliminary trial of a contextual-behavioral intervention. Unpublished manuscript: University of Washington.

Masuda, A., Hayes, S. C., Sackett, C. F., & Twohig, M. P. (2004). Cognitive defusion and self-relevant negative thoughts: Examining the impact of a ninety-year-old technique. *Behaviour Research and Therapy, 42*(4), 477–485.

McHugh, L., & Stewart, I. (2012). *The self and perspective taking: Contributions and applications from modern behavioral science.* Oakland: New Harbinger Publications.

McHugh, L., Stewart, I., & Almada, P. (2019). *A contextual behavioral guide to the self.* Oakland: Context Press.

Miller, A., Williams, M. T., Wetterneck, C. T., Kanter, J., & Tsai, M. (2015). Using functional analytic psychotherapy to improve awareness and connection in racially diverse client-therapist dyads. *The Behavior Therapist,* 150–156. doi:10.1119/1.19159

Nakash, O., Rosen, D., & Alegría, M. (2009). The culturally sensitive evaluation. In P. Ruiz & A. Primm (Eds.), *Disparities in psychiatric care: Clinical and cross-cultural perspectives* (pp. 225–235). Bethesda, MD: Lippincott Williams & Wilkins.

Norcross, J. C. (2011). *Psychotherapy relationships that work: Evidence-based responsiveness,* 2nd Edition. New York, NY: Oxford University Press.

Okech, J. E. A., & Champe, J. (2008). Informing culturally competent practice through cross-racial friendships. *International Journal for the Advancement of Counselling, 30,* 104–115.

Owen, J., Tao, K. W., Imel, Z. E., & Wampold, B. E., & Rodolfa, E. (2014). Addressing racial and ethnic microaggressions in therapy. *Professional Psychology: Research and Practice, 45*(4), 283–290. doi:10.1037/a0037420

Page-Gould, E., Mendoza-Denton, R., & Tropp, L. R. (2008). With a little help from my cross-group friend: Reducing anxiety in intergroup contexts through cross-group friendship. *Journal of Personality and Social Psychology, 95*(5), 1080–94.

Pettigrew, T. F., & Tropp, L. R. (2006). A meta-analytic test of intergroup contact theory. *Journal of Personality and Social Psychology, 90*(5), 751–783.

Reis, H., & Clark, M. (2013). *Responsiveness.* New York, NY: The Oxford Handbook of Close Relationships.

Reis, H. T., & Shaver, P. (1988). Intimacy as an interpersonal process. In S. Duck, D. F. Hay, S. E. Hobfoll, W. Ickes, B. M. Montgomery (Eds.), *Handbook of personal relationships: Theory, research and interventions* (pp. 367–389). Oxford, England: John Wiley & Sons.

Rosen, D. C., Kanter, J. W., Manbeck, K. E., Branstetter, H., Corey, & M. D., Williams, M. T. (2018, July). A contextual-behavioral intervention to improve provider empathy and emotional rapport in racially charged interactions: A randomized trial. In M. Corey (Chair), *It Is Time to Discuss Race and Politics: Applying CBS to Address Social Divisions.* Symposium presented at the Association for Contextual Behavioral Science 16th Annual World Conference, Montréal, Canada.

Rosen, D. C., Nakash, O., & Alegría, M. (2014). Disproportionality and disparities in the mental health system. In J. James, R. Fong, A. Dettlaff, & C. Rodriguez (Eds.) *Addressing racial disproportionality and disparities in human services: Multisystemic approaches* (pp. 280–311). New York, NY: Columbia University Press.

Rosen, D. C., Nakash, O., Kwong, A., & Branstetter, H. (2017). Culturally responsive assessment and diagnosis in the mental health intake. *The Behavior Therapist, 40*(3), 93–98.

Shelton, J. N., Douglass, S., Garcia, R. L., Yip, T., & Trail, T. E. (2014). Feeling (mis)understood and intergroup friendships in interracial interactions. *Personality and Social Psychology Bulletin, 40*(9), 1193–1204.

Shelton, J. N., Trail, T. E., West, T. V., & Bergsieker, H. B. (2010). From strangers to friends: The interpersonal process model of intimacy in developing interracial friendships. *Journal of Social and Personal Relationships, 27*(1), 71–90. Doi:10.11770265407509346422

Shelton, J. N., Richeson, J. A., & Salvatore, J. (2005). Expecting to be the target of prejudice: Implications for interethnic interactions. *Personality and Social Psychology Bulletin, 31*(9), 1189–1202.

Shin, R. Q., Smith, L. C., Welch, J. C., & Ezeofor, I. (2016). Is Allison more likely than Lakisha to receive a callback from counseling professionals? A racism audit study. *The Counseling Psychologist, 44*(8), 1187–1211. doi:10.1177/0011000016668814

Sprecher, S., Treger, T., Wondra, J. D., Hilaire, N., & Wallpe, K. (2013). Taking turns: Reciprocal self-disclosure promotes liking in initial interactions. *Journal of Experimental Social Psychology, 49*(5), 860–866. doi:10.1016/j.jesp.2013.03.017

Tajfel, H., & Turner, J. C. (1986). The social identity theory of intergroup behavior. In S. Worchel & W. G. Austin (Eds.), *Psychology of intergroup relations* (pp. 7–24). Chicago, IL: Nelson Hall.

Tsai, M., Kohlenberg, R. J., Kanter, J. W., Kohlenberg, B., Follette, W. C., & Callaghan, G. M. (2009). *A guide to functional analytic psychotherapy: Awareness, courage, love, and behaviorism.* New York, NY: Springer. https://doi.org/10.1007/978-0-387-09787-9

Vilardaga, R., & Hayes, S. C. (2009). Acceptance and commitment therapy and the therapeutic relationships stance. *European Psychotherapy, 9,* 1–23.

Villatte, M., Villatte, J. L., & Hayes, S. C. (2016). *Mastering the clinical conversation.* New York, NY: Guilford Press.

Wegner, D. M. (1992). You can't always think what you want: Problems in the suppression of unwanted thoughts. *Advances in Experimental Social Psychology, 25,* 193–225.

CHAPTER 9

Culturally Responsive Assessment and Diagnosis for Clients of Color

Jessica R. Graham-LoPresti,
Suffolk University

Monnica T. Williams,
University of Connecticut

Daniel C. Rosen,
Bastyr University

Introduction

Clinical assessment and diagnosis can be characterized as the foundation of effective therapy outcomes. As clinicians, we use mental health assessments to diagnose, develop effective case conceptualizations and treatment plans, examine progress in therapy, and promote positive change in our clients. While the importance of clinical assessment and diagnosis is well understood, mental health disparities in the context of clinical assessment and diagnosis continue to jeopardize the quality of mental health care for underserved and marginalized populations.

Cultural Competency and Responsiveness

Given that cultural competency and responsiveness have become benchmarks for ethical and effective clinical practice, it is of crucial importance to consider the implementation of these throughout the different stages of the therapeutic process, including assessment and diagnosis. Cultural competence and responsiveness is described as a clinician's commitment to gaining awareness, knowledge, and skills that can promote optimal functioning in diverse clients presenting with varied clinical presentations, with an understanding of the impact of societal and institutional systems (Sue & Sue, 2003). Sue and Sue (2003) described two different approaches to the counseling process, the *etic* and *emic* approaches, with the latter being a multicultural, culturally responsive approach. The *etic* approach, which is the manner in which assessment and diagnosis have been traditionally practiced, is housed in the theory of cultural universality and operates under the assumptions that assessment, diagnostic, and intervention approaches are universal. Consistently, the etic approach maintains that disorders like depression and anxiety appear similarly across cultures and the assessment, diagnostic, and treatment approaches for these types of disorders should be uniformly applied cross-culturally. Although this approach is widespread, it may impose dominant-group cultural biases upon clients from diverse backgrounds. More specifically, applying the approach of cultural universality during the assessment process can prevent clinicians from assessing for unique experiences (e.g., oppression, cultural, and familial influences) that may contribute to the development, maintenance, and expression of psychological symptoms.

The *emic* approach to assessment, diagnosis, and treatment challenges the assumptions that mental health difficulties are of the same nature and development across cultures. This approach suggests that culture and life contexts significantly influence the manifestation, course, and expression of mental health difficulties and, in turn, should influence our assessment, diagnostic, prevention, and intervention efforts. The emic approach to therapeutic processes is at the core of culturally responsive assessment and diagnosis and leads to a multidimensional model of identity development that includes individual, group, and universal level influences. This tripartite model of identity, first proposed by Kluckholn and Murray (1953), begins with the individual level of personal identity, which suggests that all individuals are, in some respect, unique due to both genetic composition and non-shared environmental experiences. At the group level, all individuals share some similarities and are like some other individuals, depending on our group memberships (e.g., race, ethnicity, gender). Each of us is born into a culture of beliefs, values, and practices that influence identity development and must play a role in our understanding of clients' presenting concerns. There are also political and sociocultural distinctions made by society that impact group membership and status. Membership in groups of race, ethnicity, gender, sexual orientation, social class, and ability status result in some shared experiences and group identification. Finally, the universal level of identity development posits that we are, in some ways, like all other individuals. For instance, we share some common experiences including biological similarities (e.g., physiological responses to threats), life experiences (i.e., interpersonal relationships), self-awareness (at varying levels), emotions, and the ability to use language and symbols as expression of thoughts and emotions.

An example of the effectiveness of the *emic* approach to assessment was presented by Fink, Turner, and Beidel (1996) in a case study exploring the treatment of social anxiety disorder experienced by a thirty-nine-year-old African American female physician. The authors discussed a course of social effectiveness therapy (SET; Turner, Beidel, Cooley, & Woody, 1994) and the ways in which the clinician included racially relevant cues in imaginal and in vivo exposures to address the client's social anxiety symptoms related to working with White male colleagues in a hospital. Specifically, after little improvement over the course of three therapy sessions, the therapist reassessed the client's core fears related to social situations and found that the client was frequently the only African American female resident in her work settings and experienced stereotype-related fears that students and faculty might view her as incompetent or unintelligent and that these fears were more intense when social encounters at work involved White males. These fears were based in a history of racial discrimination experienced by the client. The client's exposures were then tailored to include racially salient cues, including inviting a White male colleague and supervisor to lunch and going to highly avoided areas in the hospital for specific periods of time. This case points to the importance of attending to a client's unique and culturally based experiences in the assessment process in support of effective diagnostic and intervention strategies.

Multicultural Counseling Competencies

The multicultural counseling competencies (Arredondo et al., 1996) comprise a widely used model for training that consists of three developmental areas: (1) attitudes and beliefs (awareness of one's assumptions, values, and biases); (2) knowledge (understanding the world views and values of diverse clients); and (3) skills (developing relevant and appropriate assessment, diagnostic, prevention, and intervention strategies and techniques). For the purposes of this chapter, we will focus on these skills as they relate to assessment and diagnosis and how this can contribute to the development of effective therapeutic relationships and mental health treatment retention.

Awareness

The first step in engaging in culturally responsive assessment and diagnosis is developing awareness of our own assumptions, values, attitudes, and biases as they relate to our identities and those of our clients. Hays (2008) presented an acronym, the ADDRESSING framework, that helps clinicians begin to attend to their own backgrounds and the diverse backgrounds and lived experiences of clients. Specifically, this framework focuses on nine cultural factors that merit attention in the context of assessment and diagnosis (the parenthetical additions are our own expansions): Age and generational influences; Development and acquired Disabilities; Religion and spiritual orientation; Ethnicity (and race); Socioeconomic status, which includes education; Sexual orientation; Indigenous heritage; National origin (citizenship and immigrant status); and Gender. See table 1.

Table 1. The ADDRESSING Framework

ADDRESSING Definitions	Client Information	Therapist Information
Age and generational influences		
Developmental and acquired disabilities		
Religion and spiritual orientation		
Ethnicity (and race)		
Socioeconomic status		
Sexual orientation		
Indigenous heritage		
National origin and generational status		
Gender		

Similarly, D'Andrea and Daniels (2001) present the RESPECTFUL model of interviewing. This model presents ten dimensions of identity including Religion and spirituality, Economic and social class background, Sexual identity, Personal style and education, Ethnic and racial identity, Chronic and lifespan status and challenges, Trauma and crisis, Family background and history, Unique physical characteristics, and Location of residence and language differences. See table 2.

Table 2. The RESPECTFUL Interview Model

Ten Dimensions	Identify yourself as a multicultural being.	What personal and group strengths can you develop for each dimension?	How effective will you be with individuals who differ from you?
Religion and spirituality			
Economic and social class			
Sexual identity			
Personal style and education			
Ethnic and racial identity			
Chronical and lifespan status and challenges			
Trauma and crisis			
Family background and history			
Unique physical characteristics			
Location of residence, language differences			

These models present a framework for clinicians to develop both self-awareness related to their identities and to understand the contexts and identities of clients. It is important for assessing clinicians to think deeply about acculturation within the context of national origin and generational status, as these can significantly impact clients' experience of mental health symptoms and the therapeutic context.

Awareness helps guard against the imposition of clinicians' cultural values, assumptions, or biases on clients of color. Specifically, awareness facilitates a process of recognizing each client's cultural context as equally valuable and places importance on working within clients' values and belief systems in the assessment and diagnostic processes. A commitment to self-reflection and valuing the diverse cultural backgrounds of our clients of color must be unremitting and continuous to effectively develop diagnostic formulations and case conceptualizations. An example of the importance of this type of awareness can be seen in the case of a thirty-five-year-old Haitian man who came to therapy seeking counseling around his decision to attend college full-time while working sixty hours per week. Since his acceptance to an urban, commuter university one year ago, he enrolled in six courses, withdrew from two, failed two, and earned two Ds. He came to counseling to discuss ways that he can improve his academic performance while maintaining his current employment commitments. In this situation, therapists need to be aware of their own belief systems and values and not impose these beliefs on the client. The therapist, a White female, was born and raised in the United States in an individualistic culture, and her parents instilled in her the importance of prioritizing college over employment and familial obligations. However, the client, having grown up in a traditional Haitian family, values supporting his family both financially and emotionally above all, which means that he must work sixty hours per week to support his nuclear family in the United States, as well as his extended family in Haiti. In this instance, even though the therapist's value system supports the client minimizing his work obligations and prioritizing school, she must find a way to support the client in doing what is best for him in the context of his life and family values, which might involve taking some time away from school. This process begins with assessment, as the therapist must comprehensively gather pertinent information related to the client's identity and values system prior to development of a diagnostic formulation and case conceptualization. Culturally responsive assessment and diagnosis includes the development of awareness about one's own background and taking care to not impose one's particular belief system on clients, but meeting clients where they are and assessing the meaning of optimal functioning within their cultural contexts.

Throughout the process of assessment, clinicians must also attend to the therapeutic relationship with awareness of the client's racial and ethnic identity in relation to their own, and the accompanying power dynamics (Parham, Ajamu, & White, 2011; Seller, Smith, Shelton, Rowley, and Chavous, 1998). There are several models of racial identity development that describe the process for White people and people of color, and these models are directly relevant to the trust and social distance that may be generated between dyads. One of the first racial identity models was Cross's nigrescence model (Vandiver, Fhagen-Smith, Cokley, Cross, & Worrel, 2001), and this model was later expanded by others to include all people of color (e.g., Minority Identity Development Model; Atkinson, Morton & Sue, 1998; Racial and Cultural Identity Development Model; Sue & Sue, 2003). Minority development models may include stages referred to as Conformity, Dissonance, Resistance, Introspection, and Integrative Awareness. In the

Conformity Stage, people of color accept the values of the majority culture without critical analysis. In this early stage, they may value White role models and White standards of beauty and success, and they may believe it is better to be White. There may be underlying negative emotions toward the self as person of color, and consequently they may reject a same-race therapist and view the White counselor as more desirable and competent. In the Dissonance Stage, individuals begin to acknowledge the personal impact of racism when a triggering event causes them to question and examine their own assumptions and beliefs. They become more aware of racism and experience confusion and conflict toward the dominant cultural system. In the Resistance Stage, they actively reject the dominant culture and immerse themselves in their own culture. They may feel hostility toward White people in this stage and reject a White therapist. In the Introspection Stage, the person of color starts to question the values of both his or her own ethnic group and the dominant group. The person becomes more open to connecting with White people to better learn and understand differences. In the final stage, Integrative Awareness, the person develops a cultural identity based on both minority and dominant cultural values. They feel comfortable with themselves and their own identity as a person of color in a multicultural society. As clients of color reach more advanced racial identity statuses, they become more inclined to appreciate counselors of their same race. Although those with a strong positive ethnic identity will recognize they may be able to benefit from a competent therapist of any race, and the person of color has no fears about confronting racial issues with a White therapist when needed.

This analysis does not take into account the more complex picture of what may occur between client and therapist when a therapist is also struggling with his or her own identity development. For example, a Black therapist in an early stage of racial identity development may feel hostility toward a Black client, resulting in distancing and an unsuccessful therapeutic alliance. A White therapist in an early stage may become upset and defensive when confronted with racially charged material from a client of color. Assumptions should not be made about goodness of fit based on race in advance of an assessment of racial identity development in both the client and therapist (Helms, 1984).

The models and the exercises presented above can aid the clinician in developing an effective therapeutic alliance and contribute to a more comprehensive understanding of the client's presenting concerns and subsequent diagnoses. Conversations about a client's many identities and their importance (or lack thereof) are encouraged early in the assessment process as part of an ongoing conversation that values these contextual frames throughout psychotherapy.

Clinicians should also attend to the contextual issues of power, privilege, and marginalization in clients' lives. The impact of these constructs on the lived experiences of clients from diverse backgrounds, which often includes intersections of multiple marginalized identities, as well as the impact of these constructs within the therapy space, is yet another level of culturally responsive assessment. *Power* is described as the ability to decide who has access to resources, while *privilege* gives unearned advantages and benefits to members of dominant groups in society.

Culturally responsive assessment and diagnosis for clients of color begins with self-reflection and awareness of one's own cultural values and belief systems and respecting the values and belief systems of clients of color. Through self-reflection, clinicians must develop an awareness of the ways they may have benefited from individual, systemic, institutional, and cultural privilege and recognize that clients of color may not have experienced these same advantages. Through recognition of privilege, clinicians are better able to assess the ways in which marginalization and oppression of clients of color contribute to their experiences of mental health difficulties and diagnostic presentation. In addition, awareness of the power that we hold as clinicians to decide the resources our clients have access to contributes to our ability to ensure access to evidence-based, quality assessment tools, diagnostic formulations, and effective interventions. Moreover, awareness of privilege in the context of assessment and diagnosis assists us, as clinicians, in developing a therapeutic space for clients to discuss their life experiences, including racial oppression, and to begin to address these inequities with clients of color (inclusive of intersecting identities) through the assessment process.

Potential cultural biases that can impact therapy with clients of color include prejudices and pathological stereotypes that clinicians may be socialized to hold in reference to any particular racial or ethnic minority group. Clinicians must work hard to gain awareness of and defuse from such stereotypes to ensure they refrain from applying inaccurate universal labels and stereotypes (e.g., intellectual inferiority, criminality, oversexualization, laziness) onto their clients in the assessment and diagnostic process (Williams, Gooden, & Davis, 2012). These forms of stereotypes have contributed to lack of access to resources and opportunities for clients of color and have a direct, negative impact on the assessment and diagnostic processes. Research indicates that prejudice dissipates as individuals gain knowledge of diverse cultures and recognize individuals for having multiple intersecting identities and group memberships (i.e., the ADDRESSING framework; Hays, 2008). It is of crucial importance that clinicians examine their own biases related to racial and ethnic groups, and that they engage in a continuous and persistent process of disallowing these to impact their behavior in assessment, diagnosis, and access to quality care for clients of color (for helpful thought and growth questions, see Miller, Williams, Wetterneck, Kanter, & Tsai, 2015).

Knowledge

Assessment and diagnostic processes are most effective when clinicians are able to connect with clients in ways that are congruent with client cultural values and belief systems. To this end, clinicians must educate themselves about the modal experiences of clients from different cultural backgrounds, while remaining open to each client's unique experiences and life contexts, given that modal experiences do not describe the full range of varied experiences within any racial or ethnic group. This education begins with clinicians learning about the history, beliefs, values, and experiences of oppressed racial and ethnic groups in society to enable clinicians to connect with clients from diverse backgrounds and be more effective in their assessment and diagnostic approaches. In this context, clinicians also need to educate themselves about the historical views of medicine, psychology, and therapy from different cultural perspectives, which includes knowledge about institutional and systemic barriers to mental health treatment that clients of color may experience.

Part of this education includes understanding the ways that racial and ethnic minorities experience marginalization and oppression within one's societal context. These groups are often set apart and perceived negatively or "less than" in society. Marginalized populations often experience barriers to health care and jobs and experience social injustices and threats to their civil liberties. One example of a threat to the civil liberties of a marginalized group can be seen in women receiving unequal pay for doing the same work as their male counterparts, and receiving even lower pay when they are women of color. In addition, we have seen systemic efforts to disenfranchise voters of color across the United States, including closing specific polling stations and heightening regulations related to voter identification. These are just a few examples of the oppression and marginalization that clients of color may experience based on multiple marginalized statuses (intersectionality). These experiences often play a significant role in clinical presentations and must be attended to during the assessment and diagnostic phases of mental health treatment, and clinicians are advised to stay well informed of such policies and practices.

In addition, it is crucial that clinicians work to become educated about the different forms of discrimination that marginalized groups experience, including both overt and covert forms of discrimination. Racial microaggressions have been described as intentional or unintentional disparaging comments, slights, or environmental indignities based on an individual's marginalized group status (Pierce, 1970). For people of color, microaggressions can occur in many different forms. For example, a racial microaggression may be a White woman clutching her purse as she walks past a Black man on the sidewalk. Additional examples are a Chinese American woman being asked what country she is from, or a White clinician making the statement "I do not see color."

Clinicians must not adhere to ideas of colorblindness and sameness, but should acknowledge and appreciate cultural differences in the therapy room with their clients of color. While "color-blind" approaches to assessment and diagnosis are meant to reduce biases, they actually serve to ignore important lived experiences of clients (e.g., exposure to racism) and can lead to ineffective diagnostic formulations and case conceptualizations, impacting the overall success of the therapeutic process (Terwilliger, Bach, Bryan, & Williams, 2013). While subtle or covert, these microaggressions often serve to demean or invalidate certain groups and have deleterious effects on mental health and well-being (Brondolo et al., 2008; Franklin, 2004). Therefore, clinicians must gain awareness and knowledge of these types of indignities in order to both assess for their impact on mental health difficulties as well as avoid engaging in these types of behaviors with clients of color. It is important for clinicians to communicate that they value their clients and their differences.

Discrimination and Assessing the Impact of Race-Based Discrimination

As discussed in chapter 5, an abundance of research finds that racial discrimination is experienced with frequency and persistence for people of color in the United States and that these experiences have a profoundly negative effect on the genesis, expression, and maintenance of mental health difficulties. Studies have linked both macro- and microaggressive experiences of racial discrimination to psychological distress, decreased treatment seeking, and mental health disparities in care for racial and ethnic minorities (Freimuth et al., 2001; Snowden, 2001; Williams, Printz, & DeLapp, 2018b).

Given this evidence, it is of crucial importance for clinicians to address the impact of racism on clients of color during the assessment and diagnostic phases of mental health treatment. Clinicians should introduce issues of marginalization early in the assessment process, and they should assess for the experience, frequency, and perceived impact of experiences of race-based discrimination and marginalization based on the clients' intersecting identities. When introducing experiences of marginalization with clients of color, it is important to understand that people of color often get the message that discussing race-based discrimination across difference (e.g., with folks who racially identify as White) can be dangerous, threatening, or lead to negative consequences (e.g., loss of employment, social ostracism, or isolation). Therefore, clinicians who introduce these issues early in the assessment process might think about checking in with clients of color related to their fears of discussing these issues in the context of therapy and across difference. For instance, an assessing clinician might ask the question, "What is it like for you to discuss experiences of racism with me?" Introducing these issues, as a clinician, early in the assessment process can send a message to clients of color that therapy is an appropriate and safe space to discuss experiences of race-based discrimination and their impact on mental health struggles, which contributes to effective diagnostic and case formulations.

Measures of Race-Based Discrimination

Therapists without much experience having discussions about race often wonder how they can start the conversation with clients. There are a number of scales that have been developed to assess experiences and impact of racial discrimination on mental health symptoms. The Race-Based Traumatic Stress Symptom Scale (RBTSSS; Carter et al., 2013) is a fifty-two-item self-report measure that assesses the psychological and emotional stress reactions one has to racial discrimination. Landrine and Klonoff (1996) developed an eighteen-item self-report inventory, the Schedule of Racist Events (SRE), that assesses the frequency of racist events experienced for African Americans in an individual's past year and across their lifetime, as well as the extent to which the discrimination was perceived as stressful. The General Ethnic Discrimination Scale (GEDS;

Landrine, Klonoff, Corral, Fernandez, & Roesch, 2006) is an eighteen-item measure that assesses perceived ethnic discrimination among different ethnic groups and was developed with a specific focus in health research, examining frequency and stress resulting from discriminatory experiences. The Racial and Ethnic Microaggressions Scale (REMS; Nadal, 2011) measures the frequency of which individuals experience different types of microaggressions. Similarly, the Racial Microaggressions Scale (RMAS; Torres-Harding, Andrade, & Romero Diaz, 2012) is a thirty-two-item scale that assesses the occurrence and distress elicited by incidents of racial microaggressions. Finally, the Trauma Symptoms of Discrimination Scale (TSDS; Williams, 2018b) is a twenty-one-item questionnaire of discriminatory distress, measuring anxiety-related trauma symptoms. Therapists can administer these or similar measures before the first meeting and use the results as a springboard for further conversations.

Williams et al. (2018a) designed an instrument (UConn Racial/Ethnic Stress and Trauma Survey; UnRESTS) to explore racial stress and trauma that guides clinicians in asking clients difficult questions about their experiences surrounding race. The survey includes questions to assess ethnoracial identity development, a semi-structured interview to probe for a variety of racism-related experiences, and a checklist to help determine whether the individual's racial trauma meets DSM-5 criteria. The format of the UnRESTS is modeled after the DSM-5 Cultural Formulation Interview (CFI; American Psychiatric Association [APA], 2013). Unfortunately, neither the CFI nor its supplementary modules examine racism or discrimination, despite the CFI having been developed as a cultural assessment. Therefore, it may be necessary for clinicians to also have access to an interview, such as the UnRESTS, specifically designed for the assessment of discrimination and its impact. The interview is available in both English and Spanish (Williams, Peña, & Mier-Chairez, 2017).

The Role of Stereotype Threat

Clinicians must also be aware of the role of stereotype threat in maintaining disparities in seeking and engaging in mental health treatment. Stereotype threat is defined as cues in the environment that make salient negative stereotypes held about one's marginalized group status. These cues often trigger physiological and psychological processes that undermine performance and success and that contribute to mental health difficulties (Steele & Aronson, 1995). In mental health settings, stereotype threat can be described as things in the mental health setting that make salient negative stereotypes held about people of color as unintelligent or unworthy of quality care. One example can be walking in to a mental health clinic and not seeing any people of color on staff or as mental health providers. An important thing to keep in mind is that stereotype threat can occur regardless of the prejudices held by particular clinicians. Stereotype threat can affect clients of color in a number of ways, including triggering difficulties with cognitive processing, lowered self-esteem, lack of self-efficacy, disengagement with the therapeutic process, difficulties with communication, and struggles related to identity (Burgess, Warren, Phelan, Dovidio, & Van Ryn, 2010). Clinicians must be aware of the potential for stereotype threat to become a barrier to effective care for people of color. In fact, it could be helpful for clinicians to discuss with clients the ways in which stereotype threat can impact quality care and engage in discussions related to stereotype threat during the assessment process.

Role of Assessment and Diagnosis in Therapy Retention

Numerous studies have highlighted the difficulties in therapy retention for people of color (see chapter 2). For example, Freimuth et al. (2001) conducted focus groups with sixty African Americans and found that the majority of participants were aware of the Tuskegee Syphilis Study and cited this as representative of medical research and as a reason for distrusting mental health care services. In addition, racial biases contribute to misdiagnosis of psychological disorders as well as mistreatment of racial and ethnic minorities based on these biases (Snowden, 2001). For instance, historically, Black Americans have been disproportionately overdiagnosed, and misdiagnosed, with schizophrenia, which has been attributed to clinician biases as well as misinterpretation of mood disorder symptoms (Coleman & Baker, 1994; Schwartz & Blankenship, 2014). Thompson, Brazile, and Akbar (2015) used focus groups to explore perceptions of psychotherapy, psychotherapists, and barriers to treatment in a sample of Black American adults. Results indicated that participants highlighted mental health stigma (e.g., shame and embarrassment associated with seeking mental health services), cultural barriers (e.g., personal issues should be resolved within the family), lack of trust, lack of knowledge about mental health issues (e.g., symptoms or signs of mental illness; lack of knowledge about resources), lack of affordability, and impersonal services as barriers to mental health treatment engagement. In addition, study participants often believed that psychotherapists were insensitive to experiences tied to their Black American identities.

Given these findings, during the assessment process, it is essential for clinicians to assess past therapy experiences, expectations related to the therapy process, and ideas related to mental health stigma for clients of color. For instance, clients who have experienced racial macro- or microaggressions in the context of a previous therapeutic relationship might be reluctant to provide pertinent information during the assessment process to protect themselves from further harm. This type of reluctance can lead to misdiagnosis or ineffective case conceptualization, contributing to early termination. Clinicians might directly ask clients of color about past therapy experiences to get a sense of both positive and negative aspects of those experiences. In addition, clinicians can ask directly about experiences of racism in the context of therapy by saying, "Given how often people of color experience racism in our society, I am wondering if you have had these experiences in you, past therapy experiences?" Assessing for past therapy experiences, both negative and positive, can signal to the client that you, as the clinician, care about tailoring the assessment, diagnostic, and intervention experience to their individual needs.

The Effects of Mental Health Stigma

Clinicians should determine the impact of mental health stigma for clients of color to aid in case conceptualization. Sources of this stigma are widespread, including media and societal messages as well as cultural and familial influence (Corrigan, 2004; Rao, Feinglass, & Corrigan, 2007). Among some communities of color, mental illness can be perceived as contagious, chronic, genetic, a personal weakness, a curse, or a sin (Mishra, Luckstead, Gioia, Barnet, & Baquet, 2009). Mental health stigma is higher among racial and ethnic minority groups compared to White Americans (Rao et al., 2007), and this is a significant barrier to treatment engagement and retention for individuals of color. It is important for clinicians to understand clients' views of others who experience mental illness as well as clients' perceptions of their own experience with mental illness. Through the assessment process, clinicians must ask direct questions related to clients' perception of their struggles generally (e.g., "How did you learn about mental health struggles?" "How are mental health struggles viewed by family members, friends, community?") The DSM-5 Cultural Formulation Interview (APA, 2013) is a good guide for asking these questions. In addition, there are other mental health stigma assessment measures that may assist in the assessment effort (e.g., the Endorsed and Anticipated Stigma Inventory; Vogt et al., 2014).

Culturally Responsive Diagnostic Process

Diagnosis is a fundamental piece of effective mental health treatment. For this reason, many clinicians adhere to evidence-based treatments that have been shown to be effective for specific mental health disorders (Proctor, 2002), which suggest that diagnosis is of crucial importance in the context of utilizing appropriate evidence-based strategies.

To that end, mental health practitioners have a responsibility to inform themselves as to whether or not the measures they use to assess clients are culturally appropriate and normed and validated in those specific populations. There is now a wealth of evidence that indicates strong cultural biases in many of our "gold standard" assessment tools. This includes popular IQ tests (e.g., Thaler, Thames, Cagigas, & Norman, 2015), diagnostic interviews (e.g., Chasson, Williams, Davis, & Combs, 2017), and self-report measures (e.g., Williams, Davis, Thibodeau, & Bach, 2013). The potential for lasting harm based on improper diagnoses is great. For example, incorrect intellectual assessment could result in improper educational placement, a wrong psychotic disorder diagnosis could result in inappropriate medications, and a misplaced personality disorder diagnosis could lead to long-lasting stigma and barriers to care. To ensure the measures chosen for the purpose of assessment are appropriate for clients of color, it is important to consult the literature outlining research related to the validity and reliability of a particular measure and whether or not a given assessment tool has been used and validated with clients of color specifically. Validation on a "representative US sample" is not adequate to ascertain if a given measure is appropriate for any specific ethnic group unless subgroup analyses have been conducted.

Culturally Responsive Diagnostic Formulation

The process by which clinicians develop a diagnostic formulation is directly tied to cultural responsiveness. Specifically, given the history of cultural mistrust of medical providers among people of color stemming from past and current exploitative practices (e.g., Tuskegee Syphilis Study, eugenics), clinicians must think deeply about the development of a collaborative diagnostic formulation in which the client feels part of the diagnostic process as well as the outcome. For clients of color, it can be helpful for clinicians to be transparent about the diagnostic process. For instance, clinicians should have an open conversation with clients about the diagnostic criteria related to their mental health struggles and check in with clients to make sure that diagnostic conclusions match with their perspectives related to their struggles. Culturally responsive assessment also includes openness and transparency on the clinician's part about how diagnoses will be portrayed in the client's chart and who will have access to it. Specifically, in many clinics, other physical and mental health providers may have access to clients' mental health diagnoses, and it is important for clients to be aware of this. Finally, clinicians must be willing to process and discuss clients' reactions and responses to their diagnosis. The basis of culturally responsive diagnosis is collaboration and trust.

Conclusion

Culturally responsive assessment and diagnosis have become a top priority for the governing bodies of psychology. While the research, training, and application of culturally responsive assessment and diagnosis have increased over the last several decades, there is a continued need for a focus on training culturally responsive clinicians. For clinicians working to enhance their cultural responsiveness, Hays (2008) noted that the skills of a culturally responsive clinician are similar to those of an effective clinician more broadly— developing cultural humility (to avoid mistaking difference for inferiority), compassion (for self and others), and critical thinking skills (the process of continually questioning one's assumptions and biases). Clinicians who attend to these principles achieve the overarching goal of every clinician: client well-being.

KEY POINTS FOR CLINICIANS

- Cultural competency and responsiveness have become a benchmark for ethical and effective assessment and diagnostic processes.

- The first step is to develop awareness of our own assumptions, values, attitudes, and biases as they relate to our identities and those of our clients.

- Each client's cultural context is equally valuable, and it is important to work within clients' values and belief systems in the assessment and diagnostic processes.

- Clinicians should attend to the contextual issues of power, privilege and marginalization in clients' lives.

- Clinicians should use properly validated measures to help assess cultural constructs for diverse clients.

References

American Psychiatric Association. (2013). *Diagnostic and statistical manual of mental disorders* (5th ed.). Arlington, VA: American Psychiatric Publishing.

Arredondo, P., Toporek, R., Brown, S. P., Jones, L., Locke, D. C., Sanchez, J., & Stadler, H. (1996). Operationalization of the multicultural counseling competencies. *Journal of Multicultural Counseling and Development, 24*, 42–78.

Atkinson, D., Morten, G., & Sue, D. (1998). *Counseling American minorities*. New York, NY: McGraw Hill.

Baldwin, S. A., & Imel, Z. E. (2013). Therapist effects: Findings and methods. In M. J. Lambert (Ed.), *Bergin and Garfield's handbook of psychotherapy and behavior change* (6th ed.) (pp. 258–297). Mahwah, NJ: Wiley.

Brondolo, E., Daniel, L., Denton, E., Thompson, S., Beatty, D., Schwartz, J., Sweeney, M., Tobin, J., Cassells, A., Pickering, T., & Gerin, W. (2008). Racism and ambulatory blood pressure in a community sample. *Psychosomatic Medicine, 70*, 49–56. doi:10.1097/PSY.0b013e31815ff3bd

Burgess, D., Warren, J., Phelan, S., Dovidio, J., & Van Ryn, M. (2010). Stereotype threat and health disparities: What medical educators and future physicians need to know. *Journal of General and Internal Medicine, 25*, 169–177. doi:10.1007/s11606-009-1221-4

Carter, R. T., Mazzula, S., Victoria, R., Vazquez, R., Hall, S., Smith, S., ... & Williams, B. (2013). Initial development of the Race-Based Traumatic Stress Symptom Scale: Assessing the emotional impact of racism. *Psychological Trauma: Theory, Research, Practice, and Policy, 5*(1), 1–9. doi:10.1037/a0025911

Chasson, G., Williams, M. T. Davis, D. M., & Combs, J. Y. (2017). Missed diagnoses in African Americans with obsessive-compulsive disorder: The Structured Clinical Interview for the DSM-IV Axis I Disorders (SCID-I). *BMC Psychiatry, 17*, 258. doi:10.1186/s12888-017-1422-z

Coleman, D., & Baker, F. (1994). Misdiagnosis of schizophrenia among older black veterans. *Journal of Nervous and Mental Disease, 182*, 527–528.

Corrigan, J. (2004). How stigma interferes with mental health care. *American Psychologist, 59*, 614–625. doi:10.1037/0003-066X.59.7.614

D'Andrea, M., & Daniels, J. (2001). RESPECTFUL Counseling: An integrative model for counselors. In D. Pope-Davis, & H. Coleman (Eds.), *The interface of class, culture and gender in counseling* (pp. 417–466). Thousand Oaks, CA: Sage.

Fink, C., Turner, S., & Beidel, D. (1996). Culturally relevant factors in the behavioral treatment of social phobia: A case study. *Journal of Anxiety Disorders, 10*, 201–209.

Franklin, A. J. (2004). *From brotherhood to manhood: How Black men rescue their relationships and dreams from the invisibility syndrome.* Hoboken, NJ: Wiley.

Freimuth, V., Quinn, S., Thomas, S., Cole, G., Zook, E., & Duncan, T. (2001). African Americans' views on research and the Tuskegee Syphilis Study. *Social Science Medicine, 52*, 797–808.

Hays, P. (2008). *Addressing cultural complexities in practice: Assessment, diagnosis, and therapy.* Washington, DC: American Psychological Association.

Helms, J. (1984). Toward a theoretical explanation of the effects of race on counseling: A black and white model. *The Counseling Psychologist, 12*, 4.

Jensen, K., & Kelley, J. M. (2016). The therapeutic relationship in psychological and physical treatments, and their placebo controls. *Psychology of Consciousness: Theory, Research, and Practice, 3*, 132–145. doi:10.1037/cns0000057

Kluckholn, C., & Murray, H. A. (1953). Personality formation: The determinants. In H. A. Murray & C. Kluckhohn (Eds.), *Personality in nature, society, and culture* (pp. 53–72). New York, NY: Alfred A. Knopf.

Landrine, H., & Klonoff, E. (1996). The schedule of racist events: A measure of racial discrimination and a study of its negative physical and mental health consequences. *Journal of Black Psychology, 22*, 144–168. doi:10.177/009579849602220022.

Landrine, H., Klonoff, E. A., Corral, I., Fernandez, S., & Roesch, S. (2006). Conceptualizing and measuring ethnic discrimination in health research. *Journal of Behavioral Medicine, 29*, 79–94.

Miller, A., Williams, M. T., Wetterneck, C. T., Kanter, J., & Tsai, M. (2015). Using functional analytic psychotherapy to improve awareness and connection in racially diverse client-therapist dyads. *The Behavior Therapist, 38*(6), 150–156.

Mishra, S., Luckstead, A., Gioia, D., Barnet, B., & Baquet, C. (2009). Needs and preferences for receiving mental health information in an African American focus group sample. *Community Mental Health, 45*, 117. doi.org/10.1007/s10597-008-9157-4

Nadal, K. L. (2011). The racial and ethnic microaggressions scale: Construction, reliability, and validity. *Journal of Counseling Psychology, 58*, 470–480.

Parham, T. A., Ajamu, A., & White, J. L. (2011). Mental health issues among African-American People. In Parham et al. (Eds.), *Psychology of Blacks: Centering our perspectives in the African consciousness* (4th ed.) (pp. 138–163) New York, NY: Pearson

Pierce, C. (1970). Offensive mechanisms. In F. B. Barbour (Ed.), *In the Black seventies* (pp. 265–82). Boston: Porter Sargent.

Proctor, E. K. (2002). Quality of care and social work research. *Social Work Research, 26*, 195–197.

Rao, D., Feinglass, J., & Corrigan, P. (2007) Racial and ethnic disparities in mental illness stigma. *Journal of Nervous Mental Disorders, 195*, 1020–1023.

Schwartz, R. C., & Blankenship, D. M. (2014). Racial disparities in psychotic disorder diagnosis: A review of empirical literature. *World Journal of Psychiatry, 4*, 133–140. doi:10.5498/wjp.v4.i4.133

Seller, R., Smith, M., Shelton, J., Rowley, S., & Chavous, T. (1998). Multidimensional model of racial identity: A reconceptualization of African American racial identity. *Personality and Social Psychology Review, 2*, 18–39.

Snowden, L. (2001). Barriers to effective mental health services for African Americans. *Mental Health Services Research, 3*(4), 181–187.

Steele, C., & Aronson, J. (1995). Stereotype threat and the intellectual test performance of African Americans. *Journal Personality Social Psychology, 69,* 797–811.

Sue, D. W., Capodilupo, C., Torino, G., & Bucceri, J. (2007). Racial microaggressions in everyday life: Implications for clinical practice. *American Psychologist, 62,* 271–286. doi:10.1037/0003-066X .62.4.271

Sue, D. W., & Sue, D. (2003). *Counseling the culturally diverse: Theory and practice* (4th ed.). New York, NY: Houghton Mifflin.

Sue, W. (2010). *Microaggressions and Marginality.* Hoboken, NJ: John Wiley and Sons.

Terwilliger, J. M., Bach, N., Bryan, C., & Williams, M. T. (2013). Multicultural versus colorblind ideology: Implications for mental health and counseling. In A. Di Fabio (Ed.), *Psychology of counseling* (pp. 111–122). Hauppauge, NY: Nova Science Publishers.

Thaler, N. S., Thames, A. D., Cagigas, X. E., & Norman, M. A. (2015). IQ testing and the African American client. In L. T.Benuto & B. D. Leany (Eds.), *Guide to psychological assessment with African Americans* (pp. 63–78). New York, NY: Springer.

Thompson, V., Brazile A., & Akbar M. (2015). African Americans' perceptions of psychotherapy and psychotherapists. *Professional psychology: Research and practice, 35,* 19–26. doi:10.1037/0735-7028 .35.1.19

Torres-Harding, S., Andrade, A., & Romero Diaz, C. (2012). The racial microaggressions scale (RMAS): A new scale to measure experiences of racial microaggressions in people of color. *Cultural Diversity and Ethnic Minority Psychology, 18,* 153–164. doi:10.1037/a0027658

Turner, S., Beidel, D., Cooley, M., & Woody, S. (1994). A multicomponent behavioral treatment for social phobia: Social effectiveness therapy. *Behaviour Research and Therapy, 32,* 381–390. doi:10 .1016/0005-7967(94)90001-9

Vandiver, B., Fhagen-Smith, P., Cokley, K., Cross, W., & Worrel, F. (2001). Cross's nigrescence model: From theory to scale to theory. *Journal of Multicultural Counseling and Development, 29,* 174–200.

Vogt, D., Di Leone, B., Wang, J., Sayer, N., Pineles, S., & Litz, B. (2014). Endorsed and anticipated stigma inventory (EASI): A tool for assessing beliefs about mental illness and mental health treatment among military personnel and veterans. *Psychological Services, 11,* 105–113. doi:10.1037 /a0032780

Williams, M. T., Davis, D., Thibodeau, M., & Bach, N. (2013). Psychometric properties of the obsessive-compulsive inventory revised in African Americans with and without obsessive-compulsive disorder. *Journal of Obsessive-Compulsive & Related Disorders, 2*(4), 399–405.

Williams, M. T., Gooden, A. M., & Davis, D. (2012). African Americans, European Americans, and Pathological stereotypes: An African-centered perspective. In G. R. Hayes & M. H. Bryant (Eds.), *Psychology of culture,* (pp. 213–221). Hauppauge, NY: Nova Science Publishers.

Williams, M. T., Metzger, I., Leins, C., & DeLapp, C. (2018a). Assessing racial trauma within a DSM-5 Framework: The UConn Racial/Ethnic Stress & Trauma Survey. *Practice Innovations, 3*(4), 242–260. doi:10.1037/pri0000076

Williams, M. T., Peña, A., & Mier-Chairez, J. (2017). Tools for assessing racism-related stress and trauma among Latinos. In L. T. Benuto (Ed.), *Toolkit for counseling Spanish-speaking clients* (pp. 71–98). New York, NY: Springer. doi:10.1007/978-3-319-64880-4_4

Williams, M. T., Printz, D., & DeLapp, R. C. T. (2018b). Assessing racial trauma in African Americans with the Trauma Symptoms of Discrimination Scale. *Psychology of Violence, 8*(6), 735–747. doi:10.1037/vio0000212

CHAPTER 10

Supervising Therapist Trainees of Color

Linda A. Oshin,
University of Connecticut

Terence H. W. Ching,
University of Connecticut

Lindsey M. West,
The Medical College of Georgia and Augusta University

Introduction

While many have called for increasing the number of trainees from underrepresented groups in psychology (Stewart, Lee, Hogstrom, & Williams, 2017), less attention has been paid to underrepresented trainees' unique needs and challenges. Clinical supervision has the potential to either support trainees of color (TOC), or be a source of discouragement and discomfort. *Supervision*, by definition, is an evaluative process and relationship between a clinical or counseling psychology trainee and a professional, where it is the professional's responsibility to provide education, evaluation and monitoring, and gatekeeping to the profession (Bernard & Goodyear, 1998). Like with all professional relationships, several challenges can arise between the supervisor and the supervisee. One such challenge is the issue of TOC experiences of microaggressions. Microaggressions have been defined as "everyday insults, indignities and demeaning messages sent to people of color by well-intentioned White people who are unaware of the hidden messages being sent to them" (Sue, quoted in DeAngelis, 2009, p. 42; see also Pierce, 1970; Sue et al., 2007). This chapter reviews research and theory about supervising TOC and offers specific skills and common challenges that supervisors encounter.

First, it is important to acknowledge that there are many forms of diversity. For example, students have multiple identities, many of which might be minority identities, resulting in a unique experience of inequality and access to power (Else-Quest & Hyde, 2016). While this chapter will focus specifically on TOC, we will attempt to take an intersectional viewpoint. We hope that the topics discussed will also be useful for supervisors working with trainees with other marginalized identities.

Background

The rates of students of color in psychology have been steadily increasing (American Psychological Association, 2016). Although increased attention has been paid to improving cultural competency within graduate school curricula, less thought has been paid to educating supervisors, who may have graduated prior to the recent focus on cross-racial dyadic supervision (Chang, Hays, & Shoffner, 2004; Constantine & Sue, 2007; Duan & Roehlke, 2001; Falendar & Shafranske, 2004; Gatmon et al., 2001). Early research has found that TOC report negative experiences in clinical supervision, often due to issues related to ethnoracial differences in dyads with White supervisors (Chang et al., 2004, Falendar & Shafranske, 2004; Garrett et al., 2001, Jernigan, Green, Helms, Perez-Gualdron, & Henze, 2010).

Many supervisors may assume that a solution to optimal training outcomes for TOC would be to match them with a supervisor of the same ethnoracial background. In addition to this being perceived by some as a segregationist training policy, being a supervisor of color does not ensure that one can effectively supervise a TOC. In fact, Jernigan et al. (2010) found in a qualitative study that some TOC who were paired with supervisors of color often felt invalidated and frustrated by their supervisors' discomfort with or lack of education regarding race and culture. A plausible reason is that a supervisor of color may not have sufficient knowledge about other races and ethnicities to facilitate a culturally attuned supervisory relationship. Another important consideration is that although the supervisor and the trainee may be matched ethnoracially, there is often a mismatch in their ethnoracial identity development process (Jernigan et al., 2010). In other words, there may be a difference in the extent to which each person has processed his or her attitudes and beliefs about race and gained awareness of racism and oppression. Ethnoracial identity development, therefore, may be a better proxy for supervisor-trainee matching (Williams, Duque, & Wetterneck, 2015). Finally, supervisors of color are still embedded in a structurally racist system that may have failed to adequately prepare them to work with people of color, and may be themselves in need of education and training in this area.

Studies on supervisory dyads show that TOC with more advanced ethnoracial identity development are often the ones to bring up race most often (i.e., "regressive dyads") (Bhat & Davis, 2007; Jernigan et al., 2010; Ladany, Brittan-Powell, & Pannu, 1997). On the other hand, in "progressive dyads," in which the supervisor was more advanced in their ethnoracial identity development, the supervisee perceived that there was plenty of space for conversations about cultural issues in supervision. These findings make clear the importance of training in the area of ethnoracial identity development for all supervisors in order to work effectively in cross-racial dyads.

The Supervisor

One of the most effective actions supervisors can take to competently supervise TOC is to increase awareness of their own identities (American Psychological Association, 2017).

Understanding one's identity does not simply mean knowing one's category, but rather learning and engaging with one's history and culture. Supervisor ethnoracial identity has been shown to influence alliance with and multicultural competence in supervisees (Ladany et al., 1997). Engaging with one's identity also includes understanding one's relative position of privilege, particularly in relation to one's supervisee. Privilege comes from multiple identities, including race or ethnicity, but also positionality as a supervisor, which often includes socioeconomic status and age. It is important for supervisors to understand their privilege in relation to each of their supervisees and how this privilege may be a context that affects the supervisory relationship. For example, supervisors can engage in an exercise using Pamela Hays's ADDRESSING Framework (Hays, 2001), in which the supervisor and the supervisee go through each of their identities within the framework (i.e., Age, Developmental and acquired Disabilities, Religion, Ethnicity and race, Social class, Sexual orientation, Indigenous heritage, Nationality, and Gender), noting one's areas of privilege and oppression. In supervision, supervisor and supervisee can engage in an open conversation about their areas of difference and similarities, and can better discuss the role of clients' identities using the ADDRESSING framework.

Awareness of Issues of Power and Privilege

A supervisor is always in a position of evaluative power over a supervisee, but other identities can add different dimensions of power to the relationship, such as race (e.g., a White supervisor with a Native American trainee). In these cross-racial supervisory relationships, the TOC may need to manage racial microaggressions, discomfort around discussion of cultural differences, and other factors that come with being a minority in a majority-White field. Due to their privilege, it is important for supervisors to make an explicit effort to establish a safe space for TOC. McNeill, Hom, and Perez (1995) posit that TOC will avoid bringing up issues of race and ethnicity to supervisors for fear that they fulfill stereotypes, or that they will receive a response that will make them feel uncomfortable or invalidated. This can result in TOC feeling confused and inadequate in their abilities as new clinicians. This discomfort is ultimately detrimental to the supervisory relationship and to TOC education. It is therefore supervisors' responsibility to educate themselves on supervising TOC and interventions for minority clients. The supervisor should be the first to explicitly bring up these issues, in order to set an understanding and communicative tone for the relationship. This is similar to conducting therapy with a client of a different cultural background, where the explicit acknowledgement and sensitivity to ethnoracial and cultural differences can set a tone of comfort and inclusivity in the relationship (Miller, Williams, Wetterneck, Kanter, & Tsai, 2015; Cardemil & Battle, 2003). For example, one could say, "I want to acknowledge that we are from different ethnoracial groups, and that is an important part of our lives, as well as an important part of being a clinician. If you are comfortable with it, I would like for us to be able to talk openly about how this difference may affect supervision, or how you see it affecting how you work with your clients."

In addition to explicitly discussing ethnoracial identity differences with a supervisee, a supervisor should make ongoing efforts to create a welcoming environment for the TOC. Some supervisors say something along the lines of, "Please feel free to let me know if I ever say anything to offend you or if you have any concerns." While this is a nice statement, it ignores the reality that the supervisor is in a position of power, while the TOC is in a vulnerable position by being the only person to bring up such concerns. Instead, a supervisor should occasionally check in with the TOC about their relationship, including any issues that may come up due to the trainee's ethnoracial minority status (e.g., inaccurate assumptions of similarities between the TOC and a client of a similar background, feeling ignored or having one's competence questioned, feeling lonely or overwhelmed as a minority student). Supervisors should check in with their supervisees regardless of their minority status, but they should also make a point to address any difficulties a TOC may be having as a result of issues related to identity differences. Of course, if a supervisee does bring up an issue, the supervisor should be open and curious, attempt to understand what the supervisee is feeling, and make any necessary changes. In ideal circumstances, the supervisor is being mindful and paying attention to issues of diversity within the dyad and with respect to clients. In these circumstances, the supervisor can then model and repair his or her mistake. For example, the supervisor might say, "I just realized that I made an assumption about this client's behavior, and I'm realizing that I am placing my worldview on this client's experience." The supervisor may also want to thank the supervisee for any part they played in bringing this to the supervisor's attention, as this communicates receptivity to feedback and reinforces constructive criticism.

Furthermore, the supervisor should make it clear to the TOC that collaborative dialogue and troubleshooting will occur where difference in opinions and perspectives arise, without instilling fear of retaliation in the TOC. For example, the supervisor can say, "Let's think carefully together about how we can find a compromise for what we think can and should be done in this situation. As we do this, I want you to rest assured that I will respect and not punish you for your opinions. If I feel like there might be some gaps in knowledge that I can fill, or strong no-no's that I think we should discuss, I will speak my mind, but with utmost respect for you and the autonomy that I believe you deserve as a trainee." This is important, because trainees may fear a negative consequence in the future as a result of the conversation. On the other hand, there may be circumstances in which the TOC has failed to meet clearly defined expectations, and remediation is necessary. In this circumstance, the expectations should have been communicated early on in supervision, the fact that the expectations are not being met should have been clearly communicated to the TOC, and a plan to help the TOC meet these expectations (along with possible consequences if the TOC does not follow the plan) should have been collaboratively instituted. In other words, remediation in the event of unmet expectations should never be a surprise for any trainee, but it is important to acknowledge that poorly handled remediation may be particularly damaging for a TOC as they may be questioning their ability to belong in their program. There may even be other situations—for example, in regards to a TOC working with a client of color (particularly from their own ethnoracial group)—in which a supervisor misjudges the way in which the TOC interacts with a similar-group client, due to the supervisor's lack of understanding about the style of communication between members of that particular cultural group. In these situations, the supervisor should be willing to practice cultural humility in being curious and respectful about how the communication style in question can actually be adaptive in better serving the needs of clients of color (i.e., a characteristic of cultural competence in the TOC), much like how experienced clinicians often adapt empirically supported treatments to the needs of each client.

Supervisors should display the ability to incorporate and guide considerations of ethnoracial identity in the case formulation process, in order to model such thinking for supervisees (Greene & Blitz, 2012). It is also important for supervisors to initiate and explicitly encourage such discussions even if the TOC fails to do so, particularly due to the power differential. In modeling an open, honest, nonjudgmental, and highly communicative supervisory atmosphere, TOC are likely to connect with the supervisor. Many supervisors may not feel adequately trained for these conversation, based on their past training experiences, and will need to make education in these topics a priority.

Increasing Comfort and Skills

Seeking cross-racial relationships is an often overlooked method of expanding one's cultural competence in clinical practice (Okech & Champe, 2008). Supervisors should seek to increase cross-racial relationships. Of course, supervisors should not do so for the sole purpose of increasing their own comfort with diverse groups at the expense of others, as these relationships would lack the authenticity that is important to developing meaningful friendships. Genuinely maintaining a diverse personal network of relationships allows for the eventual discussion of issues related to ethnoracial identity, racism, and stereotypes within the context of an interpersonal relationship.

Supervisors can also increase their comfort in addressing issues related to ethnoracial differences by engaging with these issues in the media and community. This may include consuming media about race and ethnicity or those targeted at a different ethnoracial group, attending community meetings or rallies about minority issues, and so forth. By engaging with these issues outside of clinical work, supervisors can increase their awareness and understanding of differences in perspectives and worldviews. It is important for supervisors to maintain an attitude of humility and curiosity to learn about differences in experiences and to never treat such experiences as mere "cultural voyeurism or tourism." For example, when discussing a Black client who was struggling to pay for car insurance, the student supervisor of the first author of this chapter (LO) suggested that this financial stressor may have added stress for the client because of the history of police brutality of Black people and the recent high-profile killings of unarmed Black people. Not only did this information help the first author to approach this topic with her client in a culturally sensitive way, but it also signaled to her that this supervisor cared about problems that affected Black people.

A supervisor must also be able to effectively incorporate information about ethnoracial identity into supervision. Many supervisors may dedicate one session to discussing issues of diversity, but this can send the message to TOC that such issues are peripheral, optional, or isolated to one point in time, rather than ongoing. On the other hand, integrating considerations of diversity into every supervision session can communicate to the supervisee that their multiple identities are important and do have an impact on the supervisory and therapeutic relationship. Integrating issues of diversity into all aspects of training also allows trainees to practice consistently engaging with these topics without discomfort. An example of a question that supervisors might consider regularly asking their trainees is, "Could you tell me more about how you think the differences you perceive in our cultural backgrounds might influence the ways in which I provide feedback, and the ways in which you might translate that feedback into your work with your clients? I have some thoughts about this, but I really value your perspective too."

Avoiding Color-blind Supervision

Some supervisors opt to take a color-blind approach with all trainees, or attempt to treat everyone equally without regard to ethnoracial differences, despite evidence that color-blindness can disguise inequality (Rattan & Ambady, 2013). In supervision, color-blindness can show up in several ways. For example, a supervisor may avoid discussing how a client's cultural difference may be a source of lack of engagement in therapy, or worse, the supervisor may attribute the lack of engagement to other factors (e.g., a hostile personality [stereotypes] or a symptom of depression [psychopathology]). Color-blindness may directly affect the supervisory relationship, such as an Asian trainee feeling angry and isolated because he is uncomfortable pointing out that the supervisor often mistakes him for another Asian student. An alternative to a color-blind approach is a multicultural approach, which includes considering culture in the conceptualization of all clients, and reinforcing trainees for their ability to bring a different perspective to a case (Terwilliger, Bach, Bryan, & Williams, 2013). By taking a multicultural perspective, a supervisor can better recognize the pain microaggressions can cause, and they can also be more open to joining with TOC in fighting inequalities that they may face, while affirming aspects of their cultural backgrounds that can be a strength in the face of adversity.

Racism and Supervision

Racism is an inescapable part of being a person of color in the United States. This section details how supervisors can help TOC mitigate the effects of racism that they may encounter from various sources. It is important to note that racism can appear in several ways, from more explicit to more implicit.

From Clients

In addition to the several ways racism may show up in everyday life, there are unique ways that racism can show up in a therapy setting. First, it is important for the supervisor to become familiar with ways racism can manifest in an inter-ethnoracial dyad. While a TOC may be familiar with identifying and responding to everyday racism, racism within a therapy dyad may be particularly disorienting and upsetting (Bartoli & Pyati, 2009). While a full discussion of the ways racism manifest in therapy is outside the scope of this chapter (see Bartoli & Pyati, 2009), this section details common experiences a TOC may experience and how a supervisor can help.

Racism may be highlighted in therapy in the differences in experiences between the TOC and client. The role of racism in the life of the TOC may make it difficult for the TOC to maintain a nonjudgmental stance when faced with clients of different world-views. For example, a Black male trainee might feel like a White female client's irrational anxiety about having a minor car accident is trivial in comparison to his experiences of being racially profiled by police. The supervisor can intervene in these situations by recommending introspective awareness of TOC biographical differences from clients as reasons for their difficulties in relating to clients' issues. Supervisors can also make sure that TOC understand that their internal experiences are valid and important and might even in some abstract manner be relatable to client. The supervisor can say to him, "I want you to feel supported in feeling that way, and I also want to help you recognize your professional obligation not to compromise the therapeutic services. I understand that your client's concerns feel trivial given what you are dealing with, and I agree that these situations are not equivalent. I wonder if it might be helpful to explore similarities in the function of the anxiety you both might experience despite incredibly different contexts, as well as ways to cope with the sense of apprehension about something bad happening while driving."

Another common experience of therapists of color is having their authority or competence questioned due to stereotypes that their ethnoracial group is uneducated, lazy, or submissive (Comas-Díaz & Jacobsen, 1995), such as an Asian woman receiving a critical response from a client for being directive because this contradicts the stereotype that Asian women are quiet and docile. Questioning their own competence as a result of such situations is particularly difficult for TOC, as they may be questioning their own competence as a part of their training. A supervisor has the unique position to encourage the TOC in their competence. The supervisor should take the responsibility to explicitly bring up race by postulating whether the TOC believes her client's doubts about her ability are due to race. If the TOC believes so, the supervisor should not only underscore the TOC's competence, but also help the TOC to process her feelings about this experience with racism and make a plan to address it with her client. This plan will vary, depending on the situation. For example, a TOC may wish to simply model effective communication by asserting her credibility to her client or discuss her client's concerns without explicitly discussing race (e.g. "I'm getting the feeling that you're not sure I will be able to help you. Tell me more about that.") On the other hand, the TOC and a supervisor may decide that race needs to be directly discussed to improve the working relationship. This discussion should be role played with the supervisor and tailored to the specific situation. In this example, the therapist could say, "It is important to note some of our visible and invisible differences and the ways in which these differences may be impacting our working relationship. I, as an Asian female therapist, and you, as a White male, are two of the more salient differences between us, and I am wondering if you have any thoughts, feelings, or concerns about how these differences may have an influence on how much you get out of therapy."

From Peers

While trainees' relationships with their peers are outside of the responsibilities of a supervisor, TOC may experience racism from their peers that may affect their comfort in their program and their ability to do clinical work. Racism may occur in group supervision, such as peers being dismissive of a TOC's contributions, questioning the TOC's competence, tokenism, or other microaggressions toward the TOC. For example, a peer may ask a Colombian trainee to speak about the culture of a Mexican client. A supervisor should take responsibility for naming and responding to any perceived racism that occurs in group supervision. In this example, the supervisor could step in and establish that there is vast diversity among Hispanic and Latinx people, the supervisor does not expect the trainee to be an expert in all of their cultures, and open up processing and discussion of the microaggression. Alternatively, the supervisor could ask the peer why they thought the Colombian trainee should answer a question about Mexican culture and use this opportunity to engage in a discussion around the topic. A supervisor's ability to help a TOC deal with racism from peers depends on the ability of the supervisor to identify racial microaggressions. For example, a supervisor might not be able to understand why a Black female trainee feels targeted by a peer calling her "angry" without understanding the stereotype of the Angry Black Woman. The most important takeaway from these examples in clinical settings is that the supervisor is paying attention to these forms of racial microaggressions in order to acknowledge them and create a space for the TOC to discuss the experience.

Supervisors can also be effective in mitigating the effects of racism they do not directly witness. The TOC may feel safe with the supervisor and tell the supervisor about the TOC's experiences with racisms from peers. Supervisors should use their privilege to help the TOC as much as possible in this situation. It can be very damaging for a TOC to tell a supervisor about an experience with racism from a peer and for this disclosure to lead to inaction on the supervisor's part (e.g., "I'm sure they didn't mean it that way."). In addition, the supervisor should communicate any actions that they plan to take to ensure consent from the TOC. For example, the TOC may simply want a supportive listener and may be concerned about retribution.

Beyond verbal disclosure, a TOC also may exhibit more subtle cues that something is wrong. For example, a TOC may underperform, be quiet, or be hostile in group supervision. These warning signs may be due to other causes (e.g., family issues, general difficulties of being a graduate student, etc.) and one should not assume that a TOC struggling is directly due to their minority status. It would be ignorant, however, to not consider that a TOC may be struggling because of difficulties being a minority in a high-performance, predominantly White context. For a supervisor with sufficient rapport with the TOC and a demonstrated comfort in discussing ethnoracial differences, it may be exceptionally helpful to have a genuine conversation about the role of racism from peers as a possible reason for this behavior. There are two important points for supervisors to make in this conversation. First, they should not assume that the TOC is struggling due to racism. Second, they should make it clear they do not think the TOC is struggling *because* the trainee is a person of color. Many TOC have encountered stereotypes that they are less prepared for their field than their White counterparts, that they are in graduate school only because of affirmative action, that people of color have lower IQs, and so forth.

From Supervisors

The experience of racism from an individual of immediate authority (i.e., one's clinical or research supervisor) can be especially damaging to the psychological health of TOC, since the supervisor is often the one person a TOC would expect to trust to turn to for help in personal and professional development. Constantine and Sue (2007) found seven ways Black counseling or clinical psychology supervisees experience racism from White supervisors: (1) invalidation of racial or cultural issues (e.g., "I don't think this is a race thing; maybe they're just sensitive"); (2) stereotypical assumptions about Black clients (e.g., calling a client with an advanced graduate degree "surprisingly articulate"); (3) stereotypical assumptions about Black supervisees (e.g., "Don't be late for supervision.... I don't want this to turn into some kind of cultural thing"); (4) reluctance to provide performance feedback for fear of being viewed as racist (e.g., "I felt like she was more concerned with being viewed as a good liberal White supervisor working with a Black supervisee"); (5) overemphasis of clinical weaknesses or lack of conformity to White normativity (e.g., "My supervisor just kept harping on the fact that I was not doing things the 'traditional way' with clients"); (6) blaming clients of color for problems stemming from oppression (e.g., "[Black people] need to stop playing the race card"); and (7) providing culturally insensitive treatment (e.g., "My supervisor never even considered that my client's family was an important part of his support system.... It was so racially insensitive and off target"). Additionally, graduate students of color have endorsed more subtle experiences of racism from faculty, such as feelings of tokenization, hypervisibility, invisibility, and accompanying dismissal by faculty members, whether due to racism, lack of cultural competence, or, more specifically, disdain at the notion of affirmative action (Linder, Harris, Allen, & Hubain, 2015).

I (LW) remember a time when I was working with a White, female client, and I felt as if she perceived me as less smart. I remember feeling a pull to assert my "smarts" in session. I brought this experience to supervision with a White supervisor, and just like Constantine and Sue's (2007) theme of invalidation, I felt as if I was being perceived as too sensitive.

As mentioned previously, supervisors should be aware of the ways racism may manifest in their relationship with TOC in order to avoid or self-correct when it happens without defense and with humility. Additionally, it is recommended that supervisors should establish group norms when beginning individual and group supervision, emphasizing mutual respect in the training context, particularly around topics related to cultural diversity (Linder et al., 2015). By compassionately facilitating "hard conversations" and inviting further exploration or clarification from trainees with the goal of deepening mutual understanding and connection, faculty can help TOC feel more willing to correct misinformation, particularly in group supervision, and to challenge notions of privilege without shutting down White trainees. Whether as a means of preventing microaggressions or defensiveness from White trainees around conversations around diversity, or to repair "ruptures" or misunderstandings in the supervisory relationship and setting, faculty should consistently convey a sense of authenticity to cultivate an enriching, inclusive, and positive learning environment (Linder et al., 2015). For example, TOC are more likely to share their experiences of discrimination for the sake of mutual learning when faculty authentically relate their own personal struggles related to experiences of exclusion from various settings. Furthermore, faculty should remain aware of the impact of current events on TOC—and that diversity topics are not an isolated academic bubble.

From Institutions

A difficult source of racism to address for both supervisors and supervisees is institutional racism. Institutional racism refers to formal or informal structural mechanisms (e.g., official policies and bureaucratic procedures) that systematically place ethnoracial minority groups in subordinate, marginalized, and alienated positions, and it is key to understanding why racism persists as a function of their embeddedness within major social, political, educational, and health care institutions (Marable, 2002). It is important to acknowledge that the field of psychology, as currently recognized, was established in a culture that was predominately White and that theories of change in psychotherapy are also based in a Western and White point of view (Sue & Sue, 2013). This has several implications for TOC, who may feel out of place as they attempt to succeed in a field that was not built for them. A full discussion of institutional discrimination and psychology is outside the scope of this chapter and will be presented in chapter 13 ("Promoting

Diversity and Inclusion on College Campuses"). As part of the institution of psychology, however, the supervisor has an important role in challenging and helping dismantle the barriers TOC face, with actions such as acknowledging the presence of racial microaggressions as they may come up in trainee evaluation meetings, pushing back when colleagues use stereotypical language, advocating for racial diversity among trainees, and standing up for TOC if there is an injustice.

Some have suggested that the education of TOC requires the trainee to acculturate to the culture of psychology (McNeill et al., 1995). This may make it difficult for a trainee to feel comfortable in the training program, and it takes their energy away from their studies in order to adjust to this new culture. A supervisor can assist in this process by validating their experiences and helping the trainees to incorporate their culture into their clinical work. This may be through encouraging the TOC to decorate their shared spaces or offices with symbols from their cultures, to dress in ways that allow them to bring their full authentic selves to the therapy room, and to welcome their perspectives and worldviews into the supervision dialogue. Clearly more work needs to be done to make institutional climate and cultural changes in our field, but any effort in the supervision relationships with TOC to acknowledge institutional issues, while making concerted efforts with the client-, peer-, and supervisor-level considerations is important.

Conclusion

In this chapter we aimed to cover research and theory about supervising TOC. In addition, through examples from clients, peers, supervisors, and institutions, it is our hope that we have offered the reader relevant common challenges and scenarios with specific suggestions and skills for addressing supervision considerations with TOC. We conclude with the following summary.

Summary

- Supervision is an evaluative, professional relationship in which power dynamics are important considerations, especially power dynamics that are related to multiple, intersecting ADDRESSING identities.

- Racial microaggressions and racism-related stress are pervasive, common experiences for TOC.

- When approaching multicultural considerations in supervision, it is important to acknowledge the limitations in the research on ethnic matching and the disservice to the field when White trainees are not exposed to clients of color. Considering racial identity development may be a more fruitful construct for thinking through trainee needs.

- When TOC are working with clients, supervisors should anticipate (not assume) the possible experiences that their TOC might encounter. When TOC are working with clients from different backgrounds, supervisors should initiate a dialogue that acknowledges awareness of this difference and pauses to invite the TOC to share their experience in working with the client, if appropriate. If your TOC are experiencing discomfort due to racial microaggressions, validate this experience and collaborate to assess the ways in which you can be helpful to your TOC.

- When TOC are working alongside peers, supervisors must navigate the dynamics among the trainees and invite dialogues across difference early on in the training experience. Supervisors should model self-awareness and reflection, awareness of their own cultural "missteps," and their commitment to ensuring that multicultural considerations are integrated throughout the training experience.

- When TOC are working with supervisors individually, supervisors will consider all of the aforementioned points, with the additional suggestion of reading relevant literature and not burdening the TOC with having to explain or justify his experience of racism.

- When TOC are working within an institution, supervisors, even though they may be limited in power, can still acknowledge the systemic barriers and issues, can be an ally for their TOC, and can strategize advocacy tactics that aim to work toward changes.

KEY POINTS FOR CLINICIANS

- Racial and ethnic matching of clients or supervisors with TOC may not always result in positive training experiences.

- An effective way to ensure TOC feel safe and empowered in a supervisory relationship is for the supervisor to engage with their own identity, including developing awareness of their privilege and power.

- Supervisors should explicitly address issues of race and ethnicity in the supervisory relationship rather than waiting for the TOC to address it, and should approach these issues with openness and curiosity.

- Issues of race and ethnicity should be actively integrated in all parts of supervision, rather than simply treating it as an optional topic.

- Supervisors should make a point to learn about issues of race and ethnicity both generally and as it pertains to therapy by educating themselves and engaging with these issues in their personal lives.

- It is important for supervisors to be aware of the subtle ways racism can manifest in therapy, in relationships with peers, and in their institution to be prepared to support the TOC when they do arise.

References

American Psychological Association. (2016). *Graduate study in psychology summary report: Student demographics.* Retrieved from https://www.apa.org/education/grad/survey-data/2017-student-demographics.pdf

American Psychological Association. (2017). *Multicultural guidelines: An ecological approach to context, identity, and intersectionality, 2017.* Retrieved from http://www.apa.org/about/policy/multicultural-guidelines.pdf

Bartoli, E., & Pyati, A. (2009). Addressing clients' racism and racial prejudice in individual psychotherapy: Therapeutic considerations. *Psychotherapy: Theory, Research, Practice, Training, 46*(2), 145–157. doi:10.1037/a0016023

Bernard, J. M., & Goodyear, R. G. (1998). *Fundamentals of clinical supervision* (2nd ed.). Needham Heights, MA: Allyn & Bacon.

Bhat, C. S., & Davis, T. E. (2007). Counseling supervisors' assessment of race, racial identity, and working alliance in supervisory dyads. *Journal of Multicultural Counseling and Development, 35*(2), 80–91. https://doi.org/10.1002/j.2161-1912.2007.tb00051.x

Cardemil, E. V., & Battle, C. L. (2003). Guess who's coming to therapy? Getting comfortable with conversations about race and ethnicity in psychotherapy. *Professional Psychology: Research and Practice, 34*(3), 278–286. https://doi.org/10.1037/0735-7028.34.3.278

Chang, C. Y., Hays, D. G., & Shoffner, M. F. (2004). Cross-racial supervision: A developmental approach for White supervisors working with supervisees of color. *The Clinical Supervisor, 22,* 121–138.

Comas-Díaz, L., & Jacobsen, F. M. (1995). The therapist of color and the White patient dyad: Contradictions and recognitions. *Cultural Diversity and Mental Health, 1,* 93–106.

Constantine, M. G., & Sue, D. W. (2007). Perceptions of racial microaggressions among Black supervisees in cross-racial dyads. *Journal of Counseling Psychology, 54,* 142–153. doi:10.1037/0022-0167.54.2.142

DeAngelis, T. (2009). Unmasking "racial microaggressions." *Monitor on Psychology, 40,* 42.

Duan, C., & Roehlke, H. (2001). A descriptive snapshot of cross-racial supervision in university counseling center internships. *Journal of Multicultural Counseling and Development, 29,* 131–146. doi:10.1002/j.2161-1912.2001.tb00510.x

Else-Quest, N. M., & Hyde, J. S. (2016). Intersectionality in quantitative psychological research: I. Theoretical and epistemological issues. *Psychology of Women Quarterly,* 1–16. https://doi.org/10.1177/0361684316629797

Falendar, C. A., & Shafranske, E. P. (2004). *Clinical supervision: A competency-based approach.* Washington, DC: American Psychological Association.

Garrett, M. T., Borders, L. D., Crutchfield, L. B., Torres-Rivera, E., Brotherton, D., & Curtis, R. (2001). Multicultural superVISION: A paradigm of cultural responsiveness for supervisors. *Journal of Multicultural Counseling and Development, 29,* 147–158. doi:10.1002/j.2161-1912.2001.tb00511.x

Gatmon, D., Jackson, D., Koshkarian, L., Martos-Perry, N., Molina, A., Patel, N., & Rodolfa, E. (2001). Exploring ethnic, gender, and sexual orientation variables in supervision: Do they really matter? *Journal of Multicultural Counseling and Development, 29,* 102–113. doi:10.1002/j.2161-1912.2001.tb00508.x

Greene, M. P., & Blitz, L. V. (2012). The elephant is not pink: Talking about White, Black, and Brown to achieve excellence in clinical practice. *Clinical Social Work Journal, 40,* 203–212. doi:10.1007/s10615-011-0357-y

Hays, P. A. (2001). *Addressing cultural complexities in practice: A framework for clinicians and counselors.* Washington, DC: American Psychological Association.

Hays, P. A. (2009). Integrating evidence-based practice, cognitive–behavior therapy, and multicultural therapy: Ten steps for culturally competent practice. *Professional Psychology: Research and Practice, 40,* 354–360. https://doi.org/10.1037/a0016250

Jernigan, M. M., Green, C. E., Helms, J. E., Perez-Gualdron, L., & Henze, K. (2010). An examination of people of color supervision dyads: Racial identity matters as much as race. *Training and Education in Professional Psychology, 4*(1), 62–73. https://doi.org/10.1037/a0018110

Ladany, N., Brittan-Powell, C. S., & Pannu, R. K. (1997). The influence of supervisory racial identity interaction and racial matching on the supervisory working alliance and supervisee multicultural competence. *Counselor Education and Supervision, 36,* 284–304. https://doi.org/10.1002/j.1556-6978.1997.tb00396.x

Linder, C., Harris, J. C., Allen, E. L., & Hubain, B. (2015). Building inclusive pedagogy: Recommendations from a national study of students of color in higher education and student affairs graduate programs. *Equity & Excellence in Education, 48,* 178–194. doi:10.1080/10665684.2014.959270

Marable, M. (2002). *The great wells of democracy: The meaning of race in American life.* New York, NY: Basic Books.

McNeill, B. W., Hom, K. L., & Perez, J. A. (1995). The training and supervisory needs of racial and ethnic minority students. *Journal of Multicultural Counseling and Development, 23*(4), 246–258.

Miller, A., Williams, M. T., Wetterneck, C. T., Kanter, J., & Tsai, M. (2015). Using functional analytic psychotherapy to improve awareness and connection in racially diverse client-therapist dyads. *The Behavior Therapist, 38*(6), 150–156.

Okech, J. E. A., & Champe, J. (2008). Informing culturally competent practice through cross-racial friendships. *International Journal for the Advancement of Counselling, 30*(2), 104–115. https://doi .org/10.1007/s10447-008-9049-x

Rattan, A., & Ambady, N. (2013). Diversity ideologies and intergroup relations: An examination of colorblindness and multiculturalism. *European Journal of Social Psychology, 43*(1), 12–21.

Pierce, C. (1970). Offensive mechanisms. In F. Barbour (Ed.), *In the Black seventies* (pp. 265–282). Boston, MA: Porter Sargent.

Stewart, C. E., Lee, S. Y., Hogstrom, A., & Williams, M. T. (2017). Diversify and conquer: A call to promote minority representation in clinical psychology. *The Behavior Therapist, 40*(3), 74–79.

Sue, D. W., Capodilupo, C., Torino, G., Bucceri, J., Holder, A., Nadal, K., & Esquilin, M. (2007). Racial microaggressions in everyday life: Implications for clinical practice. *American Psychologist, 62*, 271–286. doi:10.1037/0003-066X.62.4.271

Sue, D. W., & Sue D. (2013). *Counseling the culturally diverse: Theory and practice* (6th ed.). Hoboken, NJ: John Wiley & Sons.

Terwilliger, J. M., Bach, N., Bryan, C., & Williams, M. T. (2013). Multicultural versus colorblind ideology: Implications for mental health and counseling. In A. Di Fabio (Ed.), *Psychology of counseling* (pp. 111–122). Hauppauge, NY: Nova Science Publishers.

Williams, M. T., Duque, G., & Wetterneck, C. T. (2015, November). Ethnic identity and regional differences as buffers against anxiety and depression in a national sample of African American young adults. In B. A. Feinstein & T. A. Hart (Chairs) & D. Rosmarin (Discussant), *The role of resilience in the health and well-being of minority populations*. Symposium conducted at the Association of Behavioral and Cognitive Therapies, Chicago, IL.

CHAPTER 11

White Parents Raising Black Kids

Anne Blakely Steketee,
Chapman University

Introduction

Mental health professionals treat every cultural group, not just White Americans; because of this, a culturally relevant understanding is needed for specific populations. Race and ethnicity are often specialized issues on the periphery of both training and the practice of psychotherapy (Murry, Smith, & Hill, 2001). As a result, the specific needs of the blended, multicultural family are not a prominent feature in these discussions; therapists counseling White parents who are raising Black children might require specialized support to navigate that particular family paradigm. To address these additional goals, therapists can turn to professional literature analyzing the voice and experience of the White parent in this situation (Rauktis, Goodkind, Fusco, & Bradley-King, 2016; Stone & Dolbin-MacNab, 2017). Allowing lived experiences to inform therapeutic practice allows the various voices of White parents raising Black children to be an added narrative stream. Family history, contextual information for family of origin, and relationships with significant others are necessary components of the counseling intake, which forms the basis for alliance and treatment. Although every family story or parent story might be salient, it is possible that the issues in biracial or multicultural families in America, especially those with White parents, are additionally complex, due to mechanisms of systemic and institutional racism that have formed the dominant parenting paradigm. More than the therapist asking parents to talk about their experiences, there are specific issues that need to be named as racialized, often a problematic undertaking for many of us White parents raised with a Eurocentric outlook.

Multicultural families with White parents are formed in several different ways—through birth, adoption, foster care, or step-parenting—and each way uniquely impacts the dynamics of the family. The issues in narratives of biracial couples who give birth to children differ considerably from foster parents who persevere to maintain placement with an older child. The medical quagmire of infertility treatment lining the path toward certain transracial adoptions impacts families physically and psychologically in ways that differ from the adjustments necessary in families formed by remarriage or re-partnership. In addition, within each family constellation, there can exist numerous other issues of intersectionality; class, gender, ethnicity, citizenship, sexuality, ability, religion, and age are additional areas to consider in addition to race. With this diversity and complexity, how can one story possibly inform therapists about the dynamics that shape transracial family life behind closed doors? It can't. One story cannot possibly stand at the crossroads of all of these dynamics in hopes of speaking for White parents, advocating for Black youth, or allying with ideas that could shift some of the current parenting dilemmas. One story of a White mother who, through adoption, raised a Black son can only hope to introduce this conversation, with some of the attendant themes and issues.

This chapter will feature a story focused on adoption, but it is important for therapists to note that family formation with regard to the White parent–Black child family is likely to add an additional and layered level of complexity as the American family continues to evolve (Potter & Potter, 2016; Smith, Juárez, & Jacobson, 2011). This narrative will intersperse research-based considerations to anchor examples to best practices, as told from the voice of the author, a White mother who is a parent of a Black child and also an educational advocate, university professor, and educational researcher. Although only one story among many, it is part of an important and complex discourse. It is also worth noting that although this chapter is focused on White parents and Black children, many of the issues discussed here could apply to families with other blended racial configurations as well.

Purpose of the Chapter

Each section in this chapter will start with a glimpse into our life as White parents raising a Black child. Balancing these narratives are paired sections with therapeutic considerations drawn from the themes introduced by the family issues—therapeutic recommendations that could be applied in a variety of family circumstances. After a brief introduction to our family, the chapter is divided into these sections: family formation and early development; school issues; complexity of social issues; developing identity; and transition into adulthood. In this way, both the narrative and the analysis move chronologically through the life of the family. The therapeutic strategies are written with a broad hand: they could apply to family therapy with siblings and extended family; many are applicable for parents in dyads or singles; often the strategies could apply to the Black child, youth, or adult. I trust that clinicians will be able to pull from these stories and the accompanying research the information that they will need to assist the families who come to them for culturally responsive help.

Our Adoption Story: Setting the Stage

Because of endometriosis that was not responsive to numerous surgeries and medical interventions, we formed our family through adoption. In its final form, our adopted family included three children: the eldest, a daughter, Asian-Pacific Islander and White;

the middle child, a son, Black and White; and the youngest, a daughter, Latina. Both my husband and I are White, with my husband having immigrated from Holland as a toddler. As part of the arduous adoption process, we were required to attend pre-parenting classes as well as extra classes for transracial adoption and parenting. At various stages in the process, social workers continued to ask us if we were "open" to adopting children who were not White. Because we consider all children equally valuable, to us this question seemed inappropriate.

With all three children, we were very aware of the way that society saw us, saw them, and saw our family. We were often cast as "saviors," with friends and strangers alike exclaiming how wonderful we were to adopt "these" children. People commented on their skin color, wondered about their intelligence, noted Cory's athleticism and remarked that it was because of his race. Our family was seen as strange and different. When we would attend a new event, the people of color had questions ("What are you doing with these children?") and the White public kept a polite distance. We decided early in the life of our family that we would remain in California and not relocate to Texas near family because there were no transracial families in the small southern towns we visited. At least in this geographic location, the children would see families like their own.

When our first daughter was two years old, we adopted our son, Cory. His birth-mother is White; his birthfather, Black. Like many African Americans of mixed heritage, we consider him Black and always have. We met several times with his birthmother and her family. After some legal challenges with Cory's family of origin, we attempted to meet with his birthfather and family several times. This was crucial to us, that both of these families remain an active and present part of Cory's life. Our first daughter's birth-mother lived with us, so we were very comfortable with extended family contact. Unfortunately, adoptive parents cannot control how everyone feels in the adoptive tri-angle, and we were unable to maintain this important link contact with Cory's birthpar-ents. This means that Cory, as a Black child, was raised completely by White adoptive parents. He was raised in a multicultural family; he had immigrant adoptive grandpar-ents who spoke both English and Dutch; he had numerous school placements with many White teachers; he participated in AAU sports much of his childhood, sustaining inju-ries that come from high activity that necessitated medical care from primarily White medical professionals; he lived in an urban setting within walking distance of a public high school with over 80 percent students of color, over 50 percent eligibility for free lunch, and years of not meeting "adequate yearly progress" (AYP—an indicator of aca-demic achievement of students on standardized tests). He is an amazing, intelligent, complex, dynamic young person whom the world sees as a Black man.

Family Formation and Early Development

For the clinician, narratives from all types of families could offer insight for partnering with these families by utilizing specific therapeutic tools. But this chapter cannot encapsulate, nor does it attempt to synopsize, the parenting paradigm of all White families raising Black children; it can, however, offer two benefits by utilizing a narrative lens. First, for clients who are moving slowly toward racial awareness, the use of story can be an effective tool for building awareness and developing identity (Bell, 2010). Second, because some families are not as prepared to acknowledge and discuss racism overtly, clinicians can use narratives to highlight the distinction between reactive parenting and creative parenting, especially with regard to racial socialization (Snyder, 2011; Stevenson, 1995). White families raising Black children have been shown to differ in the communication pattern when processing incidents of racism (reactive socialization), and there is a noted need for White parents to increase both reactive and creative (proactive) socialization practices (McKinney, 2016).

Narrative Reflection

The amount of preparation required when adding a baby to the family is excessive, especially for first-time parents. At the time of adoption, we were told that contact with Cory's birth family might be possible, but when we attempted contact with Cory's birth family we were rebuffed. Looking back, I wish I had pushed the issue more for his sake. Adoptive children, in general, show some benefit from contact with their families of origin, especially if the relationship is well-negotiated (Crea & Barth, 2009; MacDonald & McSherry, 2011). The cultural richness of including more people in our community cannot be underestimated, especially people who love and care for our children. But the most important reason to have included his birth family is that this is his family, his kin. Kinship in the African American culture—a sense of community, of *we*—operates in contrast to the tenants of individualism emphasized in the White culture (Hines & Boyd-Franklin, 2005; Smith et al., 2011). No matter what we might do as a multicultural family, we are not a Black family. This is a balancing act, though, and the respect for people's privacy must be weighed against the needs of a child.

The issue of race can sometimes fade to the background or get lost in the myriad of other family formation details: White parents do not typically think about "race" when they consider parenting issues, because White people do not consider their Whiteness. In this way, Whiteness is said to be invisible (Todd & Abrams, 2011). White people are socialized not to talk about Whiteness. White families do not typically sit around the dinner table discussing issues of fairness, racism, or disenfranchisement, but these conversations about race can and should be initiated within the White community with partners, extended family, friends, circles of support, communities of faith, and neighbors. In our experience, these conversations were naturally occurring with our friends of color but were abnormal and artificial in White company. At the time of Cory's adoption, the only people in our multicultural church who discussed his race were friends of color; interestingly, White friends never commented on his race.

Along with communities of support, we attempted to seek out quality professionals. I considered looking for a Black pediatrician for Cory. Our White pediatrician seemed somewhat offended when I questioned him about his practice. As we sat in the doctor's office for visits, we were the only family of color. Questions about emotional development or reactions to community issues were never raised. As Cory grew, he seemed to feel isolated as he sensed his difference at doctor check-ups. Later we found an orthopedist who had a specialty with athletes and, as a result, worked with many Black young men. He had a natural connection with Cory; they discussed current issues in athletics with other Black men. When Cory was small, this doctor gave us his business card and told us to bypass the hospital in order to get to Cory's treatment as soon as possible. He recognized Cory's ability as an athlete and valued him as a person—even as a six-year-old child.

Although we had books, songs, artwork, holidays, food, and explicit teaching about race and adoption, it cannot be overstated that what seems explicit to adults might not be getting through to children. To hear Cory speak now, he says he did not really come to know he was Black until he was a preteen. This shocks me, and it cannot be emphasized enough. We talked about culture often, but these conversations might need to be daily, explicit conversations. Looking back, our multicultural family identity seemed to subsume his Black ethnoracial identity. A strong positive Black identity has been found to be critical for optimal development of Black children (Williams, Chapman, Buckner, & Durrett, 2016).

Therapeutic Considerations

Therapists working with families who are in the formative stages of building a family have several specific issues of focus that could present in session. Consciousness-raising for White parents of Black children is crucial. If clients who are in the planning or initial stages of family formation do not raise issues of race and ethnicity, then it is essential for therapists to mention these areas as a "check-in" to ascertain how the family is integrating these goals, as applicable, within the family structure.

FAMILY OF ORIGIN

For multiracial families formed by birth or by marriage, issues of family origin might not carry the additional complexity noted in families formed by adoption or fostering. This is not to discount or disrespect the fact that White parents raising Black children face special challenges regardless of how the family is formed. But for families formed outside of adoption, the relationships with extended family members are therapeutic issues for which there are precedents. For transracial families formed by open adoption, the literature and legal picture is not as clear: the child has dueling legal needs as both an individual with the rights that are afforded in American society and as a part of a legally formed family group (Shanley, 2003). Shanley (2003) also argued that children in transracial adoptive families would benefit from a reframe of two key philosophical misidentities: adoptive families "as if" biological families and adoptive children from "parentless" origins. The foster care system mitigates against both of these misunderstandings; foster parents are trained to understand that the origin of the family is unusual and certainly not similar to biological formation. Additionally, foster families do not attempt to maintain a parentless myth. For adoptive families that tend toward this myth, both of these reframes are exceedingly helpful for nudging the adoptive parent toward the idea that the family of origin is a part of the child's life, whether the adoptive parent addresses this reality or not. Therapists working with adoptive and foster families, in particular, might want to recognize the context-specific nature of this family system as they assist clients.

COMMUNITY OF SUPPORT

The transracial family needs additional support through the lifespan. This support often comes from extended family; friends; faith, community, and neighborhood organizations; school or work associates; and more. An obvious application of this is maintaining relationships, especially positive relationships, with people of color. Specifically, for White parents, it is helpful to build relationships with Black people. For me, this seems like a rather foreign concept to be communicating in writing, because it is a seamless part of my life. Friends, coworkers, associates—my community is now and has been one of color. But it is important for therapists to recognize that this is not the case for many White people (Jones, 2014). In fact, the vast majority of White people have no friends of color at all.

Recognizing that not all families live in an environment as ethnically diverse and culturally rich as Southern California, it might be difficult for families to cultivate friendships in communities of homogeneity. The US Census Bureau (2010) lists ten states with fewer than twenty-five thousand Black people in the entire state; five of these states report fewer than ten thousand Black people. This means that communities of support in certain areas might not be diverse ethnically or racially—but they can be diverse with regard to discourse. How we communicate about our family identity, our children's race and culture, and systemic racism in the United States can be a common bond for all types of families in all communities of support. White parents with Black children can and should develop the discourse in their families and extended communities to provide a more nuanced understanding of race in America. Frankly, this means initiating conversations about race—even if this produces feelings of discomfort, as these conversations benefit the developmental adjustment of children of color (Anderson, Rueter, & Lee, 2015).

Therapists are uniquely situated to assist families through these conversations by utilizing several different theoretical tools. Intergroup and outgroup theorizing (Soliz & Rittenour, 2012) provides both a useful framework for conceptual understanding of the many identities in families, as well as a helpful vocabulary that children and adults can use with regard to being or feeling in and out of a group. Nelson and Colaner (2017) extend intergroup work across the idea of family borders; this is especially salient in families with birthparents, stepparents, and supportive cultural or ethnic mentors and family communication theory. This means that sometimes a person appears to be inside or within a border of a family, like a birthparent, but also appears to be outside the border of the family. With cultural mentors and others, embracing the nuanced complexity of border-crossers can support the identity development of Black children (Nelson & Colaner, 2017).

MEDICAL

The therapist can and, at times, should be asking parents to think through issues like medical care. In this way, therapists are encouraging multicultural families to use preventative strategies as opposed to reactive strategies. White families raising Black children need to consider a broader range of medical issues that might be involved than ones in their general experience, such as lactose intolerance, skin rashes, increased risk of sickle cell anemia, and higher levels of infant mortality (Office of Minority Health, 2017). African Americans also experience increased levels of stress due to racial discrimination (Berger & Sarnyai, 2015), which may be compounded further by issues of intersectionality, such as sexual orientation (Cook, Juster, Calebs, Heinze, & Miller, 2017). It can be important that parents find pediatricians who are well-versed in issues facing communities of color, as well as the other issues of intersectionality that are context-specific to the family.

EXPLICIT RACIAL TEACHING

Therapists are uniquely positioned to work with White parents in a safe and non-threatening environment to explore issues of racial construction within the family. Hagerman (2017) emphasized that while some progressive White parents might have discussions around dealing with prejudice or cultivating racial pride, many White parents do not have these same types of discussions about race explicitly, including challenging systems of White supremacy. Contrasting the explicit racial teachings of Black families with those of Whites, the White teachings are rooted in individualism, having a good reputation, and getting along with Whites (Smith et al., 2011). White parents can carefully consider their teachings and work through the underpinnings of these teachings with a trusted professional, like a therapist. In addition, there are some resources available online to assist with this. Visit http://www.newharbinger.com/41962 to download the list of resources.

School Issues

The educational landscape in the United States is pitted with obstacles for minoritized students, particularly for Black students: Black students are overrepresented in special education and in disciplinary activity, like suspensions and expulsions, while underlying theoretical assumptions leverage schools as sources of solutions while casting students and families as progenitors of problems (Haight, Kayama, & Gibson, 2016). Therapists will want to help strengthen educational advocacy strategies with White families raising Black children at every step of the educational journey.

Narrative Reflection

In our family, books, games, music, artwork, food, dolls, clothes, holidays, and magazines, along with family activities, affiliations, and social groups (friends) all became multicultural. Because the presupposition of "Whiteness" was rather pervasive, it took us a while to find an area where we could buy art, cards, games, books, toys, and décor celebrating Black culture (for example, Black Jesus, Black angels, Black children on cards, and so forth). In my practice as an educational advocate and intensive special needs tutor, I came to see that students of color had an unusually difficult time in the educational system at all levels. From kindergarten through graduation, Cory had over eight educational placements. This was not due to relocation; this was due to a confluence of societal, educational, and personal issues. It would be easy for me to spend the rest of the chapter extolling Cory's virtues—he is intelligent, with a quick wit, a compassionate heart, and a natural leadership ability. He is also tall and athletic, which, for people who do not know him, can seem imposing in today's America. We had to fight the repeated suggestion to "test him for special education" or even to consider a stronger, more medical diagnosis; and we had to contend with disengagement and pushout and dropout issues before he finally graduated. The stories that are the most disenfranchised in my repertoire from my educational practice are, in fact, my stories centering on Black youth. In education, I consider this population highly endangered by educational practices and highly undervalued.

Therapeutic Considerations

SCHOOL ISSUES

There are many books written about Black students in the educational system. Therapists working with White parents could recommend any number depending on the age of the student, the gender of the student, and the interest level of the parent (a list is available online at http://www.newharbinger.com/41962). Three key educational issues impacting Black students are implicit bias, disproportionality of special education referrals, and dropout continuum. The therapist working with a family system, with parents, or with an individual student would benefit from understanding these critical foundational issues.

Implicit bias. Social justice therapy focuses on ending oppression as an additional therapeutic objective (Sue & Sue, 2016). When confronting oppression, clinicians and parents might want to believe that teachers and the school system, especially for very young children, are open-minded and open-hearted when it welcomes all children into pre-school and kindergarten. Brown (2016) reported on a Yale study released to the US Administration for Children and Families (ACF) that highlighted that preschool teach-ers not only expected difficulties with Black children but showed particular concern about Black boys. This suggested specific implicit racial biases on the part of preschool teachers against Black boys. Research indicates that young children are aware of this bias and the stigma it implies; racialized knowledge is not *adultcentric* but is also highly mean-ingful in the social lives of children (VanAusdale & Feagin, 2001). If one goal of educa-tion is to improve the lives of students, the positive impact of best practices already is compromised when a group of students has to overcome built-in teacher biases—starting in preschool and continuing through every level of education (Rowley et al., 2014). Therapists working with parents can offer a strengths-based alternative framework and communication strategies for dealing with school personnel. Finally, bias might need to be identified and interrogated. Although such feedback may not be welcome by teachers and administrators, conflict, in these types of social justice cases, could be a natural and healthy result (Sue & Sue, 2016).

Disproportionality in special education. Students in special education are dispropor-tionately students of color (Harry & Klingner, 2014). There is no single explanation for this, but certain factors contribute to the phenomenon, including psychometric test bias; the influence of poverty; unequal opportunity in general education; inadequate special education practices in the areas of referral, assessment, and eligibility; and the misinter-pretation of behavioral issues leading to suspension or expulsion and a cultural mismatch between student and teacher (Skiba et al., 2008; Smith & Tyler, 2010). Factors impacting Black students particularly include teacher anti-Black bias (Harry & Klingner, 2014) and cultural hegemony (Gay, 2010), as well as a dearth of Black teachers who serve as support and role models (Madkins, 2011).

White parents should approach the special education system with caution. If they feel their child should not be identified or even evaluated, therapists should encourage these parents to listen carefully to that viewpoint. On the other hand, if parents feel strongly that their child would benefit from special education services, then initiating the Individualized Education Program (IEP) evaluation process is of paramount importance (US Department of Education, 2007). Support from professionals is often needed when parents are initiating this process with the school.

Dropping out as a continuum. Students who feel engaged and motivated are more likely to remain in school, while students who are disengaged are more likely to drop out (Henry, Knight, & Thornberry, 2011). Dropping out, though, is not just one discrete act that occurs because of one issue but is conceived of as a continuum with the final act—leaving school—the culmination of a long series of actions (Sweeten, Bushway, & Paternoster, 2009). These actions that end in disengagement or dropping out might begin with disciplinary referrals, low test scores, and increasing truancy. Certain external behaviors, then, become the antecedents of the actual act of dropping out or disengaging.

Black male dropouts unpacked. Student dropout rates are improving, especially for Black and Hispanic students (Fry, 2014). This means that the White-Black gap is closing, albeit slowly (Addis & Withington, 2016). However, Black students have a higher chance of dropping out than White students. Suspensions, retentions, and teacher and parental factors contribute to the gap between the two groups, with suspension the most significant contributor, which functions to push Black students from school (Suhyun, Malchow, & Jingyo, 2014). Siler (2015) described engagement, *verve* (a cultural energy reflecting the Black ethnicity), and teacher connection as important components for assisting students with staying in school. Kunjufu (2002) referred to teacher relationships as a necessary component for school success for Black males. This teaching relationship includes using classroom strategies that are community based; collectivistic Afrocentric traditions are at odds with American school traditions of competition, so the use of more cooperative methodology is a strong part of the teacher-student relationship because it opens avenues of trust (Siler, 2015).

THERAPEUTIC SUGGESTIONS FOR ADVOCACY

The counseling relationship equips individuals and families to work toward wholeness and wellness utilizing a value-neutral approach (Harrist & Richardson, 2011). There are times, though, when social issues and the need for advocacy are so compelling that they overcome the desire for "therapeutic objectivity." When confronted with the disproportionate realities of the American public school system with the concomitant life expectancy results inherent in a lack of access to a quality education, at best, and systemic racism, at worst, it is crucial that therapists adopt a social justice stance. Therapists can respond to the realities of social injustice by working with parents in the following areas: coaching parents to interact with teachers, guiding parents to gather crucial information, and equipping parents with tools for analyzing systemic racism in their child's classroom.

Coach parents with the teacher-student relationship. Until the educational picture improves in America, therapists can work with parents to strengthen or build the teacher-Black student relationship. The need for parent involvement cannot be underemphasized. Therapists can encourage parents to utilize a variety of strategies. Schedule time to meet with the teacher; utilize technology for Skype or other virtual meeting sites if parents or teachers cannot meet immediately after school (consider before school or lunch time). Share the story of family formation. Try to accentuate to the teacher one area that the child really enjoys or excels in. For example, "My son loves art! If you need any posters made for class, he can help with that!" In this way, the parent is cementing in the teacher's mind a positive (and helpful) trait. Finally, it is important for parents to remember that school is a *culture* itself. Children can learn to code-switch. There is academic or *school talk* and *school rules* and neighborhood or home talk and rules. The idea that school is a culture of its own, one that can be mastered with specific cultural rules, but one that is certainly in no way better than their community of origin, is eye- and heart-opening to students of all ethnicities and learning profiles.

Guide parents with information on the lasting impact of pushing out. In the counseling relationship, when White parents begin to describe their child's sense of disengagement and disenfranchisement from school—especially in the teacher-student relationship—this is especially problematic and an indicator that the Black student is at greater risk for *pushing out*. A parent might be in great distress at this point; much of the counseling could be focused on supporting the parent and decreasing family stress. However, there is another task for the therapist at this crucial crossroad: being an information conduit regarding the devastating lifespan impact of dropout or pushout on a person's life advantages. These may seem like "educational issues"—and statistical ones, at that—but they are truly life-long family systems issues, especially when Black children who have been pushed out of the system enter into cycles of poverty, or worse. The longer students stay in education, the more their life outcomes potentially improve (OECD, 2016). They have more job choices—couched in the terms of *considerable advantages* when it comes to job selection—earn more money, have better mental and physical health, and even live longer, not just in the United States but even internationally (Covaleskie, 2014; OECD, 2016; Pew Research Center, 2014). These advantages show that there are protective or enhancing factors that can affect a student throughout the lifespan. For Black students facing societal racism, which is institutionalized at every level, the advantages diminish quickly. White parents need therapists to arm them with clear and direct information.

Equip parents with tools for evaluating systemic school issues. Disengagement and engagement are both complex; what is clear is that there appears to be an engagement gap between White and Black students, with White students reporting more engagement (Yazzie-Mintz, 2007). Clinicians can introduce parents to the idea of vigilance in the classroom space, for example, to notice where children are sitting in the classroom. Anecdotally, Black parents tell stories about walking into their child's class and being dismayed to see that their son or daughter is sitting off in a corner or right up by the teacher (separated from the other students). Therapists with knowledge of discipline systems can explain to White parents about Positive Behavior Intervention System (PBIS), as opposed to a suspension and expulsion system (suspension and expulsion disproportionately works against students of color), and they can encourage parent-teacher meetings so White parents can meet personally with teachers to introduce their child in order to describe their child's strengths. Much of the conversation around Black students (Black males, in particular) is focused on deficits (Howard, 2014), which then normalizes racism (Duncan, 2002); this is a stepping stone toward disengagement, which often begins with overrepresentation in discipline referrals, suspensions, and expulsions.

Parents can role-play with therapists to begin to shift the conversation away from the idea that Black students are the problem.

Complexity of Social Issues

To develop an understanding or vernacular for processing social issues requires cultural socialization, not just ethnic awareness and pride, but also an acknowledgement of institutional privilege and racism (Smith et al., 2011).

Narrative Reflection

As our family developed, our need for both a conceptual understanding of social issues and a language for which to process social issues also developed. With our children, we lived through and tried to discuss the police acquittal and subsequent Los Angeles Riots in 1992; the O. J. Simpson trial in 1994–1995; 9/11; and even the beginning of the Occupy Wall Street movement in 2011. Many of these social issues leveraged a law enforcement component. When we formed our family, our view about interactions with law enforcement were naïve and simplified; they were unexplored, with untested assumptions. As the children grew, we began to note that the police became more interested in the many children of color who visited our home for tutoring or socializing. As the police interest became more specific and intrusive, our family had to find a new language to discuss our relationship with law enforcement and a new lens through which to see law enforcement. I struggled with compliance and politeness on the one hand, and injustice, hegemony, and authoritarianism on the other hand. Because we had used a simplistic "critical thinking" framework for exploring social issues, I began to apply this to our relationship with law enforcement. The method, which I describe more fully in the next section, gathers the history of an issue, explores pros and cons, and seeks to come to a new understanding.

As the police presence and rigidity increased, we experienced friction notable between people who have different worldviews. I initiated my critical thinking framework by gathering narratives of Black friends of mine and Cory's, to see how their experiences with law enforcement differed from mine. Additionally, I read some articles about policing in communities of color. Cory and I talked through the pros and cons of compliance versus noncompliance, with special emphasis on the difference between a White woman complying with the police and a Black man complying with the police. In the end, Cory understood more clearly that his response to law enforcement involved his actual safety (he was close to six feet tall at the time); for my part, I understood that, due to the history of contention in this relationship, I could modify my approach and center Cory's needs as primary when approached by law enforcement. In other words, I learned to be more cautious, with eyes more opened. I trusted the narratives I heard more and the media images I had received less.

Therapeutic Considerations

SOCIAL ISSUES

I utilized a framework for having conversations about social issues, considering four aspects: *old-pro-con-new*.

- Old: I use the word *old* to reflect the history of an issue. How far back you trace an issue is up to you. I usually am comfortable tracing an issue back far enough so that I feel like I can teach it in about five minutes to someone.

- Pro and con: This is an exploration of both sides of the issue.

- New: This is any update that might be necessary to inform your viewpoint…or even change your viewpoint. This new information might help you have continued conversations.

As an example for parents today, therapists could help families use a similar framework to process the complex racial and social issue of police shootings of young Black men. Beginning with *old*, White parents can work to trace the foundation and historicity of Black mortality through *legal intervention* (Krieger, Kiang, Chen, & Waterman, 2015). Next, therapists could guide families through the variance of opinion traced in the social development of Black Lives Matter, All Lives Matter, and Blue Lives Matter. Finally, the last step involves not only arriving at a statement of new understanding but also being able to accurately state the other person's new statement (if another person is involved). Sometimes, White parents might cycle through *old-pro-con-new* on their own, without children. Conversely, a Black youth might it useful to work through this type of strategy when faced with an unfamiliar social construction. The *old-pro-con-new* might be a cognitive framework that could shape discussions and be of benefit to the family system, especially if introduced and practiced within the safety of a caring therapeutic alliance.

Multicultural family life does not take place isolated from social issues and pressures. Therapists can assist White parents with developing a framework for conversations similar to the one above or altogether different. The important point is that White parents begin and continue the conversations, when age appropriate, with their Black children about issues like the N-word, implicit and explicit racism, police shootings of Black males, microaggressions and microinvalidations, Black Lives Matter, and more. As White parents develop these conversations about social issues within the family, they form an awareness of the differences and similarities that sometimes surface between the opinion frames of these communities, and understand fully—from an informed, historical viewpoint—the antecedents of these viewpoints.

COMMUNICATION

In America, much of the racial construction of the above social issues is formed through the use of language. We use language in school, dialog through language online, and receive our information 24/7 through a constant stream of news media, parsing every phrase, every nuance, every tweet. Clinicians can work with White parents to interrogate the roots of their beliefs about the world, because these beliefs bubble up into language every day.

Ridley, Chih, and Olivera (2000) made a strong case for therapists' clinical dispositions and therapeutic decisions being informed by their own cultural schemas. The researchers encouraged clinicians to resolve cultural schema incongruence with clients. In the same way, therapists can use these same skills to assist White clients toward cultural congruity with their Black children. Toward this end, Sleeter (2013) described a framework to explain this juxtaposition of language and worldviews based on conflict theory: in society, there are the dominant groups and the oppressed groups. The dominant groups see the *nature of society* as fair and open, while the oppressed groups see the same *nature* as unfair and rigged—completely different views, depending on the group with which you affiliate. Due to pervasiveness of the dominant cultural worldview, a racial lens or *racial frame* (Feagin, 2010) can be a useful paradigm through which to evaluate societal differences. For example, having conversations at home can prepare a child for conversations at school after an incident of police violence against Blacks, or even in response to increased bullying (US Department of Education, 2016). Therapists can work with parents to help children see that part—not all, but part—of what is happening in the public discourse and in the discourses they might face in school, in the neighborhood, and in the community is a theoretical difference; this can help ground them and give them a language for dealing with conflict. By clinicians modeling the application of a theoretical lens, clients can learn one more useful tool.

Developing Identity

A healthy identity is important for all people; for the Black community, a strong ethnic identity is positively related to mental health and may function as a protective factor (Williams, Chapman, Wong, & Turkheimer, 2012). Many White parents raising Black children are not equipped for the daily task of developing identity, especially Black identity (Smith et al., 2011).

Narrative Reflection

For our family, Black identity formation was a combination of "push" and "pull." By this, I mean that we worked hard to add positive cultural identity formation teaching, conversations, and experiences (push), and we worked equally hard at extinguishing negative cultural identity formation (racist) teaching, conversations, and experiences (pull). Because of my educational practice and family of color, I had converging interests in the issues of race. I experienced silence around issues of race in the White community, but once I started engaging in conversations with my friends of color, I realized that these families had these conversations on a daily basis—not because they chose to, but because they had to.

As our multicultural identity grew, our friendship circle included many Black friends. My home-based tutoring practice was entirely students of color. During this time, Cory and his older sister became very involved in basketball. We paved the backyard to make a half-court basketball court so he could practice out back and have friends from the team over. We read biographies of Black role models in sports, history, and public life. When I homeschooled Cory, I used curriculum that was Afrocentric. Even teaching him to read, I found readers that featured a Black cowboy. These were pushes.

The pulls are probably areas that Cory might not have been as aware of until he was older. I exited social situations when I perceived racial bias. I noticed unfair scrutiny of Cory in stores when we shopped. When I corrected the language of people with racism, I was countered with, "Can't you take a joke?" I remember telling people in my family of origin that I would have to sever contact with them if they could not adjust their attitude toward my family and toward Black people in particular. When Cory was older, we would talk about the differing treatment in stores, driving while Black, and policing reactions. These are complex pulls.

It is probable that our "family identity as multicultural" clashed with his "personal identity as Black," because even with all of our work to develop a family identity as multicultural, Cory's feelings of identity incongruence were at odds with our supposed positive family identity. Vera, Buhin, and Shin (2006) asserted that integrating culturally sensitive material into education is most effective not as an add-on or an afterthought, but rather as a persistent and ongoing exposure to positive messages in the face of institutional racism. The same is true with families; cultural identity is not formed through Black History month or Martin Luther King Jr. Day, but rather through ongoing daily lifestyle of cultural identity development.

Therapeutic Considerations

DEVELOPING IDENTITY

Clinicians are situated to support White parents with one of the most difficult yet important parenting tasks for transracial families: to help children develop a strong ethnoracial identity (Eccles, Wong, & Peck, 2006). Black parents recognize that having a strong ethnoracial identity provides a protective factor against mental health problems, which gives children tools for dealing with discrimination in society (Williams et al., 2012). The theories addressing identity for Black children, especially Black males, are numerous, complex, and—thankfully—gaining traction in research and literature (see Williams et al., 2016).

Cultural identity formation is not something that White families typically think about for their White children; because *Whiteness* is the dominant racial construction in social institutions and practices, White parents have the privilege of just *assuming* adaptive cultural formation (Hughey, 2010). For ethnoracial minority children, though, and especially Black children in America, this cultural formation cannot be taken for granted.

Black identity is complex and can be impacted by socioeconomic factors, age, family, and friends (Sullivan & Platenburg, 2017). Media images have a strong impact on Black identity, as do the lived experiences of the individuals themselves (Howard, 2014). Nobles (2013) encouraged a consideration of spiritual and family dimensions when working with Black clients. The plethora of information concerning Black identity formation is offset by a diversity within the African American culture, as identified by scholars providing information to clinicians (Hines & Boyd-Franklin, 2005). For therapists working with White parents, it is important to express to parents that identity formation is just that: formation. Parents need to take an active part, even though identity issues are multilayered and complex. Howard (2014) noted that identity development involves not just age, race, and place, but also ways of being and knowing. The daily *check-in* with the child cannot just end with, "How was school today?" or "Anything new at basketball practice?" but needs to reach beneath the surface to gently probe, in an age-appropriate way, relationships with authority, additional interactions with other groups of students, and—especially—for those narratives that sound like racism. Therapists can help White parents learn to validate and legitimate these stories as a first and necessary step toward building identity in their Black children.

Transition into Adulthood

As Black youth develop into adults, racial identity continues to be salient and protective (Stock et al., 2017). Identity formation, though, is also impacted by social issues as young people step into adult roles. Glaude (2007) described Black identity formation in America as uniquely linked not just to social issues but to ethical ones as well. Glaude reflected that it is possible, among several varying approaches to Black identity, to consider a pragmatic approach within the context of changing and developing social issues, like racialized experiences with law enforcement.

Narrative Reflection

If White parents are raising Black boys, they are going to need to address the issue of contact with the police as the boys develop. Because of police stereotypes about Black men, any encounter with police is potentially life-threatening—whether or not the target is involved in any wrongdoing. My son is large. I had to talk to him about lowering his voice; complying with law enforcement immediately; using eye contact; speaking before moving; and, in certain situations, asking permission before moving. And under no circumstances was he to turn his back and run from the police or make a sudden movement to put his hand in his pocket. These are life-and-death conversations, but these are not typically White dinner conversations, because this issue does not typically pertain to

White people. These conversations are not one-time conversations; they are lifespan issues that require numerous conversations. I think of this as a "cycle" issue—we will cycle through this conversation at just about every developmental milestone.

Therapeutic Considerations

DEALING WITH POLICE INTERACTIONS

Regardless of White parents' viewpoints toward the issue of police brutality, Black Lives Matter, and the subsequent protests that have followed in the public sphere and in sports, there are links between police brutality and decreased health outcomes for Black people (Alang, McAlpine, McCreedy, & Hardeman, 2017). The definition of police brutality is hard to agree upon but, regardless of the definition, Feldman, Chen, Waterman, and Krieger (2016) found that incidents of violence from police, noted in the literature as *legal intervention*, is 4.9 times more likely for a Black person as for a White person. Additionally, when society as a whole underreacts to these injuries and deaths, this increases stress in communities of color, which, in turn, decreases productivity and economic viability in these same communities. White communities see police action in completely different ways from communities of color (AP-NORC Center for Public Affairs Research, 2017). Therapists can not only provide updated public health information to White parents but also share with parents the discrete differences between the viewpoints about law enforcement that are likely, especially from their White family of origin and their children's developing peer- and community-support system. By sharing information, White parents have a glimpse into the stressors that their children will grow to face within American society.

Conclusion

As a White parent of a Black child, I share my experience with the therapeutic community in hope that there might be some usefulness here for clients who are part of families raising Black children. From the early development of the family, specific issues of race and ethnicity can be supported in therapeutic milieus. Adoptive families might benefit from reframes of the adoptive experience (Shanley, 2003). While White parents might seem overwhelmed with the details of family formation, therapists can provide support and information about the differences in medical and explicit racial differences between White and Black communities.

As children progress through the educational system, clinicians will be aware of how implicit bias, disproportionality of special education referrals, and the dropout continuum particularly impact Black children. Therapists can encourage parents to be active participants and advocates with the educational system. In addition to educational role-playing, clinicians can initiate conversations with White parents around social issues and language-based strategies for discussing oppression. This therapeutic alliance will be of benefit to White parents who will need guidance with strengthening Black identity in their children at every stage of development (Sullivan & Platenburg, 2017).

Although families with White parents and Black children are formed in a variety of ways, there are some issues that appear to be universal. Children need access to quality medical treatment, they require equitable schooling, and they deserve protection within society from fear of brutality. Children, regardless of family formation or other issues of intersectionality, will face systemic racism through the lifespan. And families or individuals who are seeking assistance from therapists will benefit from a therapeutic alliance formed on a foundation of culturally inclusive information, strategies, and practices. The more context-specific this alliance can be, the more responsive to the particular issues that could arise in the moment. In one brief chapter, there is no way to anticipate all of the possible issues with every family constellation in this transracial paradigm; it is possible, however, to frontload the idea that White parents, no matter how progressive or attuned to cultural issues, will continually need to develop strategies to mitigate the effects of White racial socialization (Hagerman, 2017). By working together, therapists and parents can fine-tune the interventions needed to take the next step, both for transracial families and, hopefully, for our multiracial society.

KEY POINTS FOR CLINICIANS

- Tease out which issues are adoption or fostering issues, extended family acceptance issues, community acceptance issues, or racial identity issues.

- Teach White families how to have explicit conversations about race that are race-intentional and not race-avoidant, by utilizing explicit teaching and then fading supports as White parents develop their own language.

- Introduce parents to the idea of "racialized habits" to help families take a smaller step into conversations about racism, especially if racism is too hard for White parents to deal with at first.

- Reflect a clear picture of educational inequities and serve as a resource provider for White parents who lack exposure to this important information.

- Encourage parents to consider a broad range of educational placements for students who are disengaged, such as online, continuation, independent, alternative, community college, correspondence, and blended options to help students reengage.

- Advocate for parents to carefully weigh all options before accepting a special education placement, due to racial disproportionalities inherent in the special education system.

References

Addis, S., & Withington, M. C. (2016). Improving high school graduation rates among males of color. *National Dropout Prevention Center/Network*. Princeton, NJ: Robert Wood Johnston Foundation

Alang, S., McAlpine, D., McCreedy, E., & Hardeman, R. (2017). Police brutality and Black health: Setting the agenda for public health scholars. *American Journal of Public Health, 107*(5), 662–665. doi:10.2105/AJPH.2017.303691

Anderson, K. N., Rueter, M. A., & Lee, R. M. (2015). Discussions about racial and ethnic differences in internationally adoptive families: Links with family engagement, warmth, & control. *Journal of Family Communication, 15*(4), 289–308. doi:10.1080/15267431.2015.1076420

AP-NORC Center for Public Affairs Research. (2017). *Law enforcement and violence: The divide between Black and White Americans. Issue brief.* The Associated Press-NORC Center for Public Affairs Research at the University of Chicago. Retrieved from http://www.apnorc.org/projects/

Bell, L. A. (2010). *Storytelling for social justice: Connecting narrative and the arts in antiracist teaching.* New York, NY: Routledge.

Berger, M., & Sarnyai, Z. (2014). "More than skin deep": Stress neurobiology and mental health consequences of racial discrimination. *Stress, 18*(1), 1–10. doi:10.3109/10253890.2014.989204

Brown, E. (2016, September 27). Yale study suggests racial bias among preschool teachers. *The Washington Post.* Retrieved from http://www.highbeam.com/doc/1P2-40085621.html?refid=easy_hf

Cook, S. H., Juster, R., Calebs, B. J., Heinze, J., & Miller, A. L. (2017). Short communication: Cortisol profiles differ by race/ethnicity among young sexual minority men. *Psychoneuroendocrinology, 75,* 1–4. doi:10.1016/j.psyneuen.2016.10.006

Costello, M. B. (2016). *The Trump effect: The impact of the presidential campaign on our nation's schools.* Montgomery, AL: Southern Poverty Law Center.

Covaleskie, J. F. (2014). What good is college? The economics of college attendance. *Philosophical Studies in Education, 45,* 93–101. Retrieved from http://ovpes.org/journal

Crea, T. M., & Barth, R. P. (2009). Patterns and predictors of adoption openness and contact: 14 years postadoption. *Family Relations, 58*(5), 607–620. doi.org/10.1111/j.1741-3729.2009.00578.x

Dei, G. J. (2005). An introduction. In G. J. Dei & G. Johal (Eds.). *Critical issues in anti-racist research methodologies* (pp. 1–27). New York, NY: Lang.

Duncan, G. A. (2002). Beyond love: A critical race ethnography of the schooling of adolescent Black males. *Equity & Excellence in Education, 35*(2), 131–143. doi.org/10.1080/713845286

Eccles, J. S., Wong, C. A., & Peck, S. C. (2006). Ethnicity as a social context for the development of African American adolescents. *Journal of School Psychology, 44,* 407–426. doi:10.1016/j.jsp.2006.04.001

Feagin, J. R. (2010). *The White racial frame: Centuries of racial framing and counter-framing.* New York, NY: Routledge.

Feldman J. M., Chen, J. T., Waterman, P. D., Krieger, N. (2016). Temporal trends and racial/ ethnic inequalities for legal intervention injuries treated in emergency departments: US men and women age 15–34, 2001–2014. *Journal of Urban Health, 93*(5), 797–807. doi:10.1007/s11524-016-00763

Fry, R. (2014). US high school dropout rate reaches record low, driven by improvements among Hispanics, Blacks. *Pew Research Center.* Retrieved from http://www.pewresearch.org/fact-tank/2014/10/02/u-s-high-school-dropout-rate-reaches-record-low-driven-by-improvements-among-hispanics-blacks/

Gay, G. (2010). *Culturally responsive teaching: Theory, research, and practice.* New York, NY: Teachers College Press.

Glaude, E. S. (2007). *In a shade of blue: Pragmatism and the politics of Black America.* Chicago: University of Chicago Press.

Hagerman, M. A. (2017). White racial socialization: Progressive fathers on raising "antiracist" children. *Journal of Marriage & Family, 79*(1), 60–74. doi:10.1111/jomf.12325

Haight, W., Kayama, M., & Gibson, P. A. (2016). Out-of-school suspensions of Black youths: Culture, ability, disability, gender, and perspective. *Social Work, 61*(3), 235–243. doi:10.1093/sw/sww021

Harrist, S., & Richardson, F. C. (2012). Disguised ideologies in counseling and social justice work. *Counseling and Values, 57*(1), 38–44. doi:10.1002/j.2161-007x.2012.00006.x

Harry, B., & Klingner, J. K. (2014). *Why are so many minority students in special education? Understanding race and disability in schools.* New York, NY: Teachers College Press.

Henry, K. K., Knight, K., & Thornberry, T. (2012). School disengagement as a predictor of dropout, delinquency, and problem substance use during adolescence and early adulthood. *Journal of Youth & Adolescence, 41*(2), 156–166. https://doi.org/10.1007/s10964-011-9665-3

Hines, P. M., & Boyd-Franklin, N. (2005). African American families. In M. McGoldrick, J. Giordano, & N. Garcia-Preto, (Eds.), *Ethnicity and family therapy* (pp. 87–100). New York, NY: Guilford Press.

Howard, T. C. (2014). *Black male(d): Peril and promise in the education of African American males.* New York, NY: Teachers College Press.

Hughey, M. W. (2010). The (dis) similarities of white racial identities: The conceptual framework of "hegemonic whiteness." *Ethnic and Racial Studies, 33*(8), 1289–1309. doi.org/10.1080/01419870903125069

Jones, R. P. (2014, August 21). Self-segregation: Why it's so hard for Whites to understand Ferguson. *The Atlantic.*

Krieger, N., Kiang, M. V., Chen, J. T., & Waterman, P. D. (2015). Trends in US deaths due to legal intervention among black and white men, age 15–34 years, by county income level: 1960–2010. *Harvard Public Health Review, 3*, 1–5. Retrieved from http://harvardpublichealthreview.org/190/

Kunjufu, J. (2002). *Black students, middle-class teachers.* Chicago, IL: African American Images.

Lee, R. (2003). The transracial adoption paradox: History, research, and counseling implication of cultural socialization. *The Counseling Psychologist, 31*, 711–744. doi:10.1177/0011000003258087

MacDonald, M., & McSherry, D. (2011). Open adoption: Adoptive parents' experiences of birth family contact and talking to their child about adoption. *Adoption & Fostering, 35*(3), 4–16. doi.org/10.1177/030857591103500302

Madkins, T. C. (2011). The Black teacher shortage: A literature review of historical and contemporary trends. *The Journal of Negro Education, 80*(3), 417–427. Retrieved from http://www.journalnegroed.org/recentissues.htm

McKinney, N. S. (2016). *Biracial adult children raised by White mothers: The development of racial identity and role of racial socialization.* Dissertation Abstracts International: Section B: The Sciences and Engineering, Vol 77(11–B)(E). Drexel University.

Murry, V. M., Smith, E. P., & Hill, N. E. (2001). Race, ethnicity, and culture in studies of families in context. *Journal of Marriage and Family, 63*(4), 911–914. doi.org/10.1111/j.1741-3737.2001.00911.x

Nelson, L., & Colaner, L. R. (2017). Becoming a transracial family: Communicatively negotiating divergent identities in families formed through transracial adoption. *Journal of Family Communication, 18*(1), 51–67. doi:10.1080/15267431.2017.1396987

Nobles, W. W. (2013). Shattered consciousness, fractured identity: Black psychology and the restoration of the African psyche. *Journal of Black Psychology, 39*(3), 232–242. doi:10.1177/0095798413478075

OECD. (2016). Education at a Glance 2016 | OECD READ edition. doi:10.1787/eag-2016-en

Office of Minority Health (OMH). (2017, November 9). *Infant mortality and African Americans.* US Department of Health and Human Services Office of Minority Health. Retrieved from https://minorityhealth.hhs.gov/omh/browse.aspx?lvl=4&lvlid=23

Okeke-Adeyanju, N., Taylor, L. C., Craig, A. B., Smith, R. E., Thomas, A., Boyle, A. E., & DeRosier, M. E. (2014). Celebrating the strengths of black youth: Increasing self-esteem and implications for prevention. *Journal of Primary Prevention, 35*(5), 357–369. doi:10.1007/s10935-014-0356

Pew Research Center. (2014, February 11). The rising cost of not going to college. *Pew Social Trends.* Retrieved from http://www.pewsocialtrends.org/2014/02/11/the-rising-cost-of-not-going-to-college/

Potter, D., & Potter, E. C. (2016). Psychosocial well-being in children of same-sex parents: A longitudinal analysis of familial transitions. *Journal of Family Issues, 38*(16), 2303–2328. doi:0192513 X16646338.

Rauktis, M. E., Goodkind, S., Fusco, R. A., & Bradley-King, C. (2016). Motherhood in liminal spaces: White mothers' parenting Black/White children. *Affilia-Journal of Women and Social Work, 31*(4), 434–449. https://doi.org/10.1177/0886109916630581

Ridley, C. R., Chih, D. W., & Olivera, R. J. (2000). Training in cultural schemas: An antidote to unintentional racism in clinical practice. *American Journal of Orthopsychiatry,* (1), 65–72. doi.org/10 .1037/h0087771

Ross, W. (2016). *Counseling African American males: Effective therapeutic interventions and approaches.* Charlotte, NC: Information Age Publishing.

Rowley, S., Ross, L., Lozada, F., Williams, A., Gale, A., & Kurtz-Costes, B. (2014). Framing Black boys: Parent, teacher, and student narratives of the academic lives of Black boys. *Role of Gender in Educational Contexts and Outcomes, 47,* 301–332. doi:10.1016/bs.acdb.2014.05.003

Shanley, M. (2003). Toward new understandings of adoption: Individuals and relationships in transracial and open adoption. *Nomos, 44,* 15–57. Retrieved from http://www.political-theory.org /index.php?/nomos

Siler, D. S. (2015). *Voices in the hall: A Black male student centered examination of engagement in urban middle school art class* (Doctoral dissertation). Retrieved from Temple University Electronic Theses & Dissertations.

Skiba, R. J., Simmons, A. B., Ritter, S., Gibb, A. C., Rausch, M. K., Cuadrado, J., & Chung, C. (2008). Achieving equity in special education: History, status, and current challenges. *Exceptional Children, 74*(3), 264–288. doi:10.1177/001440290807400301

Sleeter, C. E. (2013). *Power, teaching, and teacher education: Confronting injustice with critical research and action.* New York, NY: P. Lang.

Smith, D. T., Juárez, B. G., & Jacobson, C. K. (2011). *White parents, Black children: Experiencing transracial adoption.* Lanham, MD: Rowman & Littlefield Publishers

Smith, D., & Tyler, N. (2010). *Introduction to special education: Making a difference.* Upper Saddle River, NJ: Merrill/Prentice Hall.

Snyder, C. R. (2011). Racial socialization in cross-racial families. *Journal of Black Psychology, 38*(2), 228–253. doi:10.1177/0095798411416457

Soliz, J., & Rittenour, C. E. (2012). Family as an intergroup arena. In H. Giles (Ed.), *Handbook of intergroup communication* (pp. 331–343). New York, NY: Routledge.

Stevenson, H. C. (1995). Relationship of adolescent perceptions of racial socialization to racial identity. *Journal of Black Psychology, 21*(1), 49–70. doi:10.1177/00957984950211005

Stock, M. L., Gibbons, F. X., Beekman, J. B., Williams, K. D., Richman, L. S., & Gerrard, M. (2017). Racial (vs. self) affirmation as a protective mechanism against the effects of racial exclusion on negative affect and substance use vulnerability among Black young adults. *Journal of Behavioral Medicine, 41*(2), 195–207. doi:10.1007/s10865-017-9882-7

Stone, D., & Dolbin-MacNab, M. (2017). Racial socialization practices of White mothers raising Black-White biracial children. *Contemporary Family Therapy: An International Journal, 39*(2), 97–111. doi:10.1007/s10591-017-9406-1

Sue, D. W. (2010). *Microaggressions in everyday life: Race, gender, and sexual orientation.* Hoboken, NJ: John Wiley & Sons.

Sue, D. W., & Sue, D. (2016). *Counseling the culturally diverse: Theory and practice.* Hoboken, NJ: John Wiley & Sons.

Suhyun, S., Malchow, A., & Jingyo, S. (2014). Why did the Black-White dropout gap widen in the 2000s? *Educational Research Quarterly, 37*(4), 19–40. Retrieved from http://erquarterly.org/

Sullivan, J. M., & Platenburg, G. N. (2017). From Black-ish to blackness: An analysis of Black information sources' influence on Black identity development. *Journal of Black Studies, 48*(3), 215–234. doi:10.1177/0021934716685845

Sweeten, G., Bushway, S., & Paternoster, R. (2009). Does dropping out of school mean dropping into delinquency? *Criminology, 47*(1), 47–91. doi:10.1111/j.1745-9125.2009.00139.x

Tatum, B. D. (2008). *Can we talk about race? And other conversations in an era of school resegregation.* Boston, MA: Beacon.

Todd, N. R., & Abrams, E. M. (2011). White dialectics: A new framework for theory, research and practice with White students. *Counseling Psychologist, 39,* 353–395. doi.org/10.1177/001100 0010377665

US Census Bureau (2011). *The Black Population: 2010. 2010 Census Briefs.* Retrieved from https://www .census.gov/prod/cen2010/briefs/c2010br-06.pdf

US Department of Education. (2007). *Guide to the Individualized Education Program.* Retrieved from https://www2.ed.gov/parents/needs/speced/iepguide/index.html

US Department of Education, National Center for Education Statistics. (2017). *The NCES Fast Facts Tool provides quick answers to many education questions.* Retrieved from https://nces.ed.gov/fast facts/display.asp?id=719

VanAusdale D., & Feagin, J. (2001). *The first R: How children learn race and racism.* Lanham, MD: Rowman & Littlefield.

Vera, E. M., Buhin, L., & Shin, R. Q. (2006). The pursuit of social justice and the elimination of racism. In M. G. Constantine and D. W. Sue (Eds.), *Addressing racism: Facilitating cultural competence in mental health and educational settings* (pp. 271–287). Hoboken, NJ: John Wiley & Sons.

Williams, M. T., Chapman, L. K., Buckner, E., & Durrett, E. (2016). Cognitive behavioral therapy. In A. Breland-Noble, C. S. Al-Mateen, & N. N. Singh (Eds.), *Handbook of Mental Health in African American Youth.* Cham, Switzerland: Springer.

Williams, M. T., Chapman, L. K., Wong, J., & Turkheimer, E. (2012). The role of ethnic identity in symptoms of anxiety and depression in African Americans. *Psychiatry Research, 199*(1), 31–36. doi.org/10.1016/j.psychres.2012.03.049

Yazzie-Mintz, E. (2007). *Voices of students on engagement: A report on the 2006 High School Survey of Student Engagement.* Bloomington, IN: Center for Evaluation and Education Policy, Indiana University.

PART 3

Structural Mental Health Disparities

Strategies for Increased Racial Diversity and Inclusion in Graduate Psychology Programs

Erin N. Arney,
Bastyr University

Sharon Y. Lee,
University of Connecticut

Destiny M. B. Printz,
University of Connecticut

Catherine E. Stewart,
University of Connecticut

Sylvie P. Shuttleworth,
Bastyr University

Introduction

The need to diversify the field of psychology has received increased attention in recent years (Stewart, Lee, Hogstrom, & Williams, 2017). Ideological commitments to equity have assisted in motivating these changes, as students, professors, and administrators recognize the benefits of a racially diverse cohort of students (Bowen & Bok, 2016). The American Psychological Association (APA) requires clinical and counseling psychology graduate programs to make efforts toward diversifying their faculties and student bodies (APA, 2016). Due to individual and systemic efforts to increase diversity, students within psychology graduate programs are more racially diverse than in previous years, and the importance of a racially diverse workforce is being recognized (National Science Foundation [NSF], 2017). However, for graduate students and faculty, it may be unclear how they can best promote diversity and inclusion within their programs and fields.

Though gains have been made over recent years, students of color (SOC) continue to be underrepresented in clinical and counseling psychology programs in comparison to United States census data, which suggests the continued existence of systemic barriers.

This problem extends throughout the academic pipeline. SOC are less likely to attend a four-year college and more likely to drop out than their White counterparts (Camera, 2015). In the field of psychology, approximately 37 percent of bachelor's degrees are conferred to SOC, while only 28 percent of doctorates are awarded to SOC (National Center for Education Statistics, 2014a, 2014b). Current racial demographics of the United States reflect that 61 percent of the population identify as non-Hispanic White (US Census Bureau, 2017), yet they account for 83.6 percent of psychologists (US Census Bureau, 2005–2013). According to the US Department of Education's most recent statistics, 84 percent of psychology faculty members and 78 percent of full-time faculty at colleges and universities identify themselves as White (National Center for Education Statistics, 2008, 2016). Within psychology, minorities are significantly underrepresented, and Whites are overrepresented relative to the national population.

Bias and discrimination may begin early in the academic experiences of SOC and may continue to follow them throughout their academic trajectories. These inequalities need to be considered within a larger social context, recognizing the roles of access to quality, early education (K-12), which is highly dependent on location, socioeconomic status, and race (Spatig-Amerikaner, 2012). In addition to economic barriers to pursuing graduate education, stereotype-driven racial bias may negatively impact how professors mentor and encourage students prior to admission (Milkman, Akinola, & Chugh, 2015) and during graduate-level education (DeLapp & Williams, 2015; Williams, Gooden, & Davis, 2012). SOC also report less satisfaction with their undergraduate psychology major than their White counterparts and sometimes report that course materials contain racial stereotypes or inaccurate information about members of a racial group (Lott & Rogers, 2011). These inaccuracies and microaggressions continue to impact SOC beyond bachelor's programs and within psychology graduate programs. Furthermore, negative experiences of discrimination, isolation, distress, devaluation, and feelings of disconnection from peers and faculty have been described by psychology graduate SOC (Clark, Mercer, Zeigler-Hill, & Dufrene, 2012; Vasquez et al., 2006). While we have witnessed some progress with racial diversification in relation to undergraduate and graduate enrollment, there remain clear disparities in racial diversity within graduate psychology programs and the broader field of psychology (NSF, 2017).

To address these challenges, this chapter will present best practices to promote diversity and inclusion in psychology graduate programs centered on effective recruitment and retention efforts, as well as honoring contextual considerations. This chapter aims to support stakeholders invested in, as well as those directly impacted by, increasing racial diversity and inclusion in graduate psychology programs, such as administrators, faculty, current and prospective students, staff, and alumni. The recruitment and retention strategies we describe below focus on how programs can cultivate a campus climate that increases SOC representation in psychology, as well as a sense of inclusion. By addressing the barriers SOC face during graduate education, psychology programs may increase racial representation, leading to more diversity in the mental health treatment workforce, and, in turn, improving treatment outcomes for racial minority clients. Visit http://www.newharbinger.com/41962 to download an outline of these best practices, as well as an annotated bibliography.

Recruiting Underrepresented Racial Minority Students

In the following sections, we present considerations and best practices for recruiting SOC. Significant work often precedes effective recruitment efforts, such as awareness of the existing campus climate and the possible need to transform the cultural climate of the institution. This campus climate is what will be marketed to potential SOC through communication and outreach efforts. We also give attention to improvements that can be made to admissions criteria to support the recruitment process of SOC.

Campus Climate

Campus climate can be defined as the current attitudes, behaviors, and standards of faculty, students, staff, and administrators regarding the level of respect for individual needs, abilities, and potential (Hart & Fellabaum, 2008). Campus climate is reflected in campus policies and practices, the demographics and values of its members, and quality of personal interactions. It is the overall environment of the institution as perceived by its members. An environment in which SOC feel safe, listened to, treated fairly, and respected is a foundational recruitment and retention tool. Assessing the campus climate is the first step to creating an inclusive and diverse learning environment that recruits, retains, and maximizes the success of SOC.

Whittaker and Montgomery (2012) suggested that institutions begin with conducting an honest campus climate assessment, as well as methods to define and measure the institution's success with improving the climate. Many major contributing factors interact to shape both the student and faculty experience, including an institution's historical legacy of inclusion or exclusion of various racial and ethnic groups, numerical representation of racial and ethnic groups, the psychological climate of perceptions and attitudes between and among racial and ethnic groups, and the behavioral climate dimension characterized by intergroup relations on campus (Hurtado, Clayton-Pedersen, Allen, & Milem, 1998). A multicampus study conducted by Gilliard (1996) found that the most significant climate measure for Black students was their perceptions of racial discrimination by college administrators. Faculty, administrators, staff, and students can play a crucial role in magnifying or diminishing the perception of a harsh campus climate for SOC. For this reason, the perspectives of all members of the campus community should be considered and institutions should establish regular and on-going assessments of the campus climate (see chapter 13; Hurtado et al., 1998).

As a response to the establishment and formal report of the Commission on Ethnic Minority Recruitment, Retention and Training, the APA accreditation standards require recruitment and retention of SOC (APA, 2015). This task force allows programs to independently determine the means by which they achieve these standards to meet respective goals and objectives. In that regard, many predominantly White institutions have primarily focused on improving structural diversity by recruiting SOC without implementing systematic, institutional changes, such as improving campus climate. To fully address campus climate, departments must work from the inside out. This can be achieved by hiring and retaining faculty who are committed to creating a culture of diversity and inclusivity (Bilimoria & Buch, 2010). Davies (2016) asserted that interventions to combat the harmful effects of implicit bias require an unwavering commitment to cultivate diversity, and cross-cultural communication can only occur if diversity already exists to enable it. Although improving structural diversity by recruiting diverse students appears to be an attractive option, due to the perception of immediate change, there will likely be challenges in retaining SOC without diversity represented among faculty, staff, and administrators.

An additional issue is the problem of racial color-blindness. Neville, Poteat, Lewis, & Spanierman (2014) described "color-blind racial ideology" (CBRI) as a worldview that stresses the importance of seeing people as individuals and not seeing skin color, resulting in the problematic rationalization of racial inequities. This CBRI mind-set may contribute to difficulties acknowledging and addressing racism as a contributing factor to bias and discrimination within an institution, and therefore may negatively impact the campus climate and psychology program's ability to achieve recruitment goals toward increased diversity (Neville et al., 2014). While many psychology faculty recognize the importance of diversity and the problems of color-blindness, less emphasis is put on social justice advocacy and other roles that psychology faculty may play as members of institutions of higher education (Shin, 2008). Awareness of racial disparities among graduate psychology programs would more easily be acknowledged and addressed if more faculty assumed roles of advocacy, employing what is known from psychological science to combat the harmful effects of CBRIs. The genuine desire to create culturally competent and representative practitioners appears to exist; and for progress to be made, all parties must be willing to confront the discomfort experienced when talking about race and one's own privilege (Sue, Torino, Capodilupo, Rivera, & Lin, 2009).

One way to constructively address the distress associated with discussing racial disparities is to consider issues of racial identity development. Helms (1992) described six stages of White identity development, as well as the confusing emotions and need for self-reflection that can come as individuals face each level of development. Such frameworks that normalize experiences and reinforce the importance of this work allow faculty, staff, and administrators to become more aware of their biases and collectively learn about White identity and privilege. This may impact SOC through an improved, less biased, and more aware White contribution to the campus climate (Sherbinin, 2004).

Psychology graduate programs can also strengthen diversity and inclusion by amplifying the voices of SOC and faculty of color. SOC who experience their voices as desired and heard on campus will feel more valued and respected. For example, space can be provided for faculty and SOC to share their perspectives and experiences during conversations inside and outside of the classroom with White students and faculty (Thomason, 1999). Faculty can take responsibility for changing the campus climate by leading discussions about decreasing biases through exposure to different cultural perspectives (Sherbinin, 2004). These changes can lay the groundwork for cultural shifts within psychology, to provide the space to promote diversity and inclusion, and, in turn, the successful recruitment and retention of SOC.

Outreach and Communication

Programs can take on a more active role in conducting outreach and communicating their investment in recruiting future underrepresented racial minority (URM) psychology graduates. Institutions with strong track records for recruiting and retaining SOC have succeeded by focusing on aggressive recruitment strategies, in lieu of affirmative action. Some faculty of color and current graduate students conduct outreach to psychology departments within their former undergraduate institutions or other institutions with high representation of SOC (e.g., historically Black colleges and universities) (Gardere, 2015). Additionally, recruitment materials tailored to prospective SOC may signal that they are welcomed and anticipated to succeed in the program. For departments that offer an undergraduate degree in psychology, efforts can also be made to recruit and retain their own undergraduate SOC for further graduate training and education.

In addition to expanding outreach efforts, programs can make deliberate efforts to engage prospective SOC once contact is established. Faculty and current graduate students can emphasize strengths of their program that have been identified as important to prospective SOC, such as senior faculty of color, faculty who conduct research on diverse populations, and programming and events dedicated to social justice issues (Ponterotto et al., 1995). Facilitating opportunities for prospective SOC to meet with current SOC on interview days and campus visits is also key. In these meetings, current SOC can share their experiences in the program and the overall campus climate, honoring the unique challenges SOC may face within a graduate program and fostering understanding that SOC are looking for an institution that values inclusivity and diversity.

Another powerful tool in recruiting SOC is to discuss the available resources within the university that are closely connected to fostering diversity on campus. Through outreach and communication efforts from faculty, staff, and current students, prospective SOC may receive information regarding centers, educational programming, research studies, and student organizations dedicated to diversity and inclusion. For example, this may include sharing with the prospective SOC (1) a university's multicultural center; (2) faculty conducting research in areas related to racial disparity and inequality; (3) trainings, certifications, or degrees related to the topic of diversity; (4) designated meeting areas on campus specifically for dialogues related to inclusion; and (5) organizations for students that identify with particular racial and ethnic backgrounds. All of these resources can demonstrate to prospective SOC that the campus climate values diversity and inclusion, an attractive quality for prospective students looking for a program that provides a sense of belonging, safety, and respect.

Programs that employ effective retention strategies can advertise these strategies to prospective SOC as a recruitment tool. Many SOC anticipate some form of discrimination when working toward professional degrees (Lewis, Chesler, & Forman, 2000). Addressing these concerns up front can ease some of the stress prospective SOC may have around the application process. By highlighting the efforts the program is making to recruit and retain SOC, prospective SOC can gain a sense of what the campus climate will be like once they are admitted.

Admissions Structures and Criteria

Part of cultivating cultural awareness includes developing an understanding of the structural barriers that perpetuate racial disparities in psychology graduate programs. A close examination of the process of deciding to pursue graduate training, applying to programs, and matriculating into a program reveals a complex system, involving multiple barriers particularly disadvantageous to SOC.

For one, the cost-prohibitive nature of psychology graduate training renders this career path as impractical or unfeasible for many SOC. The costs of graduate psychology tuition can seem exorbitant for many SOC, considering that 27.0 percent of American Indians and Alaska Natives and 25.8 percent of Blacks live below the poverty level (US Census Bureau, 2013). Even SOC who are able to shoulder the tuition costs may be deterred from graduate psychology training by its opportunity-cost of income generation. Concerns with expedient entry into the workforce are particularly relevant for SOC, who have higher debt from undergraduate education compared to White students (US Department of Education, 2006) and may also be supporting immediate and extended family.

Graduate psychology training programs may receive a more diverse pool of candidates if they acknowledge and address the financial constraints that limit this pathway. Programs can invest funds into financial aid for SOC by offering application fee waivers, as well as creating fellowships, assistantships, and awards to defray the costs of tuition or provide stipend support. Additionally, the burden of understanding the financial implications of pursuing graduate training should not be exclusively placed on prospective applicants. SOC interested in psychology graduate programs often prioritize financial aid as a major factor in their decision making about programs, but they find the information in recruitment materials to be limited (Ponterotto et al., 1995). As a result, the admissions team should make information related to financial aid and tuition costs clear and easily accessible to increase SOC recruitment.

In addition to improving clarity and comprehensiveness of financial aid and tuition information, programs can communicate transparently about the return on investment of graduate training by providing data on the jobs acquired by recent alumni and potential salaries, as well as the average time to complete the program and obtain licensure.

The more the prospective SOC feel there is transparency regarding the financial aspects of psychology graduate study and a genuine desire from the university for them to be well informed, the more SOC may feel there is an investment from the university in their success.

Even when prospective SOC are engaged, the final arbiter of access to psychology graduate programs is the admissions committee. Traditional criteria for evaluating candidates for admission, such as Graduate Record Examination (GRE) scores, tend to disadvantage SOC. Blacks, in particular, have lower mean scores on every section of the GRE (verbal, quantitative, analytic) when compared to the overall mean scores (Educational Testing Service, 2014). Therefore, emphasis on GRE scores should be reduced until such racial bias no longer exists on this exam, while greater emphasis should be placed on indicators of commitment to diversity, such as leadership roles in cultural organizations, community service, competence in several cultures, and bilingual abilities (Gardere, 2015). Removing barriers that perpetuate racial disparities in psychology graduate programs by improving admissions structures and criteria is a key component to the successful recruitment of SOC.

Retaining Underrepresented Racial Minority Students

In the section that follows, we will present considerations and best practices for retaining SOC. Beyond the admissions process, SOC face a new set of challenges when embarking upon graduate psychology training that may challenge and conflict with their cultural values (Alvarez, Blume, Cervantes, & Thomas, 2009). For example, SOC may have cultural values in which greater familial responsibility is assumed, creating competing interests for time when managing academic responsibilities and familial obligations. SOC may also have difficulty negotiating social norms in academic culture, such as debating with colleagues and questioning the views of professors, which may differ from their cultural norms of maintaining social harmony and respect for authority. This difficulty may also stem from their socialization to fear challenging White people due to their disempowered status (McGregor, 2006). Navigating these kinds of challenges can be made more manageable when appropriate mentorship is provided. Strong mentorship and support from multiple levels (faculty and peers) and channels (formal and informal) can play a major contributing role in the retention and success of SOC within psychology graduate programs.

In addition, the campus climate described previously in this chapter as critical to SOC recruitment is critical to student retention. SOC recruits are more likely to be retained if the inclusive and diverse campus climate marketed to them during recruitment exists in reality and is demonstrated through impactful interactions and mentorship experiences. Impactful interactions and mentorship create a sense of belonging and connection aligned with the collectivistic cultural values of many SOC, creating a sense of family within the academic setting (Walton & Cohen, 2011).

Impactful Interactions

The influence that faculty have on SOC has the potential to be amplified or reduced by the interactions these students have with their peers. In addition, the influence that peers have on SOC has the potential to be amplified or reduced by the interactions SOC have with their faculty. Universities can make the most of these faculty and peer group interactions by allowing diversity to be a topic of engagement. The foundation in creating impactful interactions involves educational programming on recognizing and confronting stereotypes and myths that people have about those who are different from them rather than maintaining a CBRI that dismisses the problem (Neville et al., 2014). When implemented, this approach has the propensity to positively impact both students and faculty alike, as students who complete more diversity activities report lower levels of CBRI (e.g., Spanierman, Neville, Liao, Hammer, & Wang, 2008). University faculty and staff can also benefit from these experiences by learning how cultural differences affect SOC and how graduate programs can adapt to unique cultural issues.

Meeting SOCs' needs for safety, sense of belonging, self-esteem, and self-actualization can be a successful retention strategy (Donnell, Edwards, & Green, 2002). While these needs are shared by all students, regardless of racial or ethnic background, it is likely more challenging for the needs of URM students to be met due to their minority status and perceived treatment within the academic system. Faculty can meet SOC needs by appreciating the nuanced differences between and within SOC groups, as well as at the individual level related to a student's skin tone, level of acculturation, socioeconomic status, language fluency, or amount of racial socialization (Sue et al., 2009).

By implementing activities in the classroom, such as a cultural genogram or immersion activity, professors intentionally invite cultural identities into the classroom. For example, a cultural genogram facilitates exploration of personal identity and cultural heritage, as well as how the two intersect for students and influence their future clinical practice. A cultural immersion activity can reveal students' strengths and weaknesses when fostering connection with others, as well as challenge preconceived stereotypes through direct contact. Allowing time in class to reflect upon these experiences can foster intercultural dialogue and increase cultural awareness and sensitivity. Research overwhelmingly indicates that students who participate in an educational diversity training (e.g., Soble, Spanierman, & Liao, 2011) or complete an introductory diversity course (e.g., Case, 2007) report significant decreases in CBRI, and these decreases are sustained over time (Kernahan & Davis, 2009). Facilitating racial bias awareness in psychology graduate programs can decrease implicit racial bias and enrich intercultural communication within the student cohort, which may positively impact URM student retention.

Impactful interaction is also fostered by creating and supporting the infrastructure for cultural dialogue. Designated groups and meeting areas on campus, specifically designed for dialogues related to diversity and inclusion, communicate to SOC that the university has made an investment in allocating space for safe discussions on those challenging topics. University-sponsored student organizations and clubs (e.g., American

Indian and Indigenous Student Organization, Latinx Student Organization), for students who identify with particular racial or ethnic backgrounds, is another opportunity for SOC to feel a sense of belonging that, as stated above, increases retention. Even if SOC do not participate in the student organization, the organization's existence is a representation of their race being recognized on campus, demonstrating the campus's investment in a diverse and inclusive climate.

Faculty Mentoring URM Students

The presence of mentors of color, and the availability of quality mentorship from both people of color and White faculty, are important factors that contribute to the retention of SOC (Yared, 2016). The visibility of faculty of color within the department can reinforce the ambitions of SOC, who may question their ability to succeed in predominantly White institutions. Imposter syndrome, characterized by doubting personal accomplishments or ability to succeed, is common for students entering a new academic setting (Sakulku & Alexander, 2011). This may be particularly true for SOC who are questioning if they belong or deserve to be a graduate psychology student. Having quality mentorship, particularly from faculty of color, is a powerful tool in combating imposter syndrome and retaining SOC, as they are encouraged by someone similar to themselves who has achieved their professional desires.

In some cases, sociocultural and language similarities between mentors and mentees may be appreciated, or even preferred, by mentees (Gonzáles-Figueroa & Young, 2005; Thomason, 1999). Partnerships between faculty and SOC through formal programs have been successful in equipping mentees with strong research training and professional development opportunities (Waitzkin, Yager, Parker, & Duran, 2006). Mentorship and retention of faculty members of color is a crucial component in retaining SOC, in order to have this valuable resource available.

Advantages exist for seeking mentorship both inside and outside of an individual's home institution. Mentorship at one's home institution, and ideally within one's department, is important for receiving guidance that is appropriately tailored to the given campus climate. Additional mentorship from faculty members of color at other institutions can also provide access to more senior mentors who may have resolved similar challenges within their own institutions. Seeking mentorship from faculty of color outside of one's home institution may also reduce the fear that the SOC may be negatively evaluated in discussing their concerns, as the faculty member is not in a position to evaluate the SOC directly.

Mentorship from people of color who have graduated and are now practicing within the field of psychology can also be a powerful intervention in retention. This is particularly helpful when the graduate program of SOC facilitates professional relationships in which mentors discuss their own experiences with graduate school, the licensing process, their current career, and their path prior to graduate school. In this regard, the graduate can discuss challenges they have faced and overcome, including racism, stereotyping, and prejudice. As graduate programs invite professionals of color to speak to students, programs are modeling how one can give back and make meaning out of their struggles and triumphs, creating ongoing mentoring relationships and opportunities to challenge imposter syndrome; all of which assist in student retention.

White mentors, too, can provide quality mentorship to SOC by developing awareness of the unique issues confronted by SOC and remaining receptive to their feedback. Conversely, a lack of cultural awareness from mentors that manifests as microaggressions or invalidation of discriminatory experiences, which may be further compounded by defensiveness about racism or color-blindness, can breed feelings of alienation and mistrust in mentees. These occurrences may subject SOC to the risk of dropout or underperformance. Alvarez and colleagues (2009) present several recommendations for mentors of SOC, including self-assessing for racist beliefs, learning about their mentee's culture, and seeking consultation to support mentees. Relationships between White mentors and mentees of color can be crafted such that mentors receive greater experience in mentoring SOC and mentees benefit from receiving instrumental support.

Peer Mentorship

Peer mentorship from other SOC can be a valuable adjunct to faculty mentoring relationships. Efforts to organize peer mentorship for SOC may be initiated and led by the students themselves. Student-led peer mentorship may occur through informal networks that extend beyond the academic department and involve SOC throughout the university or across several universities. Designated meeting areas on campus for dialogues related to diversity and inclusion and university-sponsored cultural student organizations are ripe opportunities for informal peer mentorship to take place. These informal and organic connections increase the sense of belonging and retention of SOC.

In addition, peer-mentorship relationships can also be organized more formally within the psychology department, with advanced students mentoring new SOC. Some mentees report additional benefits when paired with mentors matched on other characteristics, such as gender (e.g., Patton & Harper, 2003). The type of peer-mentor support received by a mentee can be variable in levels of instrumental and emotional support (Noonan, Ballinger, & Black, 2007); therefore, clarifying role expectations from the outset of the relationship is recommended.

The mentee of color may have instrumental or informational needs, such as how to navigate the logistical details of the program. Peer mentors can begin by clarifying the questions and goals of SOC to determine what information would be helpful to provide. Providing different perspectives can broaden the mentee's vision and understanding, as some SOC may be the first in their family to pursue graduate education. For example, it may be useful for the mentor to describe similar experiences and how they navigated those, while normalizing, validating, and empathizing with the mentee.

Remembering that emotional support is also a key component to the mentorship relationship, it can be helpful to take time to build rapport. Conditions that may facilitate a positive peer relationship include active listening, providing structure (e.g., meeting place and time), expressing positive expectations, and serving as an advocate for the mentee (Brown, Davis, & McClendon, 1999). Discussing one's own mentoring experiences can also assist in exploring the expectations and limitations of the formal peer-mentoring relationship. In order to best prepare the peer mentor in this new role, it may be useful to provide training regarding the peer mentorship process, as well as consultation from a faculty member regarding the mentorship relationship, roles, and approaches.

Peer mentorship can pose many benefits for SOC by equipping them with additional support, improving their sense of community, and maintaining their desire to persist with their academic training. From the perspective of URM students, peer mentors can be a resource for veteran advice about navigating conflict between cultural values and academic norms, and a sounding board for managing difficult race-related issues, such as how to address a microaggression from a faculty member or fellow student. Compared to the hierarchical relationship of faculty mentorship, peer mentorship provides an outlet for SOC to candidly discuss their experiences. In addition to cultivating greater satisfaction with the graduate school experience (Clark et al., 2012), receiving peer mentorship can play a role in educational outcomes, such as academic persistence (Hernandez, 2000). When academic programs already have mentorship programs in place, intentionally pairing new SOC with an advanced standing SOC mentor may also be beneficial.

Conclusion

Research supports the need to fully embrace diversity within the field of psychology to accomplish its basic goals of describing, explaining, and predicting behavior. To facilitate the enrichment of society, innovative recruitment and retention structures are needed to broaden the conversations that dictate student success. Persisting through discomfort around diversity topics can benefit all students in peer relations and improve faculty's mentoring of SOC. By providing an academic environment that values cultural competency, diversity, and inclusion, from the systemic to the individual level, we can create equity within the psychological sciences that can strengthen the discipline as a whole. Graduate students, faculty, and administrators with privilege especially have roles to play in facilitating mentorship, awareness, and structural changes to target the goals of increased diversity. It is vital for psychology graduate programs to commit to working on addressing systemic barriers to education, access, treatment, and professional opportunity for individuals of racial minority (APA, 2000; Vasquez et al., 2006). Not only will increasing diversity and inclusion for SOC benefit individuals within academic fields, it will also increase cultural competence with clients and promote research to benefit a diverse population of individuals in need of evidence-based treatments.

KEY POINTS FOR CLINICIANS

- Students of color (SOC) continue to be underrepresented in clinical and counseling psychology programs, suggesting the existence of systemic barriers. They report experiences of discrimination, isolation, devaluation, and disconnection from peers and faculty.

- In recruiting SOC, an awareness of the existing campus climate and the possible need to transform the cultural climate of the institution is key. Experiences of racism reported by SOC are often a reliable predictor of the campus racial climate.

- SOC who experience their voices as desired and heard on campus undoubtedly will feel more valued and respected within the institution's community, improving their sense of belonging, self-esteem, and sense of belonging.

- SOC interested in psychology graduate programs often prioritize financial information as a major factor in their decision making, but find limited information provided in recruitment materials. Programs should make information related to financial aid, tuition costs, and potential future salaries clear and easily accessible.

- SOC may face demands and expectations during graduate education that challenge their cultural values. Appropriate mentorship is needed; mentorship can pose many benefits by equipping students with additional support, improving their sense of community, and maintaining their desire to persist with their academic training.

References

Alvarez, A. N., Blume, A. W., Cervantes, J. M., & Thomas, L. R. (2009). Tapping the wisdom tradition: Essential elements to mentoring students of color. *Professional Psychology: Research and Practice, 40*(2), 181–188.

American Psychological Association. (2000). *Model strategies for ethnic minority recruitment, retention, and training in higher education.* Washington, DC: Office of Ethnic Minority Affairs, American Psychological Association.

American Psychological Association. (2015). *Standards of accreditation for health service psychology.* Washington, DC: Author.

American Psychological Association. (2016). *Quick reference guide to accreditation guidelines for doctoral programs.* Retrieved from http://www.apa.org/ed/accreditation/about/policies/doctoral.aspx

Bilimoria, D., & Buch, K. K. (2010). The search is on: Engendering faculty diversity through more effective search and recruitment. *Change: The Magazine of Higher Learning, 42*(4), 27–32.

Bowen, W. G., & Bok, D. (2016). *The shape of the river: Long-term consequences of considering race in college and university admissions.* Princeton, NJ: Princeton University Press.

Brown, M. C., Davis, G. L., & McClendon, S. A. (1999). Mentoring graduate students of color: Myths, models, and modes. *Peabody Journal of Education, 74*(2), 105–118.

Camera, L. (2015, November 6). Native American students left behind. *US News and World Report.* Retrieved from: https://www.usnews.com/news/articles/2015/11/06/native-american-students -left-behind

Case, K. A. (2007). Raising white privilege awareness and reducing racial prejudice: Assessing diversity course effectiveness. *Teaching of Psychology, 34*(4), 231–235.

Clark, C. R., Mercer, S. H., Zeigler-Hill, V., & Dufrene, B. A. (2012). Barriers to the success of ethnic minority students in school psychology graduate programs. *School Psychology Review, 41*(2), 176–192.

Davies, S. L. (2016). Driving campus diversity one decision at a time. *Liberal Education: Association of American Colleges & Universities, 102*(4). Retrieved from https://www.aacu.org/liberaleducation /2016/fall/davies

DeLapp, R. C. T., & Williams, M. T. (2015). Professional challenges facing African American psychologists: The presence and impact of racial microaggressions. *The Behavior Therapist, 38*(4), 101–105.

Donnell, C. M., Edwards, Y., & Green, D. (2002, July). Find them and keep them: Strategies for the successful recruitment and retention of diverse graduate students. *10th annual NAMRC Conference,* Las Vegas, Nevada.

Educational Testing Service (2014). *A snapshot of the individuals who took the GRE revised General Test.* Retrieved from https://www.ets.org/s/gre/pdf/snapshot_test_taker_data_2014.pdf

Gardere, J. (2015). *Recruiting black males into psychology doctoral programs.* Retrieved from https:// www.nationalregister.org/pub/the-national-register-report-pub/the-register-report-spring-2015 /recruiting-black-males-into-psychology-doctoral-programs/

Gilliard, M. D. (1996). *Racial climate and institutional support factors affecting success in predominantly White institutions: An examination of African-American and White student experiences* (Doctoral dissertation), University of Michigan.

Gonzáles-Figueroa, E., & Young, A. M. (2005). Ethnic identity and mentoring among Latinas in professional roles. *Cultural Diversity and Ethnic Minority Psychology, 11*(3), 213–226.

Hart, J, & Fellabaum, J. (2008). Analyzing campus climate studies: Seeking to define and understand. *Journal of Diversity in Higher Education, 1*(4), 222–234.

Helms, J. E. (1992). *A race is a nice thing to have: A guide to being a white person or understanding the white persons in your life.* Content Communications.

Hernandez, J. C. (2000). Understanding the retention of Latino college students. *Journal of College Student Development, 41,* 575–588.

Hurtado, S., Clayton-Pedersen, A. R., Allen, W. R., & Milem, J. F. (1998). Enhancing campus climates for racial/ethnic diversity: Educational policy and practice. *The Review of Higher Education, 21*(3), 279–302.

Kernahan, C., & Davis, T. (2009). What are the long-term effects of learning about racism? *Teaching of Psychology, 37,* 41–45. doi:10.1080/00986280903425748

Lewis, A. E., Chesler, M., & Forman, T. A. (2000). The impact of "colorblind" ideologies on students of color: Intergroup relations at a predominantly White university. *Journal of Negro Education, 69*(1), 74–91.

Lott, B., & Rogers, M. (2011). Ethnicity matters for undergraduate majors in challenges, experiences, and perceptions of psychology. *Cultural Diversity and Ethnic Minority Psycholgy, 17,* 201–210.

McGregor, L. N. (2006). Teaching and mentoring racially and ethnically diverse students. In W. Buskist & S. F. Davis (Eds.), *Handbook of teaching of psychology* (pp. 164–169). Malden, MA: Blackwell.

Milkman, K. L., Akinola, M., & Chugh, D. (2015). What happens before? A field experiment exploring how pay and representation differentially shape bias on the pathway into organizations.
Journal of Applied Psychology, 100(6), 1678–1712.

National Center for Education Statistics. (2008). *Full-time and part-time faculty and instructional staff in
degree-granting postsecondary institutions, by race/ethnicity, sex, and program area: Fall 1998 and fall
2003.* Retrieved from https://nces.ed.gov/programs/digest/d15/tables/dt15_315.80.asp?current=yes

National Center for Education Statistics. (2014a, August). *Bachelor's degrees conferred by postsecondary
institutions, by race/ethnicity and field of study: 2011–12 and 2012–13.* Retrieved from https://nces
.ed.gov/programs/digest/d14/tables/dt14_322.40.asp

National Center for Education Statistics. (2014b, September). *Doctor's degrees conferred by postsecondary institutions, by race/ethnicity and field of study: 2011–12 and 2012–13.* Retrieved from http://nces
.ed.gov/programs/digest/d14/tables/dt14_324.25.asp

National Center for Education Statistics. (2016, May). *Characteristics of postsecondary faculty.* Retrieved
from https://nces.ed.gov/programs/coe/indicator_csc.asp

National Science Foundation, National Center for Science and Engineering Statistics. (2017).
Doctorate Recipients from US Universities: 2015. Arlington, VA. Retrieved from https://www.nsf
.gov/statistics/2017/nsf17306/

Neville, H. A., Poteat, V. P., Lewis, J. A., & Spanierman, L. B. (2014). Changes in White college
students' color-blind racial ideology over 4 years: Do diversity experiences make a difference?
Journal of Counseling Psychology, 61(2), 179.

Noonan, M. J., Ballinger, R., & Black, R. (2007). Peer and faculty mentoring in doctoral education:
Definitions, experiences, and expectations. *International Journal of Teaching and Learning in
Higher Education, 19*(3), 251–262.

Patton, L. D., & Harper, S. R. (2003). Mentoring relationships among African American women in
graduate and professional schools. *New Directions for Student Services, 2003*(104), 67–78.

Ponterotto, J. G., Burkard, A., Yoshida, R. K., Cancelli, A. A., Mendez, G., Wasilewski, L., & Sussman,
L. (1995). Prospective minority students' perceptions of application packets for professional psychology programs: A qualitative study. *Professional Psychology: Research and Practice, 26*(2),
196–204.

Sakulku, J., & Alexander, J. (2011). The imposter phenomenon. *International Journal of Behavior
Science, 6*(1), 73–92.

Sherbinin, J. W. (2004). White professors can help uproot racism. *Chronicle of Higher Education, 50*(35),
16.

Shin, R. Q. (2008). Advocating for social justice in academia through recruitment, retention, admissions, and professional survival. *Journal of Multicultural Counseling and Development, 36*(3),
180–191.

Soble, J. R., Spanierman, L. B., & Liao, H. Y. (2011). Effects of a brief video intervention on White
university students' racial attitudes. *Journal of Counseling Psychology, 58*(1), 151–157.

Spanierman, L. B., Neville, H. A., Liao, H. Y., Hammer, J. H., & Wang, Y. F. (2008). Participation in
formal and informal campus diversity experiences: Effects on students' racial democratic beliefs.
Journal of Diversity in Higher Education, 1(2), 108.

Spatig-Amerikaner, A. (2012). *Unequal education: Federal loophole enables lower spending on students of
color.* Washington, DC: Center for American Progress.

Stewart, C. E., Lee, S. Y., Hogstrom, A., & Williams, M. (2017). Diversify and conquer: A call to
promote minority representation in clinical psychology. *The Behavior Therapist, 40*(3), 74–79.

Sue, D. W., & Sue, D. (2012). *Counseling the culturally diverse: Theory and practice.* New York, NY:
Wiley.

Sue, D. W., Torino, G. C., Capodilupo, C. M., Rivera, D. P., & Lin, A. I. (2009). How White faculty
perceive and react to difficult dialogues on race: Implications for education and training. *The
Counseling Psychologist, 37*(8), 1090–1115. https://doi.org/10.1177/0011000009340443

Suite, D. H., La Bril, R., Primm, A., & Harrison-Ross, P. (2007). Beyond misdiagnosis, misunderstanding and mistrust: Relevance of the historical perspective in the medical and mental health treatment of people of color. *Journal of the National Medical Association, 99*(8), 879–885.

Thomason, T. C. (1999). Improving the recruitment and retention of Native American students in psychology. *Cultural Diversity and Ethnic Minority Psychology, 5,* 308–316.

US Census Bureau. (2005–2013). *American Community Survey 1-Year PUMS file.* Retrieved from http://www.census.gov/programs-surveys/acs/data/pums.html

US Census Bureau. (2013). *Poverty rates for selected detailed race and Hispanic groups by state and place: 2007–2011.* Retrieved from https://www.census.gov/prod/2013pubs/acsbr11-17.pdf

US Census Bureau. (2017). *Quick facts United States race and Hispanic origin.* Retrieved from https://www.census.gov/quickfacts/fact/table/US/PST045217

US Department of Education. (2006). *Dealing with debt: 1992–93 bachelor's degree recipients 10 years later.* Retrieved from https://nces.ed.gov/pubs2006/2006156.pdf

Vasquez, M. J., Lott, B., Garcia-Vazquez, E., Grant, S. K., Iwamasa, G. Y., Molina, L. E., Ragsdale, B. L., & Vestal-Dowdy, E. (2006). Personal reflections: Barriers and strategies in increasing diversity in psychology. *American Psychologist, 61,* 157–172.

Waitzkin, H., Yager, J., Parker, T., & Duran, B. (2006). Mentoring partnerships for minority faculty and graduate students in mental health services research. *Academic Psychiatry, 30*(3), 205–217.

Walton, G. M., & Cohen, G. L. (2011). A brief social-belonging intervention improves academic and health outcomes of minority students. *Science, 331*(6023), 1447–1451.

Whittaker, J. A., & Montgomery, B. L. (2012). Cultivating diversity and competency in STEM: Challenges and remedies for removing virtual barriers to constructing diverse higher education communities of success. *Journal of Undergraduate Neuroscience Education, 11*(1), A44.

Williams, M. T., Gooden, A. M., & Davis, D. (2012). African Americans, European Americans, and pathological stereotypes: An African-centered perspective. In G. R. Hayes & M. H. Bryant (Eds.), *Psychology of culture* (pp. 25–46). Hauppauge, NY: Nova Science.

Yared, L. S. (2016, April 27). A broken pipeline: Minority students and the pathway to the Ph.D. *The Harvard Crimson.*

CHAPTER 13

Promoting Diversity and Inclusion on College Campuses

Monnica T. Williams,
University of Connecticut

Jonathan W. Kanter,
University of Washington

Introduction

Racial conflict at universities across the nation has become the focus of academic concern and media attention (Hartocollis & Bidgood, 2015). Students, student organizations, staff, and faculty are, in large numbers, complaining of widespread racism and that officials have often not responded or not responded quickly enough. One website tracked demands from students at eighty different universities who are calling for quantifiable changes in the status quo to improve the academic climate for racial minorities (The Demands, 2016). In the face of this outcry, universities would be hard pressed to ignore the common themes imbedded in these complaints, which include calls for more diverse faculty, racial sensitivity training for students and faculty, and more accountability in response to racist events (Berner, 2015). Many psychologists who work on college campuses, either in academic, clinical, or mixed settings, are faced with not wanting to ignore the situation, on the one hand, but not knowing what to do, and, as a result, they lapse into passivity that supports the status quo. This chapter presents an overview of these prominent concerns for psychologists on college campuses and concludes with action steps and ways to participate as agents of change.

Why Do Students Complain?

Research resoundingly concludes that a climate marred by racism and discrimination leads to physical and mental unwellness in ethnic and racial minorities (Berger & Sarnyai, 2015; Chou, Asnaani, & Hofmann, 2012). On campus, a negative racial environment can also be costly, resulting in disproportionate dropouts among students of color (Piotrowski & Perdue, 1998), burn out and poor retention of minority faculty (Cropsey et al., 2008), discrimination lawsuits, and even the forced resignation of officials held responsible for the unfavorable situation (e.g., Svrluga, 2015a). Victims of racially hostile environments can be left with diagnosable psychiatric symptoms that may include traumatization, anxiety, depression, and extended periods of disability (Pieterse, Carter, Evans, & Walter, 2010; Williams, Kanter, & Ching, 2018; Williams et al., 2014).

We have seen these issues play out in clinical settings and on campuses, our own included. It is discouraging to note that conditions have not substantially improved for underrepresented minorities over the last several decades and, in some respects, have worsened. For example, since the passage of the Civil Rights and Higher Education Acts of the 1960s, which led to large increases in college attendance for students of color, gaps in college attendance and success between Blacks and Whites have remained unchanged and have widened for Hispanics (Rothwell, 2015). Representation of Black males in medical schools has been declining and is now at lows not seen since 1978 (Association of American Medical Colleges, 2015). Furthermore, large disparities in school quality are observed for enrolled students (Carnevale & Strohl, 2013). The vast majority of students of color are enrolled in two-year and four-year open-access schools, which are documented to produce much less successful career trajectories for graduates.

Why Do Racial Problems Persist?

Racism in America today is harder to see than in previous eras because overt and legally codified forms of racial discrimination have been reduced or eliminated. Nonetheless, policies and practices that maintain the racial hierarchy persist and permeate nearly all sociocultural structures and institutions in America in ways that benefit and promote the well-being of Whites at the expense of people of color. These systems maintain racial inequities even though they may adapt to changing times or accommodate new ethnoracial groups. This specific manifestation of racism in America is termed "institutional racism" or "structural racism" (Lawrence, Sutton, Kubisch, Susi, & Fulbright-Anderson, 2004).

In higher education, disparities in access and outcomes are well documented, and—because of the importance in our society of higher education and the access to resources gained from a high-quality education—not only are higher educational disparities distressing, but they also create unfair labor-market advantages and perpetuate intergenerational advantages for Whites throughout the lifespan (Carnevale & Strohl, 2013). College campuses also produce repeated experiences of racism and discrimination for students of color, which are major determinants of quality of life and psychological distress for them (Solórzano, Ceja, & Yosso, 2000) and may even result in increased suicide risk (O'Keefe, Wingate, Cole, Hollingsworth, & Tucker, 2015). Thus, addressing institutional racism in higher education is a crucial goal with immediate and long-term benefits for students of color from both a social justice and public health perspective. Furthermore, these problems have trickle-down effects, contributing to mental health disparities by reducing the number of people of color in the mental health workforce as clinicians, educators, and researchers.

To combat institutional and structural racism on campuses, we must first understand both societal and individual obstacles to progress. Mainstream socialization processes, which protect White people from racist experiences and racial stress, render invisible and make it difficult for many White people to see or acknowledge racist processes and systems (Neville, Worthington, & Spanierman, 2001). At the individual level, White people tend to underestimate and minimize the degree and severity of racism in our systems and communities as a result (Carter & Murphy, 2015; Jones, Cox, & Navarro-Rivera, 2014). Thus, when people of color or victims of racism attempt to discuss or advocate for changes to reduce systemic racial discrimination, bias, and inequities, such attempts are often socially punished by being dismissed, ridiculed, or met with defensive and avoidant reactions (Sue, Rivera, Capodilupo, Lin, & Torino, 2010). This serves to perpetuate rather than solve the problem.

Additional individual factors make it likely White people on campus will perpetuate rather than solve institutional problems. People may attempt to preserve and increase their self-esteem by embracing the belief that the group to which they belong is better than others, and to believe in oneself as better typically requires also believing that the other group (the out-group) possesses inferior or negative attributes (Tajfel, 1982). In the case of stigmatized minorities, these negative attributes become pathological stereotypes that function to explain group differences at the expense of the oppressed. These are termed "pathological stereotypes" because they do not represent true characteristics of the stigmatized group and thereby perpetuate oppression (Williams, Gooden, & Davis, 2012). It is important to understand that social status or group position determines the stereotype content, not the actual personal characteristics of group members (Jost & Banaji, 1994). Groups that enjoy fewer social and economic advantages will be pathologically stereotyped in a way that helps explain inequities, for example, "laziness" or "lack of intelligence" will be advanced to explain lower college graduation rates, rather than in-group favoritism or structural racism.

Gaertner and Dovidio (2005) describe aversive racism, a type of racism seen in individuals who support racial equality but have conflicted, often unconscious, negative biases and feelings toward minorities. These attitudes result in biased (racist) behaviors in ambiguous situations, when expectations are unclear or when stigmatized minorities hold positions that violate social expectations based on the traditional racial hierarchy (e.g., an African American male provost). As noted in chapter 6, it is well known that much bias operates implicitly, without awareness (Greenwald & Krieger, 2006) and, fueled by pathological stereotypes and in-group favoritism, leads to intentional and unintentional discriminatory behaviors (Greenwald & Pettigrew, 2014). One may hope that, due to advanced education, faculty members of institutions of higher education would hold less implicit bias, but summary data from the Implicit Association Test suggest only trivial differences in bias due to educational level (Greenwald & Krieger, 2006).

One of the more common ways in which bias influences interactions with people of color on a regular basis is in a tendency for White people to engage in microaggressions—brief, everyday exchanges in the form of seemingly innocent and innocuous comments, and subtle or dismissive gestures and tones that send denigrating messages to people of color because they belong to a minority group (Pierce, 1970; Sue et al., 2007). Minority college students cite microaggressions as the primary source of racist experiences on a day-to-day, campus-life basis (Solórzano et al., 2000; Yosso, Smith, Ceja, & Solórzano, 2009), and microaggressions are also a major source of stress among minority faculty (e.g., Constantine, Smith, Redington, & Owens, 2008; DeLapp & Williams, 2015; Pittman, 2012).

As shown in figure 13.1, all of these problems (individual bias, pathological stereotypes, and microaggressions) intersect within the structures and institutions of higher education to create and maintain adverse environments for people of color. These problems also make it difficult to instigate change, as efforts to address racism on campus often seem unfair to those who have not experienced racial prejudice and have difficulty seeing the full extent of the problems, creating a sense of inequity and corresponding resistance to remediation efforts (Kravitz & Klineberg, 2000). Thus, attempts to address institutional problems must also include education about these obstacles and influences, as well as the benefits to everyone of having a diverse environment (Galinsky et al., 2015). It is important for those in leadership positions to champion this cause, as the proactive management of diversity initiatives requires the commitment of leadership with a clear purpose and vision for the organization (Ng, 2008).

Although we have some understanding of the factors that cause and maintain poor racial environments, we still do not have adequate research to instruct us on how to best remedy the situation. For example, there is no standard for what the essential elements of a "diversity program" should include, no consensus on what the goals of such programs should be, and no clear outcome measures to determine if they reduce racism on campuses (McCauley, Wright, & Harris, 2000; Paluck & Green, 2009). Additionally, interventions need to be tailored to the unique contextual features of the local environments.

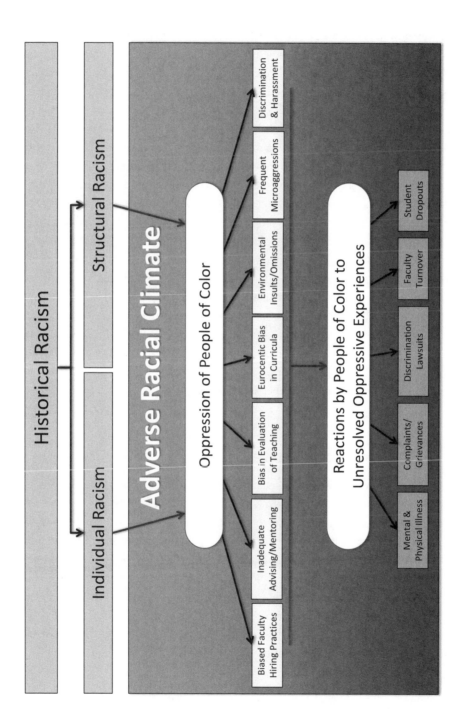

Figure 13.1.

What We Do Know

That being said, there is much we do already know, including practical actions that can be taken now in the service of equity and dismantling institutional racism in higher education. In this chapter, we offer a pragmatic list of empirically supported actions that psychologists can take to improve academic racial climates now, using examples from our own universities and others. The first author is writing from her experience as a diversity educator and African American female in a traditional department of psychology made up of mostly White males. At her prior institution, she was the only minority in the clinical division of the department and first minority woman to be tenured in the department's 108-year history. The second author is writing from his experience as a White male psychology professor and the only researcher in his previous department working in minority communities and with colleagues of color. We provide personal examples of issues experienced in our respective psychology departments to move abstract concepts into a familiar and relatable frame of reference for readers.

In terms of an adverse racial climate, much of what is presented here applies to many academic departments and probably a number of other organizations and venues as well. Although there are many forms of diversity, the interventions presented here are focused on improving racial climate. It is worth noting that many of these points could apply to other forms of diversity as well, such as gender differences, sexual orientation, national origin, and disability. These are all important areas of concern, and rather than weakly address all forms of diversity, we focus on a single yet critical form of diversity that lies squarely within our experience and expertise.

Improving Campus Climate

In the sections that follow, we will discuss how psychologists on college campuses can participate in efforts to improve recruitment and retention of minority faculty and academic advisors, academic diversity course offerings, integration of diversity issues into existing courses, conversations about inequity, diversity trainings for faculty, environmental microaggressions, and use of student course evaluations. Additionally, we will encourage psychologists on campuses to advocate for conducting departmental or unit climate assessments, to respond directly to the experiences of those suffering as a result of an adverse climate, and to appreciate the importance of disciplining as needed. We end with additional discussion of what psychology has to offer in addressing these problems on college campuses, broadly defined.

Recruit and Hire More Ethnically and Racially Diverse Faculty

Real commitments to improving the ethnic and racial diversity of the faculty should be the first order of business in addressing institutionalized racism in higher education (Turner, González, & Wood, 2008). At the very least, the faculty composition should reflect the diversity of the local community and the student body. Research suggests that a critical mass of 20 percent to 35 percent minorities is needed to produce beneficial effects in the environment, such as greater tolerance of difference among Whites and increased feelings of inclusion among people of color (Berrett & Giorgi, 2015). Nationally, only 6 percent of higher education faculty are Black and only 5 percent are Latinx (Kena et al., 2015). Through conversations with undergraduate research assistants, I (first author) was dismayed to discover that many of my students had never had the experience of being instructed by a person of color (e.g., Bradley, 2005), and I found this to be true at both elite and less-competitive institutions. Thus the students had no schema for academic learning from a person like myself, a member of a stigmatized ethnic group at the bottom of the racial social hierarchy. A lack of minority educators gives the false impression that scholarly knowledge comes from White people alone, which is not the message we want to transmit at an institution of higher learning. Diversity improves the learning experience of all concerned, as it introduces new perspectives, disrupts stereotypes, and facilitates appreciation of differences (Galinsky et al., 2015). Additionally, the presence of greater numbers of faculty of color improves academic performance among students of color (Hagedorn, Chi, & Cepeda, 2007). However, numerical representation is not enough; diverse faculty must be present in adequate numbers at every level of the university system—as junior faculty, senior faculty, deans, and top officials. Faculty of color are overrepresented in the lower ranks, such as assistant professor, but underrepresented as full professors, which limits their power and influence (Turner et al., 2008; Kena et al., 2015).

Adequate numbers of diverse faculty are important for effectively mentoring students of color. I (second author), a White male professor, have mentored several students of color. Even though I have done the best I can to be the best mentor possible for them, we have lamented together over the fact that they have not had clear role models of professors who shared their lived experiences *and* their research interests, who could talk to them about their experiences, understand the nuances that sometimes eluded me, and advise them as a complement to my efforts. Thus, it should be no surprise that many students of color prefer mentors who understand their cultural concerns (Maton et al., 2011), and many experience racism, intentional or unintentional, with their White mentors. McCoy, Winkle-Wagner, and Luedke (2015) documented a pattern in which White mentors of Black students used race-neutral, color-blind language that allowed them to ignore structural racism and avoid accusations of racial bias while describing their Black students as academically inferior, less prepared, and less interested in pursuing research and graduate studies. Graduate students, in particular, require a close relationship with faculty, and research indicates that the mentoring relationship and perceptions of diversity within the academic environment are critical for recruitment, retention, and satisfaction among minority graduate students (Rogers & Molina, 2006; Maton et al., 2011).

As a field, psychology is not producing enough psychologists of color to completely meet the need in our universities, and so some might argue that there are simply not enough psychologists of color to hire, or that those who are available are "not good enough" (Gasman, 2016). About 78 percent of faculty in accredited doctoral psychology programs are White (Smith, 2015), which is about the same percentage of White US citizens and permanent residents being awarded doctoral degrees (76.6 percent in 2014; National Science Foundation, 2016), although only 63.7 percent of the US population is White.

Faculty of color should not simply be hired as "token" or so-called diversity hires. Although 58 percent support affirmative action for minorities, that leaves 37 percent who do not (and 6 percent with no opinion; Gallup, 2015), which makes this quite a divisive issue, with potential repercussions for new hires of color. "Diversity hires" may evoke negative reactions and (mis)perceptions of unfairness among others, resulting in backlash (social punishment) directed toward the new faculty member (Kravitz & Klineberg, 2000), marginalization (Niemann, 2003), and even stereotype threat, which can cause decreased performance (Leslie, Mayer, & Kravitz, 2014). Furthermore, when faculty of color are underrepresented, they may feel isolated, and they are more likely to face "cultural taxation," which includes doing a disproportionate amount of unrecognized diversity-related work and more mentoring of students of color compared to their White peers (Joseph & Hirshfield, 2011).

For these reasons, "diversity hires" should be avoided except under the most desperate circumstances. Rather than hiring a token or even a quota of minority faculty or being resigned to the notion that minority faculty cannot be found (which are actual sentiments expressed by faculty at department meetings), the best solution is a campus-wide effort at reform. That means working harder to find solutions (see Cross & Slater, 2002; McMurtrie, 2016). One noteworthy example of this is provided by the University of Michigan's ADVANCE program, which comprehensively addresses diversity recruitment, retention, campus climate, and leadership (Linderman, 2015).

At the department level, one approach could be to create a subdivision within the department dedicated to cultural diversity science that includes a critical number of faculty numerically on par with other psychology departmental divisions. This would likely result in a number of ethnically diverse faculty but not be exclusive to people of color, as qualification would be based on area of expertise rather than dependent on the race of the applicant. Departments also may consider creating joint appointments with diverse faculty from other departments or bringing in new faculty as joint hires between psychology and disciplines that enjoy more diversity, such as Pan-African or Hispanic and Latino Studies. This practice can be misleading, because it makes a department appear larger and more diverse than it actually is, but it can be an excellent place to start in the face of real shortages of faculty of color.

Hire a Person of Color as an Academic Advisor for Your Department

High-quality academic advising, free from bias and stereotypes, is crucial for students of color, especially for first-generation students without a familial history of higher educational achievement from which to learn (Strayhorn, 2013). Extant research supports the importance of an "intrusive" advising style, which involves a more proactive and involved role of the advisor in the personal and academic affairs of the student (Earl, 1988). Intrusive advising has been shown to improve retention rates, GPA, and graduation rates among at-risk students, including students of color (Glennen, Baxley, & Farren, 1985; Molina & Abelman, 2000).

Our experiences talking with students and advisors at our institutions, however, is that White advisors overwhelmingly favor a color-blind, more detached, and more formal approach to advising. This is supported by the publication record of the advising field's major journal, which published only one article on Black student advising issues (Guiffrida, 2004) and no articles on Latinx student issues over a fifteen-year period (Shaffer, 2010). More publications in this journal discuss issues of "at-risk" students, which is often coded language to describe students of color. Our experience is that this publishing trend of minimizing race and racism while emphasizing other variables is consistent with mainstream advising practices, which fails to account for cultural differences.

Adding a person of color as a departmental academic advisor was a suggestion from one of our students, and we think it is an important idea, because we have noticed that our Black undergraduates are not getting the messages they need about how to best prepare to further their education. They often come to us during their final year of college for advice about how to get into a clinical psychology doctoral program, and at that point it is too late for them to get the GPA or undergraduate experiences they need to be competitive for graduate school. Although there is not yet much research to confirm our observations, it seems that these students are not getting the same quality of advising, mentorship, and research opportunities as afforded to White students, that advisors are not able to adapt their advising practices to the needs of students of color, and that advisors may perpetuate bias and stereotypes in their advising practices (e.g., Crosby & Monin, 2007). Consistent with the need to raise the level of multicultural competence across all points of interaction with students of color (administration, staff, faculty, and students), we suggest that an important resource is access to advisors of color who understand and share their lived experiences.

Underrepresented students of color often struggle due to generations of disadvantage that place them in college while simultaneously caring for families and holding full-time jobs. Campaigns focused on increasing the graduation rate push students to take fifteen or more credits per semester, which is not beneficial for those with demanding work schedules (Attewell & Monaghan, 2016) or who have children or other family responsibilities, and can conceivably result in lower grades. We know of one faculty member who has been telling such students that they simply do not have the time to take hard classes, due to their circumstances. Students like this would most likely feel more comfortable receiving advice from someone who they perceive has a better ability to understand, empathize, and problem-solve around their real-life issues and backgrounds (Chan, Yeh, & Krumboltz, 2015; Guiffrida, 2005).

Provide Adequate and Impactful Undergraduate and Graduate Diversity Courses

Institutional racism manifests not only as who is teaching and advising students but also as what courses are offered to students. Research indicates that diversity courses reduce bias and that taking more than one diversity course improves student well-being and orientations toward diversity (Bowman, 2010; Denson, 2009). Although some sort of cultural diversity requirement is becoming the norm for colleges and universities, a national survey of one hundred institutions found that required diversity courses were less effective at teaching diversity and inclusivity than elective diversity courses that students are not required to take (Laird & Engberg, 2011). The survey also documented that 37 percent of the institutions in the sample had no diversity requirement at all.

When we evaluated the course offerings in our own psychology departments, we found diversity courses sorely lacking. Most other departments in our respective colleges of arts and sciences offered more diversity classes than we did, whereas each of our departments offered one or fewer courses per year. Additionally, both of us had been faculty in psychology departments that encouraged graduate students to take courses from other departments to meet diversity requirements—which communicates to students that these courses are not important enough to be taught in our own departments. Our experiences in departmental and committee meetings is that some faculty react with resistance to suggestions to increase diversity offerings, expressing a lack of understanding of the importance of offering more classes and a reluctance to put in the work needed to make this happen, while other faculty express a willingness to teach the courses if asked. It is a divisive issue that often results in a lack of consensus and inaction—which maintains the status quo. One way to address concerns about the importance of such courses and stimulate action is to conduct student surveys or engage in self-assessment. Research in the first author's former department showed that White and minority students alike believe these courses are important and want to see more being offered (DeLapp, DeLapp, & Williams, 2016).

There is no question that making changes to any program will require more work and effort, and diversity courses can be hard to teach and often result in lower student course evaluations if the content includes topics like racism and White privilege (Boatright-Horowitz & Soeung, 2009). Deliberate efforts will be needed to meet the important goal of fostering diversity, and it is incumbent on the department leadership to transmit this important message to the rest of the faculty (Kezar & Eckel, 2008; Ng, 2008). Departments should acknowledge the challenges of doing this work well and consider offering faculty incentives to teach these kinds of courses (i.e., higher pay, extra merit points, separate quality point cut-offs).

The content of diversity coursework matters. It has become increasingly evident that we need to shift away from teaching facts about different racial and cultural groups to including material from modern psychological science on racism, implicit bias, stereotypes, White privilege, intersectionality, microaggressions, and other topics that require more self-reflection and critical appraisal of one's self and one's role in a structurally racist society (Case, 2007). This imperative comes from both the accumulation of science and personal experience. After teaching multicultural psychology a few times, it became evident that lectures and readings were often not sufficient to bring about a multicultural shift in perspective, as we are often combatting a lifetime of learned prejudice in students, many of whom were from all-White communities in the rural South. Teaching racism to White students is tricky. In addition to expecting lower course evaluations (Boatright-Horowitz & Soeung, 2009), teachers should expect that attempts to raise awareness of bias and discuss these topics can actually increase interracial anxiety, helplessness, guilt, and fear of being misunderstood, leading to increased avoidance and defensiveness (Case, 2007; Perry, Dovidio, Murphy, & van Ryn, 2015; Sue et al., 2010).

Strategies that effectively engage White students in these topics and produce more positive outcomes are an active source of research inquiry. Denson's (2009) meta-analytic review of twenty-seven curricular interventions found that tested interventions do produce benefits. Furthermore, a significant increase in intervention effectiveness was observed when interventions included a contact component in which students engaged in interracial interactions as part of the intervention. Contact has long been heralded as an effective anti-racism interaction and appears to work through reduced anxiety and increased empathy towards the out-group (Pettigrew, Tropp, Wagner, & Christ, 2011).

Research also supports the importance of active learning, experiential strategies that put participants in contact with counter-stereotypical examples, and teaching concrete strategies for overriding bias rather than a sole emphasis on didactics (Lai et al., 2014). Consistent with these recommendations, in our diversity courses, we have found that sensitive experiential exercises that facilitate intergroup contact while allowing students to explore their biases and reactions personally and directly are powerful learning tools. As behavioral scientists, we explain to students that these experiential assignments can be thought of as "exposures" to address interracial anxieties through disconfirmation of cognitive distortions (e.g., pathological stereotypes) and habituation to feared stimuli (e.g., talking about race).

As an undergraduate psychology student, I (first author) remember participating in an exercise at the University of California at Los Angeles in which students wore a pink triangle button for forty-eight hours, then journaled about the experience of being associated with a sexual minority group (Rabow, Stein, & Conley, 1999); this exercise gave me a profound new perspective on what it meant to be stigmatized—beyond my race and gender—and so, to this day, I have a keen appreciation of the impact of experiential learning. In my graduate classes, exercises focused on race may include having a discussion with a classmate of a different race about race-related experiences, visiting a house of worship where everyone "looks different from you," or giving a clinical interview about cultural beliefs or racism (e.g., Williams, Peña, & Mier-Chairez, 2017). To facilitate processing, students write weekly reflection papers about these experiences, and we discuss them in class (i.e., Causey, Thomas, & Armento, 2000). Along those lines, the University of North Carolina has implemented a diversity program for its clinical doctoral students that includes a critical experiential component they refer to as a "cultural plunge." With the help of an advanced student facilitator, "plungees" plan an experience where they are in a stigmatized minority position rather than in a position of privilege (Bardone-Cone et al., 2016).

Better Integrate Diversity Issues into the Curriculum for All Courses

In addition to adding new courses to the curriculum that directly teach diversity and inclusiveness, existing courses across disciplines must be vetted to eradicate bias and more accurately represent our multicultural world and history. Historically, racial bias has existed in textbooks in terms of errors of omission (minimal treatment of minorities); stereotypical representations of minorities; selective interpretations of minority issues that omit minority perspectives; glossing over, simplifying, or distorting unpleasant facts to make them more palatable for White readers; isolating minority issues to special inserts, boxes, or peripheral chapters; linguistic practices; and cosmetic treatment of minorities that provide the illusion of equity (Zittleman & Sadker, 2002).

The above forms of bias exist across existing course content in current university curricula. For example, people of color are substantially underrepresented in major government and politics textbooks (Monforti & McGlynn, 2010) and general chemistry textbooks (King & Domin, 2007), negative stereotypes about Blacks and other minorities are widespread in popular nursing textbooks (Byrne, 2001), and White geologists are seventeen times more abundant than non-Whites as examples and role models in geology textbooks (Mattox et al., 2008). Psychology does not fare much better, with one recent review indicating that no brief introductory psychology textbooks include a chapter on diversity at all (Griggs & Jackson, 2013). Furthermore, I (first author) was disturbed to discover that a cross-cultural textbook that my department had been using cited racist intelligence research without any mention of the researchers' biases or deficiencies in their research methods.

Professors seem to know they should include diversity in their curricula, but many simply do not know how to do it (Causey et al., 2000). As a result, there may be social pressure to profess coverage of diversity issues, but it may be done inadequately or not at all. Faculty should look carefully at their reading materials and syllabi and solicit input from others with knowledge and expertise on cultural issues to contribute material that will help balance out the tendency to provide information from a Eurocentric perspective (Collins & Hebert, 2008). For example, we continue to be saddened and perplexed by the fact that so many students we encounter know nothing about the astounding contributions to the field of psychology by psychologists of color, such as the influential research of Drs. Kenneth and Mamie Clark, who conducted the doll studies that were later used to desegregate public schools (Clark & Clark, 1939). When I (first author) teach clinical psychopathology to graduate students, every week one of the four assigned readings is focused on mental health differences in a marginalized group (e.g., racial and ethnic minority groups, sexual minorities, low income communities, cross-cultural groups, etc.), and students tell me that they appreciate the expanded perspective beyond the DSM-5.

Provide Effective Forums for Dialogue and Increasing Awareness of White Privilege, Inequities, and Microaggressions

Students of color report that the day-to-day experience of campus life is fraught with insults, racist events, and experiences of exclusion and marginalization (e.g., Smith, Allen, & Danley, 2007; Smith, Mustaffa, Jones, Curry, & Allen, 2016). Some of these experiences may be seen as structural—being the only Black student in a class, having no Black instructors or advisors, or finding no examples incorporating realistic portrayals of Blacks in textbooks—and are addressed in our points above. Much of the problem, however, is interpersonal and involves direct interactions between students of color and others on campus. Qualitative studies of the campus-life experiences of Black students, including a recent study of our own, document that Black students experience interpersonal microaggressions and other racist interpersonal interactions on a regular basis, not just from other students, but from faculty and others on campus as well (Debreaux et al., 2015; Lewis, Chesler, & Forman, 2000; Smith et al., 2016; Solórzano et al., 2000). These microaggressions range from insults that students receive so often they have habituated to them (e.g., "Can I touch your hair?" or being ignored by the barista in the line at the cafe) to insults that shock and upset them for prolonged periods (e.g., a professor stating in a lecture that Blacks are genetically less intelligent). Research indicates that the accumulation of these experiences has deleterious effects on mental health (Carter, 2007; O'Keefe et al., 2015).

Today, many higher education institutions across the nation have hired a chief diversity officer, created a diversity office, or started a campus diversity initiative charged with improving the racial climate (Wilson, 2013). One typical product of such efforts is the provision of stand-alone or a series of workshops or dialogues for the larger campus community (faculty, staff, and students) that are intended to address the racist interpersonal interactions that students of color experience with regularity. Local diversity trainers may be hired to lead forums or dialogues, or in-house facilitators are used. Some research indicates that these dialogues are fraught with peril, as many White people have been socialized to squelch and minimize the painful realities of inequality that are shared by non-Whites in these forums (Sue, Torino, Capodilupo, Rivera, & Lin, 2009). This process may generate, during the forum, the very microaggressions the forums intend to reduce (Sue et al., 2007). Overall, however, meta-analyses of the effects of diversity trainings suggests that they produce small-to-moderate effects on measures of White attitudes and bias, and these effects can be strengthened if the dialogue lasts longer or occurs in a series rather than a stand-alone workshop (Kalinoski et al., 2013).

Our experience is that it is important to provide these forums, as they serve several important functions. In pilot research on dialogues that we have been developing using a contextual behavioral science model, White students have reported to us that they have benefited from hearing about the negative experiences of their non-White peers; this can be an important means of raising awareness, promoting empathy, and exploring what it means to be White in a social racial hierarchy (Thurston-Rattue et al., 2015). The fact that a majority of White Americans (52 percent) believe that discrimination against their group has become as big a problem as discrimination against people of color indicates widespread and massive misunderstandings regarding the racial realities of our society (Jones et al., 2014), so raising awareness of the extent of the problem is an important outcome in its own right.

A second important function of these dialogues is that they may facilitate cross-group friendships and connections. Consistent with both intergroup contact theory and intergroup process theory (MacInnis & Page-Gould, 2015), research suggests that when cross-racial participants exchange personally vulnerable details of their lives with each other, interracial anxiety decreases, and intimacy and friendship increases (Page-Gould, Mendoza-Denton, & Tropp, 2008). Thus, in our dialogues, White participants are encouraged to listen with empathy to the narratives of Black participants and also to reciprocally disclose vulnerable details from their own lives. Multiple participants from our dialogues have reported to us that cross-racial friendships have developed from this experience that have lasted beyond the workshop session (Thurston-Rattue et al., 2015). One established example of how this work can be done well is intergroup dialogue, studied extensively at the University of Michigan and picked up by many universities across the country (Dessel & Rogge, 2008; Gurin, Sorensen, Lopez, & Nagda, 2015).

Provide Diversity Training for All Faculty

At the first author's former institution, they were greatly embarrassed by a photo that emerged from a campus Mexican-themed Halloween party featuring the university president dressed in a sombrero and colorful poncho along with the whole executive staff, several sporting bushy moustaches or strange veils (Svrluga, 2015b). This picture was featured in many major media outlets, including the Associated Press, Fox News, the Washington Post, USA Today, and the Huffington Post. Although ethnically or racially themed parties have fallen out of fashion at universities all over the nation, no one in the executive office was knowledgeable enough or empowered enough to speak up to prevent this catastrophe from happening. After the event, many departments and divisions sent frantic emails to students, staff, and faculty, apologizing for what happened and attempting to make amends. I (first author) also apologized to my students on behalf of the university and subsequently utilized the event as a teaching tool, where I met with the leaders of the university and provided a training on microaggressions to the president's office. Fortunately, psychology has answers to many of these problems, and when racist events occur, faculty can use them as an opportunity for learning and growth.

The aforementioned embarrassing and hurtful incident illustrates what can happen when universities decide that isolated racial dialogues are enough and neglect to develop a comprehensive plan that includes basic diversity training to their faculty and leaders. It is critical that all faculty are able to properly interact with students of color (Delano-Oriaran & Meidl, 2012), yet one of the most consistent concerns cited by campus protesters is the need for sensitivity training for faculty to reduce racism (Berner, 2015; The Demands, 2016). Students deserve an environment free of racism, which is difficult to accomplish if faculty themselves are unwitting perpetrators (e.g., Hartocollis & Bidgood, 2015). Yet research shows that many faculty members continue to commit microaggressions and engage with minority students from a colorblind perspective (McCoy et al., 2015; Sue et al., 2007; Terwilliger, Bach, Bryan & Williams, 2013), indicating a need for increased training and growth. Our experiences are that insensitive and unaware faculty members are not uncommon and can have the effect of a bull in a China shop, leaving a trail of trampled students in their wake (Harper & Hurtado, 2007).

It is particularly difficult for students to know how to respond to racism inflicted by faculty due to traditional hierarchies that may create fear of retaliation, perceived lack of accountability, and hopelessness about change. Students may be reluctant to complain to a department chair or ombudsman, who likely also is White. If a student of color approaches the offending faculty member or a colleague about racial issues, they may find themselves misunderstood or even attacked by defensive faculty. For example, I (second author) have had several conversations with my students of color during which they revealed offensive comments or discriminatory behavior directed toward them from other faculty members. But when I suggested that I confront these faculty members directly, such was their legitimate fear of repercussions that they panicked at the thought and made me promise that I would not do anything. The structural bind was too strong for us to overcome ourselves.

Although it will be challenging, faculty must be encouraged to face their own privilege, explore their own biases, stereotypes, and behaviors, and learn how to have hard conversations in a productive way. As we discuss below, they also need to learn how to listen non-defensively and with empathy. Although some faculty may exhibit resistance toward the idea of mandatory trainings (perhaps those most in need of such trainings), consider that many departments require trainings for sexual harassment, HIPAA regulations, and IRB research ethics. Diversity issues are no less important. Mandatory trainings send the message that the organization is strongly committed to diversity, which has been hypothesized to increase the motivation to learn, and although faculty prefer and are more favorable toward voluntary training, mandatory diversity trainings are, in fact, more effective (Bezrukova, Spell, Perry, & Jehn, 2016). One solution implemented by the first author's department that circumvented this potentially thorny issue was to invite a diversity trainer to facilitate the annual department retreat, an event that all faculty already attend. We believe that mandatory trainings would have provided a safe, leadership-supported forum for a discussion of the problems raised by the second author's students above, which could not be resolved without better structures in place.

It is important that trainings be provided by individuals that faculty will respect, which in our departments would mean other academic psychologists who understand both diversity issues *and* the scientific literature. Research indicates that minorities who conduct diversity trainings are more respected than White trainers, who may be perceived to have less life experience in managing racial events (Liberman, Block, & Koch, 2011). However, White professors are perceived as more competent, at least by students, so a White trainer may be more effective in that regard (Ho, Thomsen, & Sidanius, 2009). Furthermore, it is valuable for White trainers to discuss their own emotions, struggles, and growth surrounding issues like stereotypes and White privilege to illustrate the relevance of the material to others like themselves (Sue et al., 2009). Thus, trainings may be offered by a diverse team (e.g., minority female and a White male), as this may best facilitate engagement from all faculty concerned. We conduct trainings as a diverse team whenever possible, and this seems to help engage the more resistant participants, as they see that the material is relevant to people like themselves. This also helps prevent White people and minorities alike from feeling like they are on the defensive or shamed and paralyzed. See chapter 7 for one successful approach we have used for diversity workshops.

Remove Environmental Microaggressions

Racism can be environmental in nature, such as when an academic setting assails a person's racial identity. According to Sue et al. (2007) someone's racial identity can be unintentionally minimized or made insignificant through the exclusion of decorations or literature that represent their racial group, which is referred to as an environmental microaggression. For example, in the hallways of the first author's former department are proudly displayed huge framed photos of the winners of the Grawemeyer Award in the field of psychology. These awards are annual prizes of $100,000 given in the fields of music, political science, psychology, education, and religion, founded by H. Charles Grawemeyer, to help make the world a better place. The pictures of the psychology winners transmit a major unfortunate environmental microaggression. All award-winners are White—every last one (see figure 13.2a). The message communicated to our students is that "no one of color did anything worth recognizing"—and to students of color, "and neither will you." Of course, there are many worthy psychologists of color who could have been awardees, but the system in place to elect psychology winners is heavily biased toward identifying White psychologists (e.g., Grawemeyer committee members are White, and none study diversity issues; ads soliciting nominees are placed in journals with primarily White readerships; and past winners help identify subsequent winners). In other words, the award process is biased due to structural and institutional racism, but our students do not know that; they may simply be left thinking that White people are smarter, and psychology proves it.

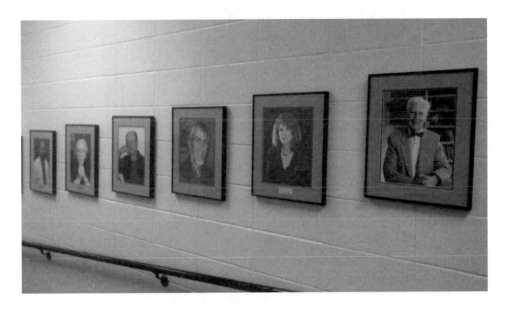

Figure 13.2a

There are also gigantic Caucasian heads placed at various places throughout the department as an ongoing art project, which amounts to an environmental microaggression of mammoth proportions (see figure 13.2b). Heads symbolize intelligence, agency, and the mind, yet gigantic East Asian or African heads are nowhere to be found. Departments should take stock of the unspoken messages transmitted by representations in the environment, as lack of diverse images can communicate prejudice and threat to people of color (Purdie-Vaughns, Steele, Davies, Ditlmann, & Crosby, 2008).

The issue of environmental microaggressions recently played out at Yale University, when, after much debate over racist imagery and building names, Corey Menafee, an African American service worker, broke a stained glass window depicting smiling slaves carrying baskets of cotton. In explanation of his actions, Menafee said, "as you look at it, it just hurts. You feel it in your heart, like, oh, man—like here in the twenty-first century, you know, we're in a modern era where we shouldn't have to be subjected to those primitive and degrading images" (Gonzalez & Goodman, 2016). University officials struggled with how to respond to the situation. Menafee was fired and charged with felony mischief, but then subsequently rehired, after some extended controversy, under the condition that he would not speak out about the case. Although the event was framed as vandalism by some and activism by others, we believe it is more accurate to conceptualize Menafee's actions as a traumatic reaction to being forced to work in a racially hostile environment (Carter, 2007; Williams, Kanter, & Ching, 2018).

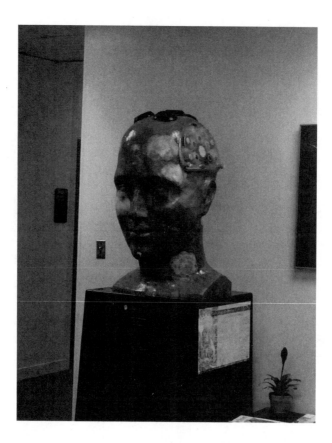

Figure 13.2b

It is possible to find peaceful and appropriate solutions for these types of problems. At my (first author's) former university, there was a similar situation in which a Confederate monument stood in the center of a busy public intersection adjacent to the campus (figure 13.3). Each day during my trek from the parking lot to my university office, I was visually assaulted by the seventy-foot-tall granite obelisk with Confederate soldiers made of bronze and dressed in war gear—the largest Civil War monument in the state. Owned by the city, the monument commemorates the "sacrifice" of Confederate veterans—soldiers who perished in a failed armed rebellion against our nation that resulted in 750,000 deaths. The monument was erected to celebrate people who were willing to die for the right to keep a whole race of people like me permanently enslaved. Many solutions had been advanced to address concerns raised by those who found the monument inappropriate and offensive, but no actions had been taken. During my afore-mentioned diversity training to the university's executive office, I explained how this monument affected me personally as an African American. I wondered aloud how toler-ant the academic community would be if this were a monument in celebration of Nazi World War II veterans, if Jewish faculty had to walk past it each day, and how Germans were rightly ashamed of their Nazi history. After the training, the university president said to me that perhaps it was time for change in regards to the monument. Shortly thereafter, the president, in partnership with the mayor, made a plan to move the monument to a more appropriate location, which was upheld, despite a lawsuit advanced by supporters of the monument to keep it at its original site (Associated Press, 2016). We believe a key factor in this positive outcome was for the president to hear first-hand about how this affected a real person at a very human level, underscoring the importance of empathy and mutual understanding in these processes (Shelton, Trail, West, & Bergsieker, 2010).

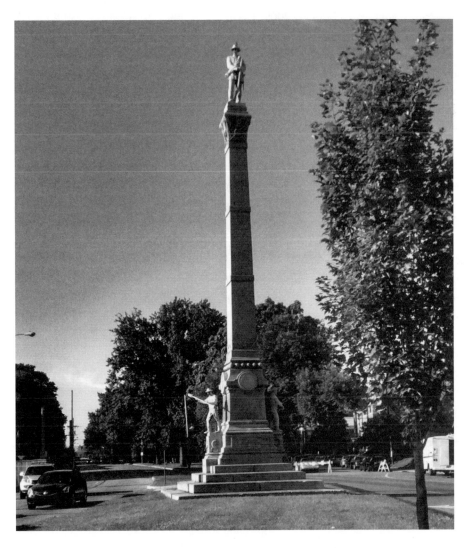

Figure 13.3

Stop Using Student Course Evaluation Scores for Raises, Promotion, and Tenure

We have known for some time that student course evaluations are sexist, racist, and a poor indicator of learning (Boring, Ottoboni, & Stark, 2016; Nast, 1999). In fact, students rate faculty significantly lower simply for being "unattractive" or having a foreign accent (Hamermesh & Parker, 2005). Students show less respect for faculty of color, and this is also manifest in lower course evaluation scores or even abusive comments rooted in negative stereotypes (Bradley, 2005; Ho et al., 2009). Despite these well-known failings, student course evaluations are retained as part of the academic tradition, with raises and promotion tied to scores as "evidence" of teaching quality. When I (first author) mentioned this to my former chair, she pointed out that my evaluations are numerically fine. However, I have to work harder when I teach multicultural psychology than when I teach other classes, like abnormal psychology, in order to keep my ratings up; and I have to work harder to overcome student biases against me as a Black female, which means I am expending much more time and energy than my White male colleagues. This is unfair, exhausting, and puts me and others in my situation at risk for burnout. This discriminatory means of evaluation will potentially decrease the number of qualified faculty of color retained by departments, contributing to a negative climate. Additionally, if we adhere to our own science, we should be assessing real learning rather than rewarding faculty for winning a rigged popularity contest that is biased against faculty who are already facing extra hurdles. Boring, Ottoboni, and Stark (2016) did an excellent study that highlighted these issues in an investigation of bias in course evaluations. They found that scores were better predictors of gender bias and grade expectations than teaching effectiveness.

There are many fairer methods that could be used to evaluate teaching effectiveness than student evaluations. For example, pre- and posttests of student knowledge would be a more objective and accurate way of determining how well professors are able to impart knowledge (Stark-Wroblewski, Ahlering, & Brill, 2007). Another technique employed in many departments is peer evaluation of teaching, which is not completely free of racial bias and may trigger stereotype threat in minority faculty (Steele & Aronson, 1995) but could be more objective, considering that observing peers have experience teaching themselves and are not being graded in the course.

Conduct a Departmental Climate Assessment

It has been said that it is hard for a fish to perceive the water it swims in. A negative racial climate may not be readily observable when a department or institution is run by people for whom White privilege is largely invisible. Furthermore, for a number of reasons having to do with power, prestige, and authority, simply asking minority faculty (who are usually lower ranked; Kena et al., 2015) and students of color what things are *really* like may not generate complete or honest answers (Stangor, Swim, Van Allen, & Sechrist,

2002). And sadly, when minorities speak up about the realities of discrimination, they are often dismissed as complainers (e.g., DeLapp & Williams, 2015; Garcia, Reser, Amo, Redersdorff, & Branscombe, 2005). Thus, an outside climate assessment of racial and ethnic diversity issues is often the only and best way to get accurate feedback on what the environment is truly like for people of color. Such an assessment, ideally conducted by psychologists who are knowledgeable in diversity and organizational issues, might include anonymous surveys, individual interviews, and focus groups to get a full picture of department strengths and weaknesses (e.g., Harper & Hurtado, 2007).

Listen

Faculty must realize that when they are approached by students, staff, or other faculty of color who describe a negative racial situation to them in confidence or who ask for support, a very important moment for healing and growth is at hand. This is a delicate moment for both parties. The person of color has chosen to engage the (typically) White person in a vulnerable interpersonal interaction and undoubtedly enters it with fears of being misunderstood (Shelton, Richeson, & Salvatore, 2005) and becoming the target of even further prejudice (Shelton, Douglass, Garcia, Yip, & Trail, 2014). Yet that person has chosen to engage nonetheless.

In this interaction, the White person may fear being seen as prejudiced and demonstrate a heightened physiological threat response, both of which make it harder for the interaction to succeed (Shelton, West, & Trail, 2010). It is crucial that the White person is able to overcome these biases and respond well in this moment. Positive intergroup interactions predict physiological recovery from stressful intergroup interactions for people of color, and the success of the interaction depends to a significant degree of the ability of the White person to listen well and demonstrate accurate empathy and understanding (Davies, Tropp, Aron, Pettigrew, & Wright, 2011; Shelton, Trail, et al., 2010).

For example, on the first author's campus, when students initially arranged a meeting with the university president to discuss their feelings about what became known as Sombrerogate, they reported that he did not seem to listen and left after only a short time because he had another appointment. This made students feel as if their concerns were unimportant, which only worsened the situation and turned what could have been a small problem into a much larger one, fueling distrust of the institution. One student said, "[the president] did not want to listen to us, and he was not interested in the context of what was going on. I feel very let down by the leader of this university" (Moody, 2015).

As clinical psychologists, we are trained to attune to issues of vulnerability and trust in our interactions, and the importance of responding with empathy and caring is key to our work, especially when a client of color is discussing racially sensitive material (Miller, Williams, Wetterneck, Kanter, & Tsai, 2015; Williams et al., 2014). However, we recognize that an administrator or faculty member outside of mental health may not naturally attune to the importance of these responses in this moment. It may be useful to note that a fundamental requirement for trust and closeness to develop is *perceived responsiveness:*

When one person engages in a vulnerable disclosure to another, the discloser must perceive the listener to respond with understanding, validation, and caring (Reis, 2007). This applies to cross-racial relationships as well (Davies, Tropp, Aron, Pettigrew, & Wright, 2011; Page-Gould et al., 2008).

Therefore, when approached by a person who is claiming to be the victim of a racially discriminatory slight, microaggression, aggressive action, or assault, the first, best, and most important thing we can do in this moment is to listen. Even if the urge is to do otherwise, and as difficult as it may sometimes be, it is imperative to resist any impulse to get defensive or make excuses for the perpetrator—especially if you are the perpetrator. Interrogating the victim through aggressive questioning about the accuracy of the event will undoubtedly lead to ruptures in the relationship and be experienced as invalidating by the person who experienced the event. The person who experienced the event is in the best position to understand the harm that it produced. It is important to empathize with the person and tell the person that you feel sorry that the event happened, even if it was not about you. It is important to explicitly recognize the larger social context of racial injustice in this moment and not be color-blind (McCoy et al., 2015). People who have suffered as a result of a poor racial climate need to feel heard, validated, and believed (DeLapp & Williams, 2015). They themselves may offer some solutions to the problem, but it is best not to require them to do so. The victim is not the cause of the problem and should not be required to fix it.

Discipline as Needed

Although most experiences of racism may be small and unintentional, sometimes they are overt and intentional. White people with a history of blindness to privilege and lack of awareness of racial issues are more likely to see events of racial harassment and discrimination as minor problems or mistakes that do not require a formal response, but Black people tend see them as severe, want a response, and feel a stronger sense of organizational justice and safety that they will not be harassed in the future if action is taken (Chrobot-Mason & Hepworth, 2005). Furthermore, many institutional obstacles exist that make it hard for victims to report problems, including fear that reporting will make things worse, not better, or result in retaliation (Chakraborti, & Garland, 2003). Thus, when such events occur, in addition to conveying empathy to victims, swift and clear responses by administration are essential to overcome institutional racism. It must be made widely known that behaviors that threaten the safety and well-being of any group will not be tolerated, that effective resources are available so people know how to report problems, that the right people are trained and in place to handle situations fully, that victims will be protected, and that disciplinary action will be implemented fully (Larsen, Nye, Ormerod, Ziebro, & Siebert, 2013; Martin, Goodboy, & Johnson, 2015).

For example, on the first author's campus, it came to light that in one of the residence halls, some students were writing derogatory messages, including racial slurs and swastikas, on a common-area whiteboard. This made many students of color upset and afraid. There was a residence hall meeting at which some suggested that upset students should just take the acts as a joke or ignore them, and still others considered it a free-speech issue. A residence hall exercise was subsequently implemented to educate students about stereotypes, and residence hall advisors were given trainings on diversity issues, but this was unsuccessful in relieving racial tensions. Concerned students were offered the opportunity to file a report or move to another residence hall, or both (Krauth, 2016).

Responses such as this one have large effects on victims, decreasing students' interest in school, reducing feelings of competence, and increasing the likelihood of dropout (Martin et al., 2015). The problem with these responses is that rather than disciplinary actions, the perpetrators were instead given a platform to continue their hurtful behaviors via group discussions. Additionally, an undue burden was placed on the victims to file reports that students worried could result in retaliation; the administration was already aware of the problems and should have investigated and disciplined those responsible when they first learned of it. Additionally, moving minority students out of the dorm should never have been advanced as a solution, as that unfairly burdens the victims and reinforces the perpetrators. Forty faculty members signed a letter to the upper administration expressing their disappointment with the way the event had been managed, and noted that "staff, faculty, and administrators have a grave responsibility to create a racially healthy climate, one where each and every student has an equitable and meaningful opportunity to flourish." Deliberate racism should never be tolerated.

What Psychologists Can Do

Psychology has already contributed a great deal to understanding and addressing the problem of racism on campuses. Excellent work has been done by social psychologists to help us understand issues like group behaviors, racism, and implicit bias. Clinical psychology has explicated the mental health consequences of a poor racial environment on people of color. Psychologists can conduct workplace assessments and give recommendations for effective changes to improve the climate, such as the interventions described in this article. Psychology has well-developed tools and research methods that allow us to design and test interventions for reducing racism, which we have been actively employing to study and ameliorate these problems. We also partner with organizational psychologists, who also have much to contribute by way of designing and implementing workplace interventions.

All of those contributions lie within our traditional spheres of influence. However, psychologists also have much to offer when we step out of our comfort zones and get directly involved as catalysts for change on campus. We can participate in campus social-justice activities, advocate for change ourselves, and solve campus problems that exist today. Much anti-racism activity is happening on campuses across our country right now, and psychologists' voices are important to these efforts. The second author's campus, for example, has established a strong campus anti-racism initiative, made up of dedicated administrative leaders and relevant staff. However, I (second author) am the only psychologist or scientist of any type on my committee, even though my department has several psychologists who study issues pertinent to the committee's mission.

Leaders within schools, departments, and divisions are needed to inspire and motivate resistant faculty and keep sympathetic faculty motivated to keep working for change, and psychologists have much to say about resistance and motivation. For example, research indicates that the inclusive ideology of multiculturalism is often not perceived as such by Whites, which may be one reason for resistance; thus, it is important to convey that diversity is not about including people of color and excluding White people, but that everyone is valued, needed, and important. Psychologists can help department chairs, deans, and presidents craft these important messages and articulate the vision for an environment that embodies a diverse and harmonious academic community.

Psychologists can volunteer for roles and provide leadership on intervening when crises occur and facilitate forums for community healing. Psychologists can provide training when needed and be agents for change, as occurred in the aftermath of the Mexican Halloween party at first author's university. Academic psychologists are often both respected by people in the community and misunderstood, and psychologists can attend community rallies, events, and protests as a way to build connections and send a message of support and understanding. I (second author) was often one of the few White people at rallies or protests about police violence in the Black community in Milwaukee, Wisconsin. As one of the only White men at these events, and a professor, I was occasionally asked to lend my voice to the rally, and I did so nervously but willingly. I received many appreciations and remarks that my presence was welcome and desired at these events, and it communicated the message that White people do, in fact, care about what happens to people of color.

Yet, as illustrated by our examples, the field of psychology and psychology departments also suffer from the many of the same institutional and structural problems that plague other departments and our campuses. This creates barriers to advancement for some of the very people who are uniquely poised to understand these difficulties and find answers (e.g., ethnic minority psychologists). We must prioritize change as a discipline if we intend to remain relevant and credible in the ongoing dialogue about our society's racial problems. This involves stepping out of our comfort zones and being willing to challenge the status quo. For example, recently a medical student at a workshop we conducted expressed reservations about telling a supervisor about a report of racist behavior perpetrated by a colleague, because, the student said, "I don't want to throw our clinic under the bus." After some brief discussion that reminded the attendee that racism is a tremendous problem in our society that affects medical clinics across the country, the attendee was able to see that change will never occur if we prioritize the image of our workplaces over institutional change. We urge all psychologists reading this to consider how they have contributed to these dysfunctional systems and ask themselves what they can do to help bring about change. We urge deans, chairs, division heads, and directors of clinical training programs to do a fearless inventory of their divisions' strengths and weaknesses, and ask themselves what steps they can take now to improve the situation for people of color, even if only by a little, with the ultimate goal of full minority participation in every facet of department life.

Conclusion

The actions proposed here will not completely eliminate racism and discrimination, but they can be important steps in making people of color feel welcome and valued, resulting in an improved learning environment for everyone. People may believe that because structural racism has evolved over decades, as policies became institutionalized, it will take decades to realize changes. However, the interventions offered here are concrete and relatively simple steps that can be taken right now, led by individuals, that can have a large impact at departmental and university levels. Many of these are top-down suggestions, but with the right level of faculty and administrative support, they are implementable.

For example, I (first author) recently witnessed a real change with respect to the removal of a significant structural barrier in a short period of time. A simple fifteen-minute discussion of the above-mentioned research, followed by a quick vote at a departmental meeting, resulted in permanent removal of course evaluation letters from merit decisions. This illustrates that some changes, including important changes, can occur quickly, if the right people with the right motivation set about the task; hopelessly believing that all structural problems are too ingrained in the system to change is simply inaccurate. While it may take years to build a wall, it can be destroyed quickly if you have the right tools. Although we have good evidence to suggest that each of these strategies can result in significant and immediate improvements to the racial climate, what remains to be seen is if there is a multiplicative benefit in implementing all of these changes at once, where needed.

One of the points we did not make, which has also been a concern at many campuses, is increasing the diversity of the student body. It is worth considering the possibility that enrolling more students of color, independent of efforts to improve the existing campus racial climate, may be problematic and unfair to those students. Much evidence, reviewed in this article, documents that students of color become disillusioned, distressed, and dissatisfied in such an environment, and that many will drop out (Cropsey et al., 2008; Piotrowski & Perdue, 1998). Indeed, the literature on recruitment of minority students and debates over affirmative action should better emphasize the need for the minority students to be received into a supportive academic environment. Although increasing the number of students of color may help with some issues (e.g., isolation), it will not help with most structural issues reviewed herein. Of course, the dynamic is transactional, in that an increased minority presence may put additional pressure on administration to create structural changes that meet their needs (Hurtado, Milem, Clayton-Pedersen, & Allen, 1998), but certainly it is unfair to place this burden on the initial cohorts of minority students.

If the needs we review above are properly addressed, we believe more students of color will be the natural results of these efforts. For example, we have paid careful attention to these issues, and as a result, we have a diverse group of graduate and undergraduates in our own labs, which includes African Americans, Hispanic Americans, Asian Americans, international students, and religious and sexual minorities. In turn, their research efforts and diverse perspectives constitute invaluable contributions to our respective departments and the field of psychology as a whole. We have not made any special efforts to recruit these students, but they apply to work with us because they perceive it to be a welcoming environment. This does not mean that recruitment efforts are not important, but if the other essential elements are in place, recruitment efforts will certainly be more successful.

Change is never easy, but these problems will not go away on their own. There is room for all of us to work harder to create nurturing and diverse academic spaces for the benefit of everyone.

KEY POINTS FOR CLINICIANS

- Students of color experience many forms of racism on campus, which contributes to poor mental health. Staff and faculty of color are also impacted.

- Much of this racism is structural in nature and self-perpetuating, requiring deliberate efforts at identifying and dismantling it.

- Attempts to bring about positive change to reduce racism and create a more inclusive environment are typically met with resistance.

- Psychology departments are not immune to these problems and can also perpetuate a negative racial climate.

- Psychologists can play a key role in facilitating change due to their understanding of human behavior and the related research base.

Acknowledgments

The authors would like to thank Ariana Levinson, JD; Lisa Hooper, PhD; Lauren Freeman, PhD; and Gareth Holman, PhD, for their insights and input into this chapter.

References

Associated Press. (2016, June 21). Judge dismisses lawsuit over Louisville Confederate monument. *Fox News US*. Retrieved from http://www.foxnews.com/us/2016/06/21/judge-dismisses-lawsuit -over-louisville-confederate-monument.html

Association of American Medical Colleges. (2015). *Altering the Course: Black Males in Medicine*. Washington, DC. Retrieved from https://members.aamc.org/eweb/upload/Black_Males_in _Medicine_Report_WEB.pdf

Attewell, P., & Monaghan, D. (2016). How many credits should an undergraduate take? *Research in Higher Education, 57*(6), 682–713. doi:10.1007/s11162-015-9401-z

Bardone-Cone, A. M., Calhoun, C. D., Fischer, M. S., Gaskin-Wasson, A. L., Jones, S. T., Schwartz, S. L., … & Prinstein, M. J. (2016). Development and implementation of a diversity training sequence in a clinical psychology doctoral program. *The Behavior Therapist, 39*(3), 65–75.

Berger, M., & Sarnyai, Z. (2015). "More than skin deep": Stress neurobiology and mental health consequences of racial discrimination. *The International Journal on the Biology of Stress, 18*(1), 1–10. doi:10.3109/10253890.2014.989204

Berner, M. (2015). When students rally for "diversity," what do they want? *Chronicle of Higher Education, 61*(27), A22.

Berrett, D. D., & Giorgi, A. (2015). Diversity's elusive number: Campuses strive to achieve "critical mass." *Chronicle of Higher Education, 62*(16), 5.

Bezrukova, K., Spell, C. S., Perry, J. L., & Jehn, K. A. (2016). A meta-analytical integration of over 40 years of research on diversity training evaluation. *Psychological Bulletin*. Advance online publication. doi:10.1037/bul0000067

Boatright-Horowitz, S. L., & Soeung, S. (2009). Teaching White privilege to White students can mean saying good-bye to positive student evaluations. *American Psychologist, 64*(6), 574–575.

Boring, A., Ottoboni, K., & Stark, P. (2016). Student evaluations of teaching (mostly) do not measure teaching effectiveness. *Science Open Research*. doi:10.14293/S2199-1006.1. SOR-EDU.AETBZC .v1

Bowman, N. A. (2010). Disequilibrium and resolution: The nonlinear effects of diversity courses on well-being and orientations toward diversity. *Review of Higher Education: Journal of the Association for the Study of Higher Education, 33*(4), 543–568. doi:10.1353/rhe.0.0172

Bradley, C. (2005). The career experiences of African American women faculty: Implications for counselor education programs. *College Student Journal, 39*(3), 518.

Byrne, M. M. (2001). Uncovering racial bias in nursing fundamentals textbooks. *Nursing and Health Care Perspectives, 22*(6), 299.

Carnevale, A. P., & Strohl, J. (2013). *Separate and unequal: How higher education reinforces the intergenerational reproduction of White racial privilege*. Georgetown Public Policy Institute: Georgetown University.

Carter, R. (2007). Racism and psychological and emotional injury: Recognizing and assessing race-based traumatic stress. *The Counseling Psychologist, 35*, 13–105.

Carter, E. R., & Murphy, M. C. (2015). Group-based differences in perceptions of racism: What counts, to whom, and why? *Social and Personality Psychology Compass, 9*(6), 269–280.

Case, K. A. (2007). Raising white privilege awareness and reducing racial prejudice: Assessing diversity course effectiveness. *Teaching of Psychology, 34*(4), 231–235. doi:10.1080/00986280701700250

Causey, V. E., Thomas, C. D., & Armento, B. J. (2000). Cultural diversity is basically a foreign term to me: The challenges of diversity for preservice teacher education. *Teaching and Teacher Education, 16*(1), 33–45.

Chan, A. W., Yeh, C. J., & Krumboltz, J. D. (2015). Mentoring ethnic minority counseling and clinical psychology students: A multicultural, ecological, and relational model. *Journal of Counseling Psychology, 62*(4), 592–607.

Chakraborti, N., & Garland, J. (2003). An "invisible" problem? Uncovering the nature of racist victimisation in rural Suffolk. *International Review of Victimology*, *10*(1), 1–17. doi:10.1177/026975800301000101

Chou, T., Asnaani, A., & Hofmann, S. (2012). Perception of racial discrimination and psychopathology across three US ethnic minority groups. *Cultural Diversity & Ethnic Minority Psychology*, *18*(1), 74–81.

Chrobot-Mason, D., & Hepworth, W. K. (2005). Examining perceptions of ambiguous and unambiguous threats of racial harassment and managerial response strategies. *Journal of Applied Social Psychology*, *35*(11), 2215–2261. doi:10.1111/j.1559-1816.2005.tb02101.x

Clark, K. B., & Clark, M. K. (1939). The development of consciousness of self and the emergence of racial identification in Negro preschool children. *Journal of Social Psychology, S. P. S. S. I. Bulletin*, *10*(4), 591–599.

Collins, J., & Hebert, T. (2008). Race and gender images in psychology textbooks. *Race, Gender & Class*, *15*(3/4), 300–307.

Constantine, M. G., Smith, L., Redington, R. M., & Owens, D. (2008). Racial microaggressions against Black counselors and counseling psychology faculty: A central challenge in the multicultural counseling movement. *Journal of Counseling & Development*, *86*(3), 348–355.

Cropsey, K. L., Masho, S. W., Shiang, R., Sikka, V., Kornstein, S. G., & Hampton, C. L. (2008). Why do faculty leave? Reasons for attrition of women and minority faculty from a medical school: Four-year results. *Journal of Women's Health*, *17*(7), 1–8. doi:10.1089/jwh.2007.0582

Crosby, J. R., & Monin, B. (2007). Failure to warn: How student race affects warnings of potential academic difficulty. *Journal of Experimental Social Psychology*, *43*(4), 663–670. doi:10.1016/j.jesp.2006.06.007

Cross, T., & Slater, R. B. (2002). A short list of colleges and universities that are taking measures to increase their number of Black faculty. *Journal of Blacks in Higher Education*, *36*, 99–103.

Davies K. R., Tropp L. R., Aron A., Pettigrew T. F., & Wright S. C. (2011). Cross-group friendships and intergroup attitudes: A meta-analytic review. *Personality and Social Psychology Review*, *15*, 332–351. doi:10.1177/1088868311411103

Debreaux, M., Mier-Chairez, O., Sawyer, B., Skinta, M., Kuczynski, A., Kanter, J. W., & Williams, M. T. (2015, November). *Promoting racial harmony: Focus groups on campus microaggressions.* Presented at the annual meeting of the *Association for Cognitive and Behavioral Therapies*, Chicago, IL.

DeLapp, C. L., DeLapp, R. C. T., & Williams, M. T. (2016, October). Making diversity matter: Comparing students' attitudes about multicultural coursework. Presented at the *2016 Association for Behavioral and Cognitive Therapies Convention*, New York, NY.

DeLapp, R. C. T., & Williams, M. T. (2015). Professional challenges facing African American psychologists: The presence and impact of racial microaggressions. *The Behavior Therapist*, *38*(4), 101–105.

Delano-Oriaran, O. O., & Meidl, T. D. (2012). Critical conversations: Developing white teachers for diverse classrooms. *Journal of Praxis in Multicultural Education*, *7*(1), Article 1.

Denson, N. (2009). Do curricular and cocurricular diversity activities influence racial bias? A meta-analysis. *Review of Educational Research*, *79*(2), 805–838.

Dessel, A., & Rogge, M. E. (2008). Evaluation of intergroup dialogue: A review of the empirical literature. *Conflict Resolution Quarterly*, *26*(2), 199–238. doi:10.1002/crq.230

Earl, W. R. (1988). Intrusive advising of freshmen in academic difficulty. *NACADA Journal*, *8*, 27–33.

Gaertner, S. L., & Dovidio, J. F. (2005). Understanding and addressing contemporary racism: From aversive racism to the common ingroup identity model. *Journal of Social Issues*, *61*(3), 615–639.

Galinsky, A. D., Todd, A. R., Homan, A. C., Phillips, K. W., Apfelbaum, E. P., Sasaki, S. J., ... & Maddux, W. W. (2015). Maximizing the gains and minimizing the pains of diversity: A policy perspective. *Perspectives on Psychological Science*, *10*(6), 742–748. doi:10.1177/1745691615598513

Gallup. (2015, August 26). Higher support for gender affirmative action than race. *Minority Rights and Relations Survey*. Retrieved from http://www.gallup.com/poll/184772/higher-support-gender-affirmative-action-race.aspx

Garcia, D. M., Reser, A. H., Amo, R. B., Redersdorff, S., & Branscombe, N. R. (2005). Perceivers' responses to in-group and out-group members who blame a negative outcome on discrimination. *Personality and Social Psychology Bulletin, 31*(6), 769–780.

Gasman, M. (2016, September 26). An Ivy League professor on why colleges don't hire more faculty of color: "We don't want them." *The Washington Post*. Retrieved from https://www.washingtonpost.com/news/grade-point/wp/2016/09/26/an-ivy-league-professor-on-why-colleges-dont-hire-more-faculty-of-color-we-dont-want-them

Glennen, R. E., Baxley, D. M., & Farren, P. J. (1985). Impact of intrusive advising on minority student retention. *College Student Journal, 19*(4), 335–338.

Gonzalez, J., & Goodman, A. (2016, July 15). Exclusive: Meet Yale dishwasher Corey Menafee, who smashed racist stained-glass window. *Democracy Now Independent Global News*. Retrieved from http://www.democracynow.org/2016/7/15/exclusive_meet_yale_dishwasher_corey_menafee

Greenwald, A. G., & Krieger, L. H. (2006). Implicit bias: Scientific foundations. *California Law Review, 94*(4), 945–968.

Greenwald, A. G., & Pettigrew, T. F. (2014). With malice toward none and charity for some: Ingroup favoritism enables discrimination. *American Psychologist, 69*, 669–684.

Griggs, R. A., & Jackson, S. L. (2013). Introductory psychology textbooks: An objective analysis update. *Teaching of Psychology, 40*(3), 163–168. doi:10.1177/0098628313487455

Guiffrida, D. A. (2004). How involvement in African American student organizations supports and hinders academic achievement. *NACADA Journal, 24*(1–2), 88–98.

Guiffrida, D. A. (2005). Othermothering as a framework for understanding African American students' definitions of student-centered faculty. *The Journal of Higher Education, 76*(6), 701–723.

Gurin, P., Sorensen, N., Lopez, G. E., & Nagda, B. A. (2015). Intergroup dialogue: Race still matters. In R. Bangs, L. E. Davis, R. Bangs, & L. E. Davis (Eds.), Race and social problems: Restructuring inequality (pp. 39–60). New York, NY: Springer Science + Business Media. doi:10.1007/978-1-4939-0863-9_3

Hagedorn, L. S., Chi, W., & Cepeda, R. M. (2007). An investigation of critical mass: The role of Latino representation in the success of urban community college students. *Research in Higher Education, 48*(1), 73–91.

Hamermesh, D. S., & Parker, A. (2005). Beauty in the classroom: Instructors' pulchritude and putative pedagogical productivity. *Economics of Education Review, 24*, 369–376.

Harper, S. R., & Hurtado, S. (2007). Nine themes in campus racial climates and implications for institutional transformation. *New Directions for Student Services, 120*, 7–24.

Hartocollis, A., & Bidgood, J. (2015, November 11). Racial discrimination protests ignite at colleges across the US. *New York Times*. Retrieved from http://www.nytimes.com/2015/11/12/us/racial-discrimination-protests-ignite-at-colleges-across-the-us.html

Ho, A. K., Thomsen, L., & Sidanius, J. (2009). Perceived academic competence and overall job evaluations: Students' evaluations of African American and European American professors. *Journal of Applied Social Psychology, 39*(2), 389–406. doi:10.1111/j.1559-1816.2008.00443.x

Hurtado, S., Milem, J. F., Clayton-Pedersen, A. R., & Allen, W. R. (1998). Enhancing campus climates for racial/ethnic diversity: Educational policy and practice. *The Review of Higher Education, 21*(3), 279–302.

Jones, R. P., Cox, D., & Navarro-Rivera, J. (2014, September 23). *Economic insecurity, rising inequality, and doubts about the future: Findings from the 2014 American Values Survey*. Washington, DC: Public Religion Research Institute (PRRI).

Joseph, T. D., & Hirshfield, L. E. (2011). "Why don't you get somebody new to do it?" Race and cultural taxation in the academy. *Ethnic and Racial Studies, 34*(1), 121–141. doi:10.1080/01419870.2010.49 6489

Jost, J. T., & Banaji, M. B. (1994). The role of stereotyping in system-justification and the production of false consciousness. *British Journal of Social Psychology, 33*, 1–27.

Kalinoski, Z. T., Steele-Johnson, D., Peyton, E. J., Leas, K. A., Steinke, J., & Bowling, N. A. (2013). A meta-analytic evaluation of diversity training outcomes. *Journal of Organizational Behavior, 34*(8), 1076–1104. doi:10.1002/job.1839

King, D., & Domin, D. S. (2007). The representation of people of color in undergraduate general chemistry textbooks. *Journal of Chemical Education, 84*(2), 342–345. doi:10.1021/ed084p342

Kena, G., Musu-Gillette, L., Robinson, J., Wang, X., Rathbun, A., Zhang, J., Wilkinson-Flicker, S., Barmer, A., & Dunlop Velez, E. (2015). *The condition of education 2015 (NCES 2015–144)*. Washington, DC: US Department of Education, National Center for Education Statistics. Retrieved from http://nces.ed.gov/pubsearch

Kezar, A., & Eckel, P. (2008). Advancing diversity agendas on campus: Examining transactional and transformational presidential leadership styles. *International Journal of Leadership in Education, 11*(4), 379–405.

Krauth, O. (2016, February 21). Racial tensions roil residence hall. *The Louisville Cardinal.* Retrieved from http://www.louisvillecardinal.com/2016/02/simmering-racial-tensions-roil-dorm

Kravitz, D. A., & Klineberg, S. L. (2000). Reactions to two versions of affirmative action action among Whites, Blacks, and Hispanics. *Journal of Applied Psychology, 85*(4), 597–611. doi:10.1037/0021 -9010.85.4.597

Lai, C. K., Marini, M., Lehr, S. A., Cerruti, C., Shin, J. L., Joy-Gaba, J. A., … & Nosek, B. A. (2014). Reducing implicit racial preferences: I. A comparative investigation of 17 interventions. *Journal of Experimental Psychology: General, 143*(4), 1765–1785. doi:10.1037/a0036260

Laird, T. N., & Engberg, M. E. (2011). Establishing differences between diversity requirements and other courses with varying degrees of diversity inclusivity. *The Journal of General Education, 60*(2), 117–137.

Larsen, S. E., Nye, C. D., Ormerod, A. J., Ziebro, M., & Siebert, J. E. (2013). Do actions speak louder than words? A comparison of three organizational practices for reducing racial/ethnic harassment and discrimination. *Military Psychology, 25*(6), 602–614. doi:10.1037/mil0000024

Lawrence, K., Sutton, S. Kubisch, A., Susi, G., & Fulbright-Anderson, K. (2004). *Structural racism and community building. Aspen Institute Roundtable on Community Change.* Washington, DC: The Aspen Institute.

Leslie, L. M., Mayer, D. M., & Kravitz, D. A. (2014). The stigma of affirmative action: A stereotyping-based theory and meta-analytic test of the consequences for performance. *Academy Of Management Journal, 57*(4), 964–989. doi:10.5465/amj.2011.0940

Lewis, A. E., Chesler, M. A., & Forman, T. A. (2000). The impact of "colorblind" ideologies on students of color: Intergroup relations at a predominantly White university. *Journal of Negro Education, 69*(1/2), 74–91.

Liberman, B. E., Block, C. J., & Koch, S. M. (2011). Diversity trainer preconceptions: The effects of trainer race and gender on perceptions of diversity trainer effectiveness. *Basic and Applied Social Psychology, 33*(3), 279–293. doi:10.1080/01973533.2011.589327

Linderman, J. J. (2015). Faculty recruitment, retention, climate and leadership development: The University of Michigan ADVANCE Program Experience. Houghton, MI: Michigan Technological University.

Martin, M. M., Goodboy, A. K., & Johnson, Z. D. (2015). When professors bully graduate students: Effects on student interest, instructional dissent, and intentions to leave graduate education. *Communication Education, 64*(4), 438–454, doi:10.1080/03634523.2015.1041995

Maton, K. I., Wimms, H. E., Grant, S. K., Wittig, M. A., Rogers, M. R., & Vasquez, M. J. T. (2011). Experiences and perspectives of African American, Latina/o, Asian American, and European American psychology graduate students: A national study. *Cultural Diversity and Ethnic Minority Psychology, 17*(1), 68–78.

Mattox, S., Bridenstine, M., Burns, B., Torresen, E., Koning, A., Meek, S. P., … & Wigent, A. (2008). How gender and race of geologists are portrayed in physical geology textbooks. *Journal of Geoscience Education, 56*(2), 156–159.

MacInnis, C. C., & Page-Gould, E. (2015). How can intergroup interaction be bad if intergroup contact is good? Exploring and reconciling an apparent paradox in the science of intergroup relations. *Perspectives on Psychological Science, 10*(3), 307–327. doi:10.1177/1745691614568482

McCauley, C., Wright, M., & Harris, M. E. (2000). Diversity workshops on campus: A survey of current practice at US colleges and universities. *College Student Journal, 34*(1), 100–114.

McCoy, D. L., Winkle-Wagner, R., & Luedke, C. L. (2015). Colorblind mentoring? Exploring white faculty mentoring of students of color. *Journal of Diversity in Higher Education, 8*(4), 225–242. doi:10.1037/a0038676

McMurtrie, B. (2016, September 11). How to do a better job of searching for diversity. *The Chronicle of Higher Education.* Retrieved from http://www.chronicle.com/article/How-to-Do-a-Better-Job -of/237750

Miller, A., Williams, M. T., Wetterneck, C. T., Kanter, J., & Tsai, M. (2015). Using functional analytic psychotherapy to improve awareness and connection in racially diverse client-therapist dyads. *The Behavior Therapist, 38*(6), 150–156.

Molina, A., & Abelman, R. (2000). Style over substance in interventions for at-risk students: The impact of intrusiveness. *NACADA Journal, 20*(2), 5–15.

Monforti, J. L., & McGlynn (2010). Aquí estamos? A survey of Latino portrayal in introductory US government and politics textbooks. *Political Science and Politics, 43*(2), 309–316.

Moody, B. (2015, November 3). Students meet with Ramsey over #Costumegate. *Louisville Cardinal.* Retrieved from http://www.louisvillecardinal.com/2015/11/students-meet-with-president-ramsey

Nast, H. J. (1999). "Sex," "Race" and Multiculturalism: Critical consumption and the politics of course evaluations. *Journal of Geography in Higher Education, 23*, 102–115.

National Science Foundation (2016). NSF doctoral recipients from US universities. Table 22. Doctorate recipients, by citizenship status, ethnicity, race, and subfield of study: 2014. Retrieved from http://www.nsf.gov/statistics/2016/nsf16300/data-tables.cfm

Neville, H., Worthington, R., & Spanierman, L. (2001). Race, power, and multicultural counseling psychology: Understanding white privilege and color blind racial attitudes. In Ponterotto, J., Casas, M., Suzuki, L., & Alexander, C. (Eds.), *Handbook of multicultural counseling* (2nd ed.) (pp. 257–288). Thousand Oaks, CA: Sage.

Ng, E. W. (2008). Why organizations choose to manage diversity? Toward a leadership-based theoretical framework. *Human Resource Development Review, 7*(1), 58–78. doi:10.1177/1534484307311592

Niemann, Y. F. (2003). The psychology of tokenism: Psychosocial realities of faculty of color. In G. Bernal, J. E. Trimble, A. K. Burlew, & F. T. L. Leong (Eds.), *Handbook of racial and ethnic minority psychology* (pp. 100–118). Thousand Oaks, CA: Sage.

O'Keefe, V. M., Wingate, L. R., Cole, A. B., Hollingsworth, D. W., & Tucker, R. P. (2015). Seemingly harmless racial communications are not so harmless: Racial microaggressions lead to suicidal ideation by way of depression symptoms. *Suicide and Life-Threatening Behavior, 45*(5), 567–576. doi:10.1111/sltb.12150

Page-Gould E., Mendes W. B., & Major B. (2010). Intergroup contact facilitates physiological recovery following stressful intergroup interactions. *Journal of Experimental Social Psychology, 46*, 854–858. 10.1016/j.jesp.2010.04.006

Page-Gould, E., Mendoza-Denton, & Tropp, L. R. (2008). With a little help from my cross-group friend: Reducing anxiety in intergroup contexts through cross-group friendship. *Journal of Personality and Social Psychology, 95*(5), 1080–1094. doi:10.1037/0022-3514.95.5.1080

Paluck, E. L., & Green, D. P. (2009). Prejudice reduction: What works? A review and assessment of research and practice. *Annual Review of Psychology, 60*, 339–367. doi:10.1146/annurev.psych.60 .110707.163607

Perry, S. P., Dovidio, J. F., Murphy, M. C., & van Ryn, M. (2015). The joint effect of bias awareness and self-reported prejudice on intergroup anxiety and intentions for intergroup contact. *Cultural Diversity and Ethnic Minority Psychology, 21*(1), 89–96. doi:10.1037/a0037147

Pettigrew, T. F., Tropp, L. R., Wagner, U., & Christ, O. (2011). Recent advances in intergroup contact theory. *International Journal of Intercultural Relations, 35*(3), 271–280. doi:10.1016/j.ijintrel.2011 .03.001

Pierce, C. (1970). Offensive mechanisms. In F. Barbour (Ed.), *In the Black seventies* (pp. 265–282). Boston, MA: Porter Sargent.

Pieterse, A. L., Carter, R. T., Evans, S. A., & Walter, R. A. (2010). An exploratory examination of the associations among racial and ethnic discrimination, racial climate, and trauma-related symptoms in a college student population. *Journal of Counseling Psychology, 57*(3), 255–263. doi:10.1037 /a0020040

Piotrowski, C., & Perdue, B. (1998). Factors in attrition of Black students at a predominantly Euro-American university. *Psychological Reports, 83*, 113–114.

Pittman, C. T. (2012). Racial microaggressions: The narratives of African American faculty at a predominantly White university. *Journal of Negro Education, 81*(1), 82–92. doi:10.7709/jnegro education.81.1.0082

Purdie-Vaughns, V., Steele, C. M., Davies, P. G., Ditlmann, R., & Crosby, J. R. (2008). Social identity contingencies: How diversity cues signal threat or safety for African Americans in mainstream institutions. *Journal of Personality and Social Psychology, 94*(4), 615–630. doi:10.1037/0022 -3514.94.4.615

Rabow, J., Stein, J. M., & Conley, T. D. (1999). Teaching social justice and encountering society: The pink triangle experiment. *Youth and Society, 30*(4), 483–514. doi:10.1177/0044118X99030004005

Reis, H. T. (2007). Steps toward the ripening of relationship science. *Personal Relationships, 14*(1), 1–23. doi:10.1111/j.1475-6811.2006.00139.x

Rogers, M. R., & Molina, L. E. (2006). Exemplary efforts in psychology to recruit and retain graduate students of color. *American Psychologist, 61*(2), 143–156. doi:10.1037/0003-066X.61.2.143

Rothwell, J. (2015, December 18). *The stubborn race and class gaps in college quality*. Brookings Institution. Social Mobility Memos. Retrieved from http://www.brookings.edu/blogs/social-mobility -memos/posts/2015/12/18-stubborn-race-class-gaps-college-rothwell

Shaffer, L. S. (2010). Cumulative subject index to volumes 16–30 of the NACADA Journal. *NACADA Journal, 30*(2), 72–102.

Shelton, N., Douglass, S., Garcia, R. L., Yip, T., & Trail, T. E. (2014). Feeling (mis)understood and intergroup friendships in interracial interactions. *Personality and Social Psychology Bulletin, 40*, 1193–1204. doi:10.1177/0146167214538459

Shelton J. N., Richeson J. A., & Salvatore J. (2005). Expecting to be the target of prejudice: Implications for interethnic interactions. *Personality and Social Psychology Bulletin, 31*, 1189–1202. doi:10.1177/0146167205274894

Shelton, J. N., Trail, T. E., West, T. V., & Bergsieker, H. B. (2010). From strangers to friends: The interpersonal process model of intimacy in developing interracial friendships. *Journal of Social and Personal Relationships, 27*, 71–90. doi:10.1177/0265407509346422

Shelton J. N., West T. V., & Trail T. E. (2010). Concerns about appearing prejudiced: Implications for anxiety during daily interracial interactions. *Group Processes & Intergroup Relations, 13*, 329–344. doi:10.1177/1368430209344869

Smith, B. (2015). New standards for psychology training. *Monitor on Psychology, 46*(5), 52. Retrieved from http://www.apa.org/monitor/2015/05/new-standards.aspx

Smith, W. A., Mustaffa, J. B., Jones, C. M., Curry, T. J., & Allen, W. R. (2016). "You make me wanna holler and throw up both my hands!" Campus culture, Black misandric microaggressions, and racial battle fatigue. *International Journal of Qualitative Studies in Education, 29*(9), 1189–1209. doi: 10.1080/09518398.2016.1214296.

Smith, W. A., Allen, W. R., & Danley, L. L. (2007). Assume the position...You fit the description: College students experiences and racial battle fatigue among African American male college students. *American Behavioral Scientist, 51,* 551–578.

Solórzano, D., Ceja, M., & Yosso, T. (2000). Critical race theory, racial microaggressions, and campus racial climate: The experiences of African American college students. *Journal of Negro Education, 69*(1–2), 60–73.

Stangor, C., Swim, J. K., Van Allen, K. L., & Sechrist, G. B. (2002). Reporting discrimination in public and private contexts. *Journal of Personality and Social Psychology, 82*(1), 69–74.

Stark-Wroblewski, K., Ahlering, R. F., & Brill, F. M. (2007). Toward a more comprehensive approach to evaluating teaching effectiveness: Supplementing student evaluations of teaching with pre-post learning measures. *Assessment & Evaluation in Higher Education, 32*(4), 403–415. doi:10.1080 /02602930600898536.

Steele, C. M., & Aronson, J. (1995). Stereotype threat and the intellectual test performance of African Americans. *Journal of Personality & Social Psychology, 69*(5), 797–811.

Strayhorn, T. L. (Ed.). (2013). *Living at the intersections: Social identities and Black collegians.* Charlotte, NC: Information Age.

Sue, D. W., Capodilupo, C. M., Torino, G. C., Bucceri, J. M., Holder, A., Nadal, K. L., & Esquilin, M. (2007). Racial microaggressions in everyday life: Implications for clinical practice. *American Psychologist, 62*(4), 271–286.

Sue, D. W., Rivera, D. P., Capodilupo, C. M., Lin, A. I., & Torino, G. C. (2010). Racial dialogues and White trainee fears: Implications for education and training. *Cultural Diversity and Ethnic Minority Psychology, 16*(2), 206–214. doi:10.1037/a0016112

Sue, D. W., Torino, G. C., Capodilupo, C. M., Rivera, D. P., & Lin, A. I. (2009). How White faculty perceive and react to difficult dialogues on race: Implications for education and training. *The Counseling Psychologist, 37*(8), 1090–1115. doi:10.1177/0011000009340443

Svrluga, S. (2015a, November 5). U. Missouri president, chancellor resign over handling of racial incidents. *Washington Post.* Retrieved from https://www.washingtonpost.com/news/grade-point/wp /2015/11/09/missouris-student-government-calls-for-university-presidents-removal

Svrluga, S. (2015b, October 30). College president apologizes for wearing stereotypical Mexican costume for Halloween party. *Washington Post.* Retrieved from https://www.washingtonpost.com /news/grade-point/wp/2015/10/30/college-president-wore-stereotypical-mexican-costume -for-halloween

Tajfel, H. (1982). Social psychology of intergroup relations. *Annual Review of Psychology, 33*(1), 1–39.

Terwilliger, J. M., Bach, N., Bryan, C., & Williams, M. T. (2013). Multicultural versus colorblind ideology: Implications for mental health and counseling. In A. Di Fabio (Ed.), *Psychology of Counseling* (pp. 111–122). Hauppauge, NY: Nova Science Publishers.

The Demands. (2016, August 6). Retrieved from http://www.thedemands.org. Last updated 12/8/15.

Thurston-Rattue, M., Kanter, J. W., Hakki, F., Kuczynski, A. M., Santos, M. M., Bailey, K., Tsai, M., & Kohlenberg, R. J. (2015, July). Increasing racially diverse social connections through contextual behavioral science. Presented at the Association for *Contextual Behavioral Science 13th Annual World Conference,* Berlin, DE.

Turner, C. V., González, J. C., & Wood, J. L. (2008). Faculty of color in academe: What 20 years of literature tells us. *Journal of Diversity in Higher Education, 1*(3), 139–168. doi:10.1037/a0012837

Williams, M. T., Gooden, A. M., & Davis, D. (2012). African Americans, European Americans, and pathological stereotypes: An African-centered perspective. In G. R. Hayes & M. H. Bryant (Eds.), *Psychology of culture* (pp. 213–221). Hauppauge, NY: Nova Science Publishers.

Williams, M. T., Kanter, J. W., & Ching, T. H. W. (2018). Anxiety, stress, and trauma symptoms in African Americans: Negative affectivity does not explain the relationship between microaggressions and psychopathology. *Journal of Racial and Ethnic Health Disparities, 5*(5), 919–927. doi:10.1007/s40615-017-0440-3

Williams, M. T., Malcoun, E., Sawyer, B., Davis, D. M., Bahojb-Nouri, L. V., & Bruce, S. L. (2014). Cultural adaptations of prolonged exposure therapy for treatment and prevention of posttraumatic stress disorder in African Americans. *Journal of Behavioral Sciences, 4*(2), 102–124.

Williams, M. T., Peña, A., & Mier-Chairez, J. (2017). Tools for assessing and treating racism-related stress and trauma among Latinos. In L. T. Benuto (Ed.), *Toolkit for Counseling Spanish-Speaking Clients* (pp. 71–96). New York, NY: Springer.

Wilson, J. J. (2013). Emerging trend: The chief diversity officer phenomenon within higher education. *Journal of Negro Education, 82*(4), 433–445.

Yosso, T. J., Smith, W. A., Ceja, M., & Solórzano, D. G. (2009). Critical race theory, racial microaggressions, and campus racial climate for Latina/o undergraduates. *Harvard Educational Review, 79*(4), 659–690.

Zittleman, K., & Sadker, D. (2002). Teacher education textbooks: The unfinished gender revolution. *Educational Leadership, 60*(4), 59–63.

CHAPTER 14

Barriers to Outpatient Psychotherapy Treatment

Camelia Harb,
Georgetown University Medical Center

Jessica Jackson,
VA Los Angeles Ambulatory Care Center

Alfiee M. Breland-Noble,
Georgetown University Medical Center

Introduction

In the area of mental health, clinical care and psychotherapy specifically, people of color have lower rates of outpatient treatment engagement, unequal access to care, and lower quality of care, and they experience more negative treatment outcomes. This chapter seeks to delineate the barriers to outpatient care and includes discussion related to practical and systemic barriers, provider bias, and cultural stigma. We suggest that health disparities in outpatient care are significant and important, and we offer suggestions for providers on how to reduce and, in some cases, overcome these barriers in their own work. In this chapter, outpatient therapy refers to services provided in primary care, community mental health clinics, solo practice, and large group practices (e.g., federally qualified health centers, community agencies, and HMOs). Further, we focus on the needs of multiple racial and ethnic groups, where possible, including African Americans and Blacks, Hispanics and Latinx, Asians and Asian Americans, and Native Americans and American Indians—whom we refer to throughout as people of color.

Our efforts focus on historical contributors to clinical care disparities (i.e., historical barriers); the role of patient and community culture (i.e., individual barriers) and their impacts on the prevalence of mental illness, manifestations of mental illness, and implications for outpatient care in racially diverse groups. Each of these topics has been described extensively in the literature but we offer a specific focus on the outpatient care setting (Breland-Noble, Al-Mateen, & Singh, 2016).

Defining Mental Health Disparities and Barriers to Care

The Institute of Medicine defines health disparities as "racial or ethnic differences in the quality of healthcare that are not due to access-related factors or clinical needs, preferences, and appropriateness of interventions" (Institute of Medicine, 2003). An extensive body of literature exists establishing the breadth and depth of differences in health outcomes, including access to and treatment within health care beyond drivers like socio-economic status (Eliacin et al., 2018). Per the seminal surgeon general's *Supplement on Mental Health Report on Culture, Race, and Ethnicity*, people of color experience mental health disparities as (1) decreased access to and less availability of mental health services; (2) reduced likelihood of receiving necessary mental health services required; (3) poorer quality of care; and (4) underrepresentation in research that seeks to build better treatments (Chung et al., 2014; USDHHS, 2001).

Epidemiological and empirical research demonstrates that despite a high prevalence of psychological disorders and distress among people of color, they are less likely to utilize mental health services (Augsberger, Yeung, Dougher, & Hahm, 2015; Caldwell, Assari, & Breland-Noble, 2016). Further, people of color demonstrate greater attrition rates and spend less time in care overall. In a mixed-method study, Augsberger and colleagues (2015) explored mental health service utilization in a large sample (N=701) of 1.5th- and second-generation Chinese American, Korean American, Vietnamese American, and mixed-race Asian American young women. Fewer than 13 percent of the participants sought mental health services in the preceding twelve months despite 43 percent being classified as medium to high risk (based on reported depressive symptoms and suicidal ideation). Family and community stigma and a lack of culturally sensitive interventions were identified as primary drivers of service underutilization.

To better engage clients of color, it is suggested that clinicians adopt a positive working alliance between provider and patient framed by openness to diverse cultures and a willingness to learn about new cultures as patients from those cultures present in treatment. We believe that these approaches can be key to better patient outcomes and perceptions of service quality and cultural competence, as providers demonstrate their willingness to be active learners. When such elements are missing, patients may become less engaged in their treatment, as evidenced by the work of Eliacin et al. (2018), who found that African American male veterans had lower levels of engagement with providers in outpatient clinics than their White male counterparts. (See chapter 16 for issues related specifically to veteran care.)

Access to Care

Defined as the "timely use of personal health services to achieve the best possible health outcomes" (Institute of Medicine, 1993, p. 33), access to care refers to an individual's ease in beginning treatment or exploring available resources. However, the phrase also encompasses an individual's experiences with practical, cultural, and psychosocial barriers to care. For many people of color, access to care can be impeded by practical issues, including limited community resources, financial constraints, and lack of information (Belgrave & Berry, 2016; Breland-Noble, 2015; Caldwell et al., 2016). Rural areas with large, racially diverse populations are often ill equipped to provide services and support, especially for mental health. This reality can mean a lack of providers overall and a significant imbalance in the representativeness of providers and services tailored to the specific experiences and needs of patients of diverse backgrounds. Further, many residents of these areas face additional difficulties accessing resources, like lack of transportation, inconvenient clinic hours, and the financial repercussions of missing work to obtain care (DeCou & Vidair, 2017).

The costs associated with outpatient care (e.g., providers who do not accept insurance or high deductibles and out-of-pocket costs even for those who are insured) can deter under-resourced people from seeking help. Additionally, given that African Americans, Latinx, and Native American populations are overrepresented among under-resourced persons, this issue is more salient for some groups of people of color (Miranda, Soffer, Polanco-Roman, Wheeler, & Moore, 2015). Though mental health parity established as part of the Affordable Care Act under President Obama has greatly improved access to basic mental health care for many, insurance companies still place restrictions on the types of mental health services covered, may limit the number of sessions available to patients, offer below-market reimbursement rates to providers, and impose high co-pays and deductibles on patients themselves.

Systemic barriers generally refer to preexisting factors within the health care system that impede or outright deny people of color full engagement in treatment. Most of the bias barriers to care are well established and include issues like assessment, lack of cultural competence, patient-provider communication problems, differing conceptualizations of mental illness, and implicit bias (Lê Cook, McGuire, Lock, & Zaslavsky, 2010). These issues can manifest themselves in ways like mistaken provider beliefs on racial differences in pain tolerance (Hoffman, Trawalter, Axt, & Oliver, 2016) or provider dismissals of patient symptoms as non-severe or not warranting further or specialty care (Huey, Tilley, Jones, & Smith, 2014; Pumariega et al., 2013).

Quality of Care

Generally, research has shown that people of color receive lower quality of care for mental health services compared to Whites, with under-resourced people of color receiving less information about symptoms, treatments, and care practices than their higher-socioeconomic-status peers (Carpenter-Song, Whitley, Lawson, Quimby, & Drake, 2011; Jimenez, Cook, Bartels, & Alegría, 2013). Patients of color often report that they feel unheard by their providers or that they feel perceived as noncooperative and unwilling to follow directions provided by clinicians. Some argue that cultural differences in communication styles (that may vary by race, gender, and socioeconomic status) and different understandings of the provider-patient relationship may impede communication and misinform provider decisions regarding treatment (Alegría et al., 2012; Barksdale, Kenyon, Graves, & Jacobs, 2014). All of these issues fit within the sphere of a pervasive issue called "implicit bias," which has been examined extensively throughout the social science literature (and is described further in chapter 6). Implicit bias is the internalization of culturally learned stereotypes about out-groups. It is recognized as a pervasive part of society and the helping professions and does indeed impact the psychotherapeutic experience (FitzGerald & Hurst, 2017). There are a few innovative ways for providers to circumvent implicit and systemic bias. For example, ethnically diverse providers can often provide guidance on the needs of patients reflecting their own cultural backgrounds and can be a good source of support via lectures, webinars, public talks, and professional talks in clinical settings (e.g., hospital-based Grand Rounds). Such training and mentoring can be especially useful for trainees, early-career clinicians, and seasoned professionals to gain insights into patients' lived experience without feeling as if they need to ask patients to serve as cultural brokers or teachers.

Manualized treatments have been developed and promoted as a means of improving the quality of care received by persons seeking psychotherapy, and they are promoted as efficacious based on findings from randomized controlled trials. While this is an important step forward for consumers and providers, patients of diverse backgrounds have been reported to view these types of treatments less than favorably. For example, research by Breland-Noble and colleagues found that African American parents reported concerns about manualized treatments as "cookie-cutter" approaches not designed to meet their individual needs or those of diverse groups (Breland-Noble, Bell, Burriss, & AAKOMA Project Adult Advisory Board, 2011). Additionally, many treatments offered in psychotherapy are perceived as incongruent with the religious beliefs, cultural values, traditional perspectives, and conceptualizations of mental health and illness held by diverse groups. For example, in a sample of African American rural mothers whose children needed mental health care, approximately one-third believed that a White professional would not understand their problems and that the resulting quality of care would therefore be poorer than that offered to a White child (Murry, Heflinger, Suiter, & Brody, 2011; Shedlin, Decena, Mangadu, & Martinez, 2011).

Overall, we recognize the importance of barriers to the quality of care in psychotherapy received by racially diverse patients and offer a few methods for assisting providers in avoiding or reducing their impacts.

Treatment Outcomes

People of color consistently experience poorer psychotherapy treatment outcomes compared to White Americans (Baglivio, Wolff, Piquero, Greenwald, & Epps, 2017; Kapke &

Gerdes, 2016). This has been suggested to be partially related to their underutilization of treatment. Therefore, it is worth noting that a key feature of clinical improvement in treatment is related to active engagement in the process. As mentioned earlier, improving the therapeutic alliance (i.e., the positive relationship between a patient and a provider) can have a significant impact on mental health service utilization, and premature treatment termination with stronger therapeutic alliance is tied to longer engagement and greater perceived benefit of treatment (Castro-Blanco, 2010; Gipson & King, 2012).

The dangers of not receiving care extend beyond the immediate consequences of untreated symptoms. It is likely that as outpatient services—including preventative care and routine visits—go underutilized, the risk of subsequent crises and need for emergency services increases. While these risks are not race specific, people of color (particularly those from under-resourced communities) with undertreated mental illness face higher risks of involuntary commitment and hospitalization, incarceration, and encounters with law enforcement (Chung et al., 2014; Lee, Goodkind, & Shook, 2017; Spinney et al., 2016), and this is due in part to underutilization of preventative and early stage clinical care. As an example, we note the oft-cited findings that indicate that African American adults are more likely to receive diagnoses of psychosis than affective disorders (Carpenter-Song et al., 2011) and are less likely to be referred for specialty care when mental illness is suspected or confirmed. Furthermore, those who do not receive care at earlier stages of their disorders face an increased risk of poorer mental health outcomes in the long term (Barksdale & Molock, 2009; Beiter et al., 2015), along with damage to daily life roles, interpersonal interactions, and social relationships (Kessler & Bromet, 2013; Miller et al., 2016).

Outpatient Treatment and Youth of Color

There are few racial differences in mental illness prevalence across youth racial groups (SAMHSA, 2015), with approximately 33 percent of adolescents in primary care settings (who screen positive for mental illness) refusing treatment referrals. Hacker and colleagues (2014) noted that despite moderate referral rates, many adolescents endorsing symptoms cancelled or did not show up for their appointments. Furthermore, over 70 percent of psychiatrically impaired youth receive no mental health care referral or follow up (Cummings & Druss, 2011; Hacker et al., 2014) and African American, Latinx and Hispanic, and Asian youth are significantly less likely to receive outpatient care compared to their White peers (32 percent, 31 percent, and 19 percent, respectively, vs. 40 percent). Also, African American youth who do enter behavioral health care are far less likely to complete treatment compared to White youth, with figures ranging from one-third to one-half the completion rates of White youth (Cummings & Druss, 2011; Merikangas, Nakamura, & Kessler, 2009).

White youth are generally more likely to receive diagnoses congruent with their presenting symptoms than are their peers of color (Baglivio et al., 2017; Lee et al., 2017).

Consequently, White children and adolescents are more likely to be referred to specialty, inpatient mental health services, while youth of color are more likely to utilize emergency services (Barksdale & Molock, 2009). Youth of color who do not access effective or appropriate care are susceptible to an increased likelihood of contact with the juvenile justice system, poorer school performance, and other punitive (as opposed to healing-focused) outcomes (Barksdale & Molock, 2009; Breland-Noble et al., 2011). In the case of youth offenders, White youth are more likely to be referred to court-ordered treatment-oriented services, while youth of color, especially African Americans, are referred to the juvenile justice system for similar offenses (Cunningham, Randall, Ryan, & Fleming, 2016; Dannerbeck & Jiahui, 2009; Kaba et al., 2015).

Cultural Stigma

Cultural factors also contribute to mental health stigma and poor treatment engagement through the promotion of negative perceptions of mental illness, mistrust of the health care system, and the perceived social consequences of seeking help (DeCou & Vidair, 2017). Overall, research indicates that people of color hold different ideas about the etiology of mental illness compared to Whites. For example, Whites are more likely to view mental illness as psychological and physiological in origin, while African Americans and Hispanics and Latinx regard mental illness as a nonmedical problem and, at times, a personal failing (Breland-Noble et al., 2011; Carpenter-Song et al., 2010; Lawton, Gerdes, Haack, & Schneider, 2014). These differing perceptions feed help-seeking stigmas and are strong deterrents to clinical care (Arora, Metz, & Carlson, 2016; Clement et al., 2015).

Stigma can influence symptom recognition and acknowledgment of illness severity, often resulting in a struggle to accept that a problem necessitates mental health treatment (Miranda et al., 2015). It is often only when the illness creates an identifiable social disturbance or risk of harm that it becomes a problem warranting professional attention. Even then, outpatient care may be bypassed in favor of confronting the problem within the family or through other socially acceptable care media (Breland-Noble et al., 2016; Han & Pong, 2015). Family and friend support systems, religious groups, and traditional prayers are heavily relied upon within communities of color and may explain some underutilization of professional treatment (Breland-Noble, Wong, Childers, Hankerson, & Sotomayor, 2015; Hankerson & Weissman, 2012; Rose, Finigan-Carr, & Joe, 2016). However, cultural support systems often come with challenges of their own that may further perpetuate mental health stigma. Breland-Noble and colleagues identified themes that speak to the nuanced relationship between African American faith communities and perceptions of mental health that may serve as barriers to treatment (Breland-Noble et al., 2015). Their qualitative study investigating the interplay between religious and spiritual beliefs and depression among twenty-eight African American youth speaks to both the supportive nature of faith communities and the rigid ideals and beliefs that

Christians should seek help only from God. It is therefore encouraged that clinicians working within African American communities be open to integrating religious beliefs and coping strategies into the treatment plan.

Strategies for Improving Access

Culturally relevant health care is key to improving access to outpatient mental health treatment and meeting the mental health needs of racially diverse groups. Cultural competence requires clinicians to consider the overlapping cultures of the patient, clinician, service provider, agency, and community (Barksdale, Kenyon, Graves, & Jacobs, 2014). The National Standards for Culturally and Linguistically Appropriate Services (CLAS; developed by the Office of Minority Health) is one tool for reducing disparities in mental health care access and service utilization for diverse people (USDHHS, 2001). The CLAS Standards provide guidance on improving quality care under three areas: *culturally competent care*, *language access services*, and *organizational supports*. Providers can use and implement CLAS to support the implementation of culturally competent care in clinical settings.

Cultural competence is also a pathway to reducing provider bias (Whaley & Davis, 2007), as it supports clinicians in learning and understanding a patient's sociocultural context. By understanding this context, providers further strengthen the patient-clinician relationship (Holden et al., 2014), resulting in patients' continued engagement in care. Providers are encouraged to evaluate markers of cultural sensitivity and cultural relevance of care within their clinical practice to determine areas in need of improvement (Alvarez, Marroquin, Sandoval, & Carlson, 2014).

Group and solo practitioners must also consider that in communities of color, multiple alternatives to care are typically pursued prior to initial consult with specialty mental health. Given this, practitioners should seek to engage within the geographic community and develop collaborative partnerships with culturally embedded community partners (churches, community centers, etc.) through community engagement activities such as mental health education and awareness campaigns (Khodyakov, Pulido, Ramos, & Dixon, 2014; Mango et al., 2014). Availability of provider services and a demonstrated willingness to understand community needs can also reduce cultural mistrust. Wells et al. (2013) examined the benefits of a community-engaged approach to care and found that collaborating with community partners improved mental health quality of life and mental wellness, and it was more predictive of positive outcomes than simply providing evidence-based practices solely in traditional clinical settings.

Additionally, new alternatives to care that extend beyond traditional forms of therapy into communities have grown in recent years. Collaborating with or training health coaches, patient navigators, *promotoras*, and other community advocates is a way for mental health clinicians to attend to barriers and simultaneously reduce disparities from a population health perspective. Faith Based Mental Health Promotion (FBMHP) is a community-engaged approach that seeks to expand upon community-based partici-patory research by making mental health interventions relevant to participants with con-nections to faith communities through an understanding and acknowledgment of the perspectives of faith communities (Breland-Noble, Wong, Harding, & Carter-Williams, 2014). Faith-based partnerships have been found helpful in screening and improving mental health access in African American communities (Breland-Noble & Board, 2012; Breland-Noble et al., 2015), improving mental health literacy (Alegría et al., 2008), and decreasing risk of mental illness (Hankerson & Weissman, 2012). Villatoro, Dixon, and Mays (2016) also suggest that utilization of faith-based organizations in the Latinx com-munity may help decrease mental health disparities and improve the efficacy of mental health care.

Researchers also suggest improving and promoting mental health literacy as a poten-tial means of reducing barriers. Mental health literacy reflects "knowledge and beliefs about mental disorders which aid their recognition, management or prevention" (Jorm, 2000). Research indicates an association between general mental health knowledge and rates of service use with poor mental health literacy having been found to increase feel-ings of stigma and decrease treatment engagement and adherence (Al-Mateen, Mullen, & Malloy, 2016; Neighbors et al., 2008). Greater knowledge of mental health has been associated with positive perception of mental health treatment and increased utilization of available services (Alegría et al., 2008; Breland-Noble & Board, 2012). One way that outpatient clinicians can foster mental health literacy in under-resourced communities, including those of color, is by using nonmedical terms (when possible) and distributing handouts written for broad readability and understanding. In integrated-care settings, clinicians also have the opportunity to advocate for the inclusion of CLAS standards and basic standards of care that promote mental health equity, including appropriate inter-preter services, documentation of patient language preferences, and flexibility in the psy-chotherapeutic encounter (i.e., clinic hours or length of sessions) (Richmond & Jackson, 2018).

Recently, newer delivery approaches have been suggested as mechanisms to increase the availability and acceptability of treatments. Examples of these approaches include behavioral health integrated into primary care settings, telehealth technologies, and school-based mental health (SBMH). When behavioral health services are integrated into the primary care setting, they are often described as primary care behavioral health (PCBH) or primary care mental health integration (PC-MHI). These approaches are not focused on specific approaches to psychotherapy per se, but they are focused on increas-ing the accessibility and acceptability of standard approaches to psychotherapy (like cog-nitive behavioral therapy (CBT) or interpersonal therapy) by including mental health care in settings where people of diverse backgrounds are already likely to be located. These approaches have a growing research base and have also shown promise for con-tributing to reduction of mental health disparities. Cognitive behavioral therapy (CBT) can be implemented in brief forms and has been tested via online platforms, smartphone apps, and integration within primary care settings for adults and youth (Arean, Raue, Sirey, & Snowden, 2012; Gladstone et al., 2014; Van Voorhees et al., 2011). Clinicians can utilize the many workbooks and findings from studies and demonstration projects that have tested and utilized these approaches to gain insights into practical application of CBT in varied formats. For example, clinicians can download CBT manuals for various delivery modes and populations online and have step-by-step guides for use in clinical outpatient settings like private and group practices (e.g., http://medschool2.ucsf.edu/latino/pdf/CBTDEN/overview.pdf).

Conclusion

It is clear via research, anecdotal evidence, and clinical reports from people of color themselves that the underrepresentation of people of color in clinical care is rooted in deep historical and current provider and systemic-level barriers. These barriers are not limited to the oft-cited factors like money and insurance status but include a host of sociocultural factors including provider bias, patient preferences, and lack of cultural relevance of present approaches to outpatient psychotherapeutic care. Future research must begin to address the malleable barriers to care via innovative means. As an example, we note throughout our discussion that the lack of perceived cultural relevance of treatments significantly negatively impacts the use of services by patients of color. We further highlight innovative means for addressing this barrier, including community partnerships and integrated-care approaches. Additionally, it is critical that the pipeline of diverse providers be increased to meet an ever-increasing demand for clinicians of varied racial and ethnic backgrounds.

Numerous studies exist that point to patient preferences for culturally competent (and culturally matched) providers. This has been demonstrated most recently in the national dialogue by college students of color demanding increased diversity in the provider setting on campus. Many campuses have responded by creating offices for diversity and inclusion and assigning persons to the role of chief diversity officer. While this approach represents one model for one setting, it has applicability across outpatient mental health. We believe that by creating a well-articulated, focused, and explicit commitment to creating a culturally relevant space for patients of diverse backgrounds, outpatient providers can take one critical step in lowering the types of nonfinancial barriers that keep people of color out of the clinical sphere.

Finally, through our focused evaluation of the existing literature on disparities in outpatient mental health care, we argue that creative strategies can ensure a more comprehensive approach toward care that accounts for the unique situations, cultural values, and socioeconomic situations of patients. Through collaborative efforts among of patients, providers, and systems, we can create a better and more impactful system of care that acknowledges and explicitly addresses the mental health needs of people of color.

KEY POINTS FOR CLINICIANS

- Recognize that few differences in the prevalence of mental illness exist across racial and ethnic groups.

- The likelihood of seeking traditional forms of care varies widely for people of color of all socioeconomic strata.

- Barriers to psychotherapy include money, but socioeconomic status is a small part of the equation. More important are the sociocultural barriers like negative perceptions of psychotherapy and fears that psychotherapy is irrelevant to the lived experience of many people of color.

- Learn key facets of cultural competence and seek to apply those learnings to all patients.

- Outcomes can be improved by personalizing and adapting psychotherapy to meet the needs of clients on a case-by-case basis.

- Helping to improve mechanisms for engagement in psychotherapy is key. Providers should identify varied ways of conducting outreach to diverse communities to share the message of the utility of psychotherapy and prepare diverse people to engage in clinical care.

References

Al-Mateen, C., Mullen, S. J., & Malloy, J. K. (2016). Pharmacotherapy. In A. M. Breland-Noble, C. Al-Mateen, & N. Singh (Eds.), *Handbook of Mental Health in African American Youth* (pp. 39–61). New York, NY: Springer.

Alegría, M., Lin, J. Y., Green, J. G., Sampson, N. A., Gruber, M. J., & Kessler, R. C. (2012). Role of referrals in mental health service disparities for racial and ethnic minority youth. *Journal of American Academy of Child and Adolescent Psychiatry, 51*(7), 703–711. doi:http://dx.doi.org/10.1016/j.jaac.2012.05.005

Alegría, M., Polo, A., Gao, S., Santana, L., Rothstein, D., Jimenez, A., … & Normand, S. L. (2008). Evaluation of a patient activation and empowerment intervention in mental health care. *Medical Care, 46*(3), 247–256. doi:10.1097/MLR.0b013e318158af52

Alvarez, K., Marroquin, Y. A., Sandoval, L., & Carlson, C. I. (2014). Integrated health care best practices and culturally and linguistically competent care: Practitioner perspectives. *Journal of Mental Health Counseling, 36*(2), 99–114.

Arean, P. A., Raue, P. J., Sirey, J. A., & Snowden, M. (2012). Implementing evidence-based psychotherapies in settings serving older adults: Challenges and solutions. *Psychiatric Services, 63*(6), 605–607. doi:10.1176/appi.ps.201100078

Arora, P. G., Metz, K., & Carlson, C. I. (2016). Attitudes toward professional psychological help seeking in South Asian students: Role of stigma and gender. *Journal of Multicultural Counseling and Development, 44*(4), 263–284. doi:10.1002/jmcd.12053

Augsberger, A., Yeung, A., Dougher, M., & Hahm, H. C. (2015). Factors influencing the underutilization of mental health services among Asian American women with a history of depression and suicide. *BMC Health Services Research, 15*, 11. doi:10.1186/s12913-015-1191-7

Baglivio, M. T., Wolff, K. T., Piquero, A. R., Greenwald, M. A., & Epps, N. (2017). Racial/ethnic disproportionality in psychiatric diagnoses and treatment in a sample of serious juvenile offenders. *Journal of Youth and Adolescence, 46*(7), 1424–1451. doi:10.1007/s10964-016-0573-4

Barksdale, C. L., Kenyon, J., Graves, D. L., & Jacobs, C. G. (2014). Addressing disparities in mental health agencies: strategies to implement the National CLAS Standards in Mental Health. *Psychological Services, 11*(4), 369–376. doi:10.1037/a0035211

Barksdale, C. L., & Molock, S. D. (2009). Perceived norms and mental health help seeking among African American college students. *The Journal of Behavioral Health Services & Research, 36*(3), 285–299.

Beiter, R., Nash, R., McCrady, M., Rhoades, D., Linscomb, M., Clarahan, M., & Sammut, S. (2015). The prevalence and correlates of depression, anxiety, and stress in a sample of college students. *Journal of Affective Disorders, 173*, 90–96. doi:10.1016/j.jad.2014.10.054

Belgrave, F. Z., & Berry, B. M. (2016). Community approaches to promoting positive mental health and psychosocial well-being. In A. M. Breland-Noble, C. S. Al-Mateen, & N. N. Singh (Eds.), *Handbook of Mental Health in African American Youth* (pp. 121–140). New York, NY: Springer.

Breland-Noble, A. M. (2015). Depressive disorders in African American youth: Historical concerns, current knowledge and future directions. In A. M. Breland-Noble, C. Al-Mateen, & N. Singh (Eds.), *Handbook of Mental Health in African American Youth* (pp. 187–199). New York, NY: Springer.

Breland-Noble, A. M., Al-Mateen, C., & Singh, N. (2016). *Handbook of Mental Health in African American Youth*. Cham, Switzerland: Springer.

Breland-Noble, A. M., Bell, C. C., Burriss, A., & AAKOMA Project Adult Advisory Board. (2011). "Mama just won't accept this": Adult perspectives on engaging depressed African American teens in clinical research and treatment. *Journal of Clinical Psychology in Medical Settings, 18*(3), 225–234. doi:10.1007/s10880-011-9235-6

Breland-Noble, A. M., & Board, A. P. A. A. (2012). Community and treatment engagement for depressed African American youth: the AAKOMA FLOA pilot. *Journal of Clinical Psychology in Medical Settings, 19*(1), 41–48. doi:10.1007/s10880-011-9281-0

Breland-Noble, A. M., Wong, M. J., Childers, T., Hankerson, S., & Sotomayor, J. (2015). Spirituality and religious coping in African-American youth with depressive illness. *Mental Health, Religion & Culture, 18*(5), 330–341. doi:10.1080/13674676.2015.1056120

Breland-Noble, A. M., Wong, M. J., Harding, C., & Carter-Williams, M. (2014). *Faith Based Mental Health Promotion for African Americans*. Paper presented at the Minority Health and Health Disparities Grantees' Conference: Transdisciplinary Collaborations: Evolving Dimensions of US and Global Health Equity, National Harbor, MD.

Caldwell, C., Assari, S., & Breland-Noble, A. M. (2016). The epidemiology of mental disorders in African American children and adolescents. In A. M. Breland-Noble, C. Al-Mateen, & N. Singh (Eds.), *Handbook of Mental Health in African American Youth* (pp. 3–20). New York, NY: Springer.

Carpenter-Song, E., Chu, E., Drake, R. E., Ritsema, M., Smith, B., & Alverson, H. (2010). Ethnocultural variations in the experience and meaning of mental illness and treatment: implications for access and utilization. *Transcultural Psychiatry, 47*(2), 224–251. doi:10.1177/1363461510368906

Carpenter-Song, E., Whitley, R., Lawson, W., Quimby, E., & Drake, R. E. (2011). Reducing disparities in mental health care: Suggestions from the Dartmouth-Howard Collaboration. *Community Mental Health Journal, 47*(1), 1–13. doi:10.1007/s10597-009-9233-4

Castro-Blanco, D. K. M. S. (2010). *Elusive alliance: Treatment engagement strategies with high-risk adolescents*. Washington, DC: American Psychological Association.

Chung, B., Ong, M., Ettner, S. L., Jones, F., Gilmore, J., McCreary, M., ... & Wells, K. B. (2014). 12-month outcomes of community engagement versus technical assistance to implement depression collaborative care: A partnered, cluster, randomized, comparative effectiveness trial. *Annals of Internal Medicine, 161*(10 Suppl), S23–34. doi:10.7326/M13-3011

Clement, S., Schauman, O., Graham, T., Maggioni, F., Evans-Lacko, S., Bezborodovs, N., ... & Thornicroft, G. (2015). What is the impact of mental health-related stigma on help-seeking? A systematic review of quantitative and qualitative studies. *Psychological Medicine, 45*(1), 11–27. doi:10.1017/S0033291714000129

Cummings, J. R., & Druss, B. G. (2011). Racial/ethnic differences in mental health service use among adolescents with major depression. *Journal of the American Academy of Child and Adolescent Psychiatry, 50*(2), 160–170. doi:10.1016/j.jaac.2010.11.004

Cunningham, C. E., Randall, P. B., Ryan, S. R., & Fleming, B. D. (2016). Conduct disorder and oppositional defiant disorder. In A. Breland-Noble, C. S. Al-Mateen, & N. Singh (Eds.), *Handbook of Mental Health in African American Youth* (Vol. 1, pp. 144–162). New York, NY: Springer.

Dannerbeck, J. A., & Jiahui, Y. (2009). Exploring patterns of court-ordered mental health services for juvenile offenders. *Criminal Justice and Behavior, 36*(4), 402–419. doi:10.1177/0093854808330799

DeCou, S. E., & Vidair, H. B. (2017). What low-income, depressed mothers need from mental health care: Overcoming treatment barriers from their perspective. *Journal of Child and Family Studies, 26*(8), 2252–2265. doi:10.1007/s10826-017-0733-5

Eliacin, J., Coffing, J. M., Matthias, M. S., Burgess, D. J., Bair, M. J., & Rollins, A. L. (2018). The relationship between race, patient activation, and working alliance: Implications for patient engagement in mental health care. *Administration and Policy in Mental Health and Mental Health Services Research, 45*(1), 186–192. doi:10.1007/s10488-016-0779-5

FitzGerald, C., & Hurst, S. (2017). Implicit bias in healthcare professionals: a systematic review. *BMC Medical Ethics, 18*(1), 19.

Gipson, P., & King, C. (2012). Health behavior theories and research: Implications for suicidal individuals' treatment linkage and adherence. *Cognitive and Behavioral Practice, 19*(2), 209–217. doi:10.1016/j.cbpra.2010.11.005

Gladstone, T., Marko-Holguin, M., Henry, J., Fogel, J., Diehl, A., & Van Voorhees, B. W. (2014). Understanding adolescent response to a technology-based depression prevention program. *Journal of Clinical Child and Adolescent Psychology, 43*(1), 102–114. doi:10.1080/15374416.2013.850697

Hacker, K., Arsenault, L., Franco, I., Shaligram, D., Sidor, M., Olfson, M., & Goldstein, J. (2014). Referral and follow-up after mental health screening in commercially insured adolescents. *Journal of Adolescent Health, 55*(1), 17–23. doi:10.1016/j.jadohealth.2013.12.012

Han, M., & Pong, H. (2015). Mental health help-seeking behaviors among Asian American community college students: The effect of stigma, cultural barriers, and acculturation. *Journal of College Student Development, 56*(1), 1–14.

Hankerson, S. H., & Weissman, M. M. (2012). Church-based health programs for mental disorders among African Americans: A review. *Psychiatric Services, 63*(3), 243–249. doi:10.1176/appi.ps.201100216

Hoffman, K. M., Trawalter, S., Axt, J. R., & Oliver, M. N. (2016). Racial bias in pain assessment and treatment recommendations, and false beliefs about biological differences between blacks and whites. *Proceedings of the National Academy of Sciences of the United States of America, 113*(16), 4296–4301. doi:10.1073/pnas.1516047113

Holden, K., McGregor, B., Thandi, P., Fresh, E., Sheats, K., Belton, A., ... & Satcher, D. (2014). Toward culturally centered integrative care for addressing mental health disparities among ethnic minorities. *Psychological Services, 11*(4), 357–368. doi:10.1037/a0038122

Huey, S. J., Tilley, J. L., Jones, E. O., & Smith, C. A. (2014). The contribution of cultural competence to evidence-based care for ethnically diverse populations. *Annual Review of Clinical Psychology, 10*, 305–338. doi:10.1146/annurev-clinpsy-032813-153729

Institute of Medicine. (1993). *Committee on Monitoring Access to Personal Health Care Services: Access to Healthcare in America.* Washington, DC: National Academies Press.

Institute of Medicine. (2003). *Unequal Treatment: Confronting Racial and Ethnic Disparities in Health Care.* Washington, DC: The National Academies Press.

Jimenez, D. E., Cook, B., Bartels, S. J., & Alegría, M. (2013). Disparities in mental health service use of racial and ethnic minority elderly adults. *Journal of the American Geriatrics Society, 61*(1), 18–25. doi:10.1111/jgs.12063

Jorm, A. F. (2000). Mental health literacy. Public knowledge and beliefs about mental disorders. *British Journal of Psychiatry, 177,* 396–401.

Kaba, F., Solimo, A., Graves, J., Glowa-Kollisch, S., Vise, A., MacDonald, R., … & Venters, H. (2015). Disparities in mental health referral and diagnosis in the New York City jail mental health service. *American Journal of Public Health, 105*(9), 1911–1916. doi:10.2105/AJPH.2015.302699

Kapke, T. L., & Gerdes, A. C. (2016). Latino family participation in youth mental health services: Treatment retention, engagement, and response. *Clinical Child and Family Psychology Review, 19*(4), 329–351. doi:10.1007/s10567-016-0213-2

Kessler, R. C., & Bromet, E. J. (2013). The epidemiology of depression across cultures. *Annual Review of Public Health, 34,* 119–138. doi:10.1146/annurev-publhealth-031912-114409

Khodyakov, D., Pulido, E., Ramos, A., & Dixon, E. (2014). Community-partnered research conference model: The experience of community partners in care study. *Progress in Community Health Partnerships-Research Education and Action, 8*(1), 83–97.

Lawton, K. E., Gerdes, A. C., Haack, L. M., & Schneider, B. (2014). Acculturation, cultural values, and Latino parental beliefs about the etiology of ADHD. *Administration and Policy in Mental Health and Mental Health Services Research, 41*(2), 189–204. doi:10.1007/s10488-012-0447-3

Lê Cook, B., McGuire, T. G., Lock, K., & Zaslavsky, A. M. (2010). Comparing methods of racial and ethnic disparities measurement across different settings of mental health care. *Health Services Research, 45*(3), 825–847. doi:10.1111/j.1475-6773.2010.01100.x

Lee, L. H., Goodkind, S., & Shook, J. J. (2017). Racial/ethnic disparities in prior mental health service use among incarcerated adolescents. *Children and Youth Services Review, 78,* 23–31. doi:10.1016/j.childyouth.2017.04.019

Mango, J., Cabiling, E., Jones, L., Lucas-Wright, A., Williams, P., Wells, K., … & Chung, B. (2014). Community partners in care (CPIC): Video summary of rationale, study approach/implementation, and client 6-month outcomes. *CES4Health. info, 2014.*

Merikangas, K., Nakamura, E., & Kessler, R. (2009). Epidemiology of mental disorders in children and adolescents. *Dialogues in Clinical Neuroscience, 11*(1), 7–20.

Miller, S., Ringeisen, H., Munoz, B., Hedden, S. L., Colpe, L. J., Rohloff, H., & Embry, V. (2016). Correlates of mental health service use among young adults with mental illness: Results from the national survey on drug use and health. *Psychiatric Services, 67*(6), 641–648. doi:10.1176/appi.ps.201400486

Miranda, R., Soffer, A., Polanco-Roman, L., Wheeler, A., & Moore, A. (2015). Mental health treatment barriers among racial/ethnic minority versus white young adults 6 months after intake at a college counseling center. *Journal of American College Health, 63*(5), 291–298. doi:10.1080/07448481.2015.1015024

Murry, V. M., Heflinger, C. A., Suiter, S. V., & Brody, G. H. (2011). Examining perceptions about mental health care and help-seeking among rural African American families of adolescents. *Journal of Youth and Adolescence, 40*(9), 1118–1131. doi:10.1007/s10964-010-9627-1

Neighbors, H. W., Woodward, A. T., Bullard, K. M., Ford, B. C., Taylor, R. J., & Jackson, J. S. (2008). Mental health service use among older African Americans: The National Survey of American Life. *American Journal of Geriatric Psychiatry, 16*(12), 948–956. doi:10.1097/JGP.0b013e318187ddd3

Pumariega, A. J., Rothe, E., Mian, A., Carlisle, L., Toppelberg, C., Harris, T., … & American Academy of Child and Adolescent Psychiatry (AACAP) Committee on Quality Issues (CQI). (2013).

Practice parameter for cultural competence in child and adolescent psychiatric practice. *Journal of the American Academy of Child and Adolescent Psychiatry, 52*(10), 1101–1115. doi:10.1016/j.jaac.2013.06.019

Richmond, A., & Jackson, J. (2018). Cultural considerations for psychologists in primary care. *Journal of Clinical Psychology in Medical Settings, 25*(3), 305–315.

Rose, T., Finigan-Carr, N., & Joe, S. (2016). Organized religious involvement and mental health among Caribbean black adolescents. *Child and Adolescent Social Work Journal,* 1–11. doi:10.1007/s10560-016-0452-6

SAMHSA. (2015). *Behavioral Health Barometer: United States, 2014.* (HHS Publication No. SMA–15–4895). Rockville, MD: Substance Abuse and Mental Health Services Administration.

Shedlin, M., Decena, C., Mangadu, T., & Martinez, A. (2011). Research participant recruitment in Hispanic communities: Lessons learned. *Journal of Immigrant and Minority Health, 13*(2), 352–360. doi:10.1007/s10903-009-9292-1

Spinney, E., Yeide, M., Feyerherm, W., Cohen, M., Stephenson, R., & Thomas, C. (2016). Racial disparities in referrals to mental health and substance abuse services from the juvenile justice system: a review of the literature. *Journal of Crime and Justice, 39*(1), 153–173. doi:10.1080/0735648X.2015.1133492

USDHHS. (2001). *Mental health: Culture, race, and ethnicity: A supplement to mental health: A report of the surgeon general.* Rockville, MD: US Department of Health and Human Services.

Van Voorhees, B. W., Mahoney, N., Mazo, R., Barrera, A. Z., Siemer, C. P., Gladstone, T. R. G., & Muñoz, R. F. (2011). Internet-based depression prevention over the life course: A call for behavioral vaccines. *The Psychiatric Clinics of North America, 34*(1), 167–183.

Villatoro, A. P., Dixon, E., & Mays, V. M. (2016). Faith-based organizations and the Affordable Care Act: Reducing Latino mental health care disparities. *Psychological Services, 13*(1), 92–104. doi:10.1037/a0038515

Wells, K. B., Jones, L., Chung, B., Dixon, E. L., Tang, L. Q., Gilmore, J., … & Miranda, J. (2013). Community-partnered cluster-randomized comparative effectiveness trial of community engagement and planning or resources for services to address depression disparities. *Journal of General Internal Medicine, 28*(10), 1268–1278. doi:10.1007/s11606-013-2484-3

Whaley, A. L., & Davis, K. E. (2007). Cultural competence and evidence-based practice in mental health services—A complementary perspective. *American Psychologist, 62*(6), 563–574. doi:10.1037/0003-066x.62.6.563

CHAPTER 15

Racial Disparities in University Counseling Centers

M. R. Natacha Foo Kune,
University of Washington

Agnes Kwong,
Interconnections Healing Center

Ellen B. Taylor,
Washington State University

Racial disparities in accessing mental health services in the college and university context have been and often continues to be an issue for students of color. In this chapter, we provide a historical overview of culturally responsive counseling practices in university settings. We then explore the scope of the problem of access and quality of care, followed by the causes of racial disparities in utilization and outcome. Finally, we provide a summary of strategies for addressing racial disparities and recommendations for future research.

Overview of Care Delivery in Counseling Centers and the Racial and Ethnic Communities Served

Throughout the first half of the twentieth century, counseling or mental health services were offered to a limited degree and in somewhat variable ways on college campuses in the United States (Kraft, 2011). The influx of students attending college at the end of World War II was accompanied by a rise in vocational counseling for this generation of students. Subsequently, the Civil Rights and feminist movements of the 1960s and 1970s brought increasing racial and gender diversity to higher education settings. From 1976 to 1999, along with changes in national demographics, the trend continued. The number of students of color on college campuses grew at more than twice the rate of White students (Anderson, 2003). In 1976, students of color represented 16 percent of enrolled undergraduates; in 2008, they represented 35 percent (National Center for Education Statistics, 2010).

With student diversity came a more complex campus environment and changing expectations for colleges and universities to better support and serve all of their students. Counseling, which had been the purview of faculty during the first part of the twentieth century, shifted to student affairs offices, and college counseling practices developed (Forrest, 1989). At the same time, counseling itself shifted toward more specialization as assessment tools and psychological interventions became both more sophisticated and more applicable to college populations. In the 1980s, counselor education and training programs emerged and counseling centers evolved into multifaceted entities at the forefront of research and practice. College mental health care became a legitimate professional specialization.

A greater developmental focus, and the notion that such development occurs along multiple dimensions, leant itself to an emphasis on the individual within context. Respect for the vast diversity of identities, backgrounds, and experiences students bring to college became, more and more, an imperative. Building on the work of Rogers (1951) and others, college counseling emphasized the uniqueness of each person while developing approaches to nurture the growth of the whole person (Williamson, 1939). A variety of models for providing mental health care developed, including prevention and education efforts designed to enhance coping (Brunner, Wallace, Reymann, Sellers, & McCabe, 2014). These models emerged from several national trends, including the development of radically more effective psychotropic medications, the rise of attention to equal access under the Americans with Disabilities Act of 1990 and its amendment in 2009, and the movement for colleges and universities to address suicide risk among their students (Brunner et. al., 2014). Still, counseling practice had largely emerged from a homogeneous worldview represented by primarily White Americans. Derald Wing Sue's seminal work, *Counseling the Culturally Diverse: Theory and Practice* (1981), heralded a virtual revolution in counseling practice by calling out the need to center culture in working with students of color. Sue's work sparked recognition that clients from differing cultural backgrounds would respond differently to psychological interventions, and that the very definitions of psychological health are based on individualistic cultural assumptions, those steeped in a White supremacist framework, that simply do not apply universally. This paradigm shift did as much to transform the approach to clinical practice as any scholarly development since psychology was established as a field of study. Perhaps because of the increasing diversity of students on American college campuses and the tradition of universities as vanguards of societal change, college counseling centers were early adopters of multicultural counseling practices.

The increasing numbers of students of color on college campuses still represent a significant underrepresentation relative to the US population. That disparity is reflected in campus politics and activism. Further, graduation rates for some groups of students of color continue to lag behind those for White students. Among students who entered college in 2010, Latinx and Black students' six-year graduation rates were 46 percent and

38 percent, respectively, while graduation rates for White students were 62 percent (Tate, 2017). Asian American students' six-year graduation rates were reported at 63 percent, but it is important to note that aggregated data about multiple ethnicities under one racial group (Asian American) can mask the fact that some groups, such as Pacific Islanders and Southeast Asian American students, have lower graduation rates (National Commission on Asian American and Pacific Islander Research in Education, 2011).

While a number of factors drive differences in graduation rates, most notably the presence of poverty and attending a high-minority high school (Flores, Park, & Baker, 2017), research reveals that stress and related mental health concerns have a strong adverse influence on academic performance and graduation rates (Barr, Rando, Krolywicz, & Winfield, 2010; Lee, Olson, Locke, Michaelson, & Odes, 2009). Only sweeping social change can truly address socioeconomic disparities that more heavily burden communities of color, but ensuring access to culturally responsive mental health services is something colleges and universities can do to support the success and graduation rates of their students of color. Indeed, providing mental health services that are responsive to cultural differences continues to be both a common institutional aspiration and an understandable demand by students. Universities are, once again, poised to serve as vanguards of broader societal change.

Scope of the Disparities and Problems

In this section, we review barriers to accessing mental health care and differential outcomes that impact students of color.

Specific Disparities Related to Access to Care

Research indicates that in most contexts, people of color access mental health care less than Whites (Smith & Trimble, 2016). However, in college populations, Hayes, Youn, Castonguay, Locke, McAleavey, and Nordberg (2011) found that students of color were utilizing counseling center services at the same rate as White students. Notably, the research also found that ethnic make-up of the counseling center staff predicted the proportion of students from those ethnic groups accessing counseling center services, underscoring the importance of diversifying the staff.

We now focus on research specific to four major ethnic groups in the United States, African Americans, Asian Americans, Latinx Americans, and Native Americans, as research often groups people of color in these four categories. It is important to keep in mind that each of these ethnic groups contains layers of diversity in terms of ethnicity, as well as other intersections of identity. Consequently, some of the general findings may not apply to the entire group or individuals within the group. Further, there is some emerging research supporting the idea that having more than one marginalized identity may be correlated with higher levels of psychological distress (Hayes, Chun-Kennedy,

Edens, & Locke, 2011) such as depression, hostility, family concerns, social anxiety, and academic issues.

Latinx (López, Barrio, Kopelowicz & Vega, 2012) and Asian American (Kim & Zane, 2016) students are less likely to seek psychological help (Smith & Trimble, 2016). Decreased likelihood to access mental health care is correlated with higher levels of psychological distress and higher levels of perceived discrimination for Latinx students (Cheng, Kwan, & Sevig, 2013). While correlation does not mean causation, we wonder if this finding suggests that someone who has experienced more discrimination is less likely to trust institutions, thus decreasing help-seeking.

When accessing counseling, Native Americans (Haviland, Horswill, O'Connell & Dynneson, 1983; Garrett et al., 2012) and Black students (Thompson & Cimbolic, 1978) have a preference for an ethnic match with counselors. This means the lack of diversity in counselors on many campuses is, in effect, a barrier.

Across groups, higher belief in both harmful and seemingly "positive" stereotypes are associated with lower help-seeking. For example, higher belief in the model minority myth for Asian Americans is linked to lower help-seeking attitudes (Kim & Lee, 2014). Similarly, belief in the "strong Black woman" was associated with lower psychological help-seeking (Watson & Hunter, 2015). These findings reinforce that all stereotypes are harmful.

Specific Disparities Related to Quality of Care

Two studies indicate students of color report lower satisfaction with quality of mental health care than White students (Neimeyer & Gonzales, 1983; Garroutte, Kunovich, Jacobsen, & Goldberg, 2004). Given clients' preference for ethnic matching, the concept has been studied as a way to improve quality of care provided to clients of color. In a meta-analysis, clients of color appear to have a moderately strong preference for ethnic matching and view ethnically matched therapists somewhat more positively (Cabral & Smith, 2011). While the prospect of ethnic matching is very important to clients, the literature does not suggest more positive treatment outcomes for ethnically matched pairs (Erdur, Rude, & Baron, 2003; Presnell, Harris, & Scogin, 2012).

The quality of any treatment depends on the assessment of the client's issue(s). Research indicates that counselors with higher color-blind attitudes (see chapter 6) assessed White students accurately but underestimated symptoms in Black students (Gushue, 2004). There is no corresponding research for other racial categories, but it does raise the question about how counselors' attitudes can impact their appraisal of the client's needs. An incorrect assessment would inevitably impact determination about treatment, appropriate fit of treatment to the underlying problem(s), and, thereby, the quality and effectiveness of that treatment.

There are also factors that were found to positively impact the quality of care for students of color. During treatment, therapist cultural competence and empathy are two key factors that predict client satisfaction at a university counseling center (Fuertes et al., 2006).

Racial Disparities in Treatment Outcomes

Many treatment outcome studies on counseling centers enrolled predominantly White student populations and did not specifically examine racial disparities (Choi, 2010; Shimokawa, Lambert, & Smart, 2010; Vermeersch et al., 2004). Some counseling center studies that examined racial disparities in treatment outcomes found no overall differences between clients of color and White clients (e.g., Hayes, Owen, & Bieschke, 2015; Hayes, McAleavey, Castonguay, & Locke, 2016; Lambert et al., 2006; Maramba & Hall, 2002), but therapists vary in their effectiveness at reducing clients' symptoms and in how quickly this change takes place. Specifically, this differential efficacy was in part due to clients' racial ethnic background (e.g., Hayes et al., 2015). This finding was replicated most recently with a large sample of 3,825 counseling center clients seen by 251 therapists across forty-five college counseling centers (Hayes et al., 2016). Here, researchers also found no overall outcome differences between clients of color and White clients. More importantly, some therapists had better outcomes with clients of color, whereas other therapists had worse outcomes with clients of color. Researchers did not find that demographics or theoretical orientation of the therapists accounted for those differences. This suggests that some therapists have better cultural competence than others. Further research is needed to understand what factors may lead some therapists to be more culturally competent.

Another measure of outcome is unilateral termination, when clients end therapy without discussing it with their therapist (Owen, Imel, Adelson, & Rodolfa, 2012). Clients who drop out of therapy have been found to have worse therapy outcomes than those who end their course of therapy or discuss termination with their therapist (Daughters et al., 2005; Masson, Perlman, Ross, & Gates, 2007; Owen, Smith, & Rodolfa, 2009). Researchers postulate that clients of color may have an increased risk for unilateral termination (Kearney, Draper, & Baron, 2005; Terrell & Terrell, 1984; Wade & Bernstein, 1991), but research on the racial disparities in therapy dropout rates has yielded mixed results. For example, Lambert and colleagues (2006) found no difference in dropout rates between clients of color and White clients with the exception of Latinx clients, who were found to have lower than expected dropout rates. On the other hand, Owen and his colleagues (2012) found that students of color were more likely to unilaterally terminate than White clients. Within those differences, therapists had differential rates of unilateral termination with their clients of color. Once again, this supports the assertion that culturally competent therapists make a difference.

Causes of the Disparity (Clinician, Cultural, Economic, Structural Issues)

Since most counseling centers are funded by tuition and student fees and, therefore, are usually free of charge to students, this removes the economic barrier. However, in recent decades, counseling centers are overstretched and underfunded in ways that make short-term counseling the norm. Many students are referred out to a community mental health provider after an initial assessment or when the upper limit in sessions has been met (Brunner et al., 2014). Under these circumstances, students of color may be disproportionately affected, given that they tend to have fewer resources to be seen in a community health agency or by a private practitioner (Quintana, Kilmartin, Yesenosky, & Macias, 1991). In more rural communities, these latter options would be even more difficult to access, especially if students of color are seeking counselors of color.

Although studies have found that students of color are utilizing counseling services at rates proportional to the enrollment rates (Hayes, Youn, et al., 2011), they also note that students of color tend to experience greater psychological distress than White students (Hayes, Chun-Kennedy, et al., 2011). If so, students of color may be underutilizing counseling center services proportional to their level of distress and need. This could be due to a number of factors, including having an insufficient number of mental health professionals of color, cultural barriers, or not providing enough culturally appropriate outreach to communities of color on campus. Clients of color tend to want to see therapists of the same race, regardless of their presenting problem (Barksdale & Molock, 2009; Haviland et al., 1983; Townes, Chavez-Korell, & Cunningham, 2009). Hayes, Youn, and colleagues (2011) have found that the higher percentage of African American therapists at a counseling center, the greater the percentage of African American students who sought services. This was also the case for Latinx, Asian Americans, and European Americans.

Although researchers have called for investigations of specific therapeutic behaviors and characteristics that contribute to successful treatment outcomes with clients of color (Hayes et al., 2015; 2016), no studies have directly examined this to date. Given the replication of findings that different therapists have differential outcomes with students of color, it is imperative that research examine what specific therapist factors lead to this difference. It is possible that those who are less effective in working with clients of color may need more training, education, or supervision to enhance their cultural competence. Indeed, the perceptions that clients of color have of their therapist's cultural competence and sensitivity predict how satisfied students are with their counseling experience (Constantine, 2002) and of their perceived gains from therapy (Owen, Leach, Wampold, & Rodolfa, 2011).

Strategies that Show Promise

Given the amount of interventions implemented on various campuses to reduce racial disparities in mental health care access, there is surprisingly little published research in the area of college counseling centers. In this section, we include strategies that are likely to be effective in a college campus, based on empirical evidence when implemented in other settings and based on anecdotal evidence in university settings.

Strategies for Increasing Access to Care and Engagement

Strategies to improve access and outcomes of counseling for students of color fall in three general categories: (1) individual-level strategies aimed at encouraging students of color to engage in help-seeking and at making counseling services more culturally relevant; (2) campus-level strategies aimed at helping faculty, staff, and peers to refer students to counseling services; and (3) campus-level strategies to improve overall student mental health by decreasing implicit bias, microaggressions, and academic distress caused by the impact of oppression.

Strategies to encourage individuals of color to seek help from counseling centers include increasing the diversity of the staff (Hayes, Youn, et al., 2011; Garrett et al., 2012; Townes et al., 2009) and expanding the languages spoken among staff. Further, Smith, Rodriguez, and Bernal (2011) recommend that therapists use culturally congruent interventions and communicate in culturally sensitive ways, ideally in the client's native language.

There is good evidence that staff diversity means students of color are more likely to come to the counseling center. Research suggests multicultural competence is also needed to improve outcomes (Hayes et al., 2015; Hayes et al., 2016; Lambert et al., 2006; Maramba & Hall, 2002) and that some counselors produce better outcomes with students of color. Larrison, Schoppelrey, Hack-Ritzo, and Korr (2011) found that the number of positive experiences and relationships that a therapist has with individuals from ethnic and racial groups dissimilar to their own predicted better outcomes with Black clients. While additional research is being conducted to provide more guidance, therapists who are more effective at working with clients of color may serve as useful role models for their colleagues.

Another area of research includes evidence-based treatments implemented on students of color, such as a cognitive behavioral skills group for students of color (Mokrue & Acri, 2013). Cultural humility is another promising concept (Comas-Diaz, 2014; Mosher et al., 2017), which emphasizes the therapist's lifelong desire to learn from others, self-reflection about cultural awareness and power imbalances, mutual partnership, interpersonal respect, and openness to new cultural information. Cultural humility has been linked to a positive working alliance and appears to be linked to the therapist committing fewer microaggressions (Mosher et al., 2017). In turn, microaggressions have been linked to decreased satisfaction with counseling services (Constantine, 2007).

Counseling centers deliver mental health services predicated on individualistic values that emphasize direct and verbal communication. Students whose cultural and familial worldviews are more collectivistic or have a different style of communication—often students of color—may not access services at a counseling center, and when they do, they may find it less helpful. As such, alternative methods of prevention and intervention are important in decreasing racial disparities. The following are strategies implemented by several campuses with good anecdotal success at increasing utilization of counseling services by students of color.

Providing outreach to communities of color across campus is one such important strategy. Outreach can take the form of culturally congruent presentations on various mental health topics, talking about services at students of color club meetings, having counseling center staff be present at different campus events for students of color, and setting up one-on-one meetings between counseling center staff and leaders of students of color groups and clubs. Central objectives of these meetings would be to establish trust, to have more informal conversations about the needs of these student groups, and to offer services in a more relationship- and community-oriented manner to help de-stigmatize mental health concerns and services. Indeed, a survey of counseling center directors (Reetz, Bershad, LeViness, & Whitlock, 2016) revealed about 12 percent of counseling centers have started to permanently situate counseling center therapists within different centers and departments across campus that are more frequented by underserved students. The hope is to increase access to mental health services after establishing a trusting relationship with the counseling center therapist. Research suggests that embedding counselors in the communities they serve is an effective way to reach clients in community settings who would not otherwise seek help (McLeod & McLeod, 2015). We expect to see a similar impact on students of color on college campuses.

Interventions aimed both at decreasing stigma and increasing tolerance to stigma show some promise in promoting help-seeking for Asian Americans (Ting & Hwang, 2009); it remains to be tested with other racial groups. Another program directed at increasing help-seeking in individual students includes an online screening tool followed by personalized feedback (Moffitt et al., 2014; King et al., 2015). A mental health counselor then reviews the results and communicates with individual students via email, using motivational interviewing principles to encourage them to make a counseling appointment. Preliminary results suggest that providing personalized feedback and offering online engagement, compared to online screening without the personalized communication, facilitates readiness to seek counseling and readiness to speak with one's support network. It also reduces stigma against seeking mental health services. There is no published research on these tools being used specifically to reach students of color, but campuses are using this tool to outreach to communities of color.

Another attempt at reaching students who may not traditionally seek counseling services is to provide drop-in consultation with a counselor outside of the counseling center. Boone and colleagues (2011) describe a program called Let's Talk, which has been implemented on multiple college campuses, with positive anecdotal reports about its ability to reach students of color as well as other student populations.

The second category of interventions includes campus-level strategies that train faculty, staff, and student employees (such as resident advisors) to recognize students in distress and refer them to counseling resources. These have often been labeled gatekeeper trainings (Goldston et al., 2010); faculty and staff have access to the gate to mental health services and can use their existing relationships with students to encourage them to seek counseling when needed. A study conducted on thirty-two campuses shows that training increased self-reported knowledge, confidence, and skills among participants, but there was no corresponding increase in mental health services utilization one semester later (Lipson, Speer, Brunwasser, Hahn, & Eisenberg, 2014). The lack of increase in demand for counseling services raises the question about whether this is an effective intervention or whether insufficient time elapsed to notice change. Further, there is no research on the effects of directing these sorts of gatekeeper training programs at those who specialize in serving communities of color. Nonetheless, given that this is a common intervention on many campuses, we are listing it as an option to consider.

In such trainings, it is important to pay attention to cultural differences when deciding on messages that will be persuasive to the faculty, staff, and students. For example, Mokkarala, O'Brien, and Siegel (2015) found that emphasizing biological origins of mental illness helped decrease shame and increase help-seeking among White students but had the opposite effect among South Asian American students.

Finally, the third category aims to improve student mental health by methods that do not involve counseling. It is worth noting that one-on-one talk therapy is rooted in individualistic, European American values, which are often in direct contrast to the values of many students of color. Exploration of interventions that do not necessitate a student's participation in traditional counseling is critical in ultimately addressing the disparities of access and the consequences in terms of academic and professional success. Given findings reviewed earlier in the chapter about how experiences of discrimination and microaggressions are correlated with depressive symptoms, Brownson, Drum, Swanbrow Becker, Saathoff, and Hentschel (2016) recommend finding strategies to reduce discrimination as a source of stressors for students of color. Based on the finding that a sense of belonging to the school is a protective factor for students of color against depressive symptoms, ensuring that efforts to promote school belonging are inclusive of the diverse student populations on campus is promising (Gummadam, Pittman, & Ioffe, 2015). This strategy extends beyond the role of the counseling center per se, but counseling centers can serve as catalysts for inclusive programming designed to promote a sense of belonging on campus.

Future Directions for Research

A number of different areas warrant further investigation, given the limited research addressing the racial disparities that exist in mental health care within universities. Understanding and addressing the factors contributing to the disparities is critical to a larger social-justice mission of ensuring success in higher education for marginalized communities.

Given that most counseling centers in the nation are moving toward a short-term model, research that examines successful referral rates for students of color and what factors contribute to a successful referral is important. Furthermore, since research has found that some therapists are more effective in working with White clients than clients of color, more research is needed in clarifying and identifying the specific factors that contribute to therapist efficacy in working with clients of color. For example, client perceptions of therapists' cultural humility has been found to foster a strong working alliance and improvement in therapy (Hook, Davis, Owen, Worthington, & Utsey, 2013). Research that examines this construct within counseling center settings in conjunction with dropout rates may help broaden our understanding of the dynamics of access, quality of care, and treatment outcomes for students of color on college campuses.

Conclusion

This chapter reviewed the history of university and college counseling centers and the importance of including culture and social justice principles in mental health services. It can be harder for students of color to access care. Diversifying the staff, increasing cultural competence, and providing services in areas of campus where students of color feel safe are ways to improve service delivery. Further, improving mental health for students of color needs to include intervention at a campus-wide level to reduce experiences of discrimination and increase a sense of belonging to the school. Much research is needed to better understand how to teach cultural competence and to help determine which campus-level interventions are effective for students of color. Finally, for there to be increased racial equity, we believe it is imperative that counseling centers and universities self-examine what it means to promote and value racial justice and to make organizational decisions that center racial justice over, or at least alongside, other important values. It is from this position that racial disparities can continue to be understood and dismantled.

KEY POINTS FOR CLINICIANS

- It is harder for students of color to access care, and they experience higher levels of distress due to discrimination and other systemic factors.

- Increasing the racial diversity of the counseling center staff helps students of color seek mental health services.

- Cultural competence, cultural humility, and empathy contribute to better quality of care for students of color.

- Within the counseling center, strategies to improve the mental health of students of color on campuses include increasing therapist cultural competence, increasing tolerance to stigma among students, providing culturally congruent psychoeducational programs, and providing care in areas of campus where students feel safe.

- On a broader campus level, strategies to improve mental health for students of color include gatekeeper trainings that address the needs of students of color, ways to reduce experiences of discrimination, and inclusive ways to increase sense of belonging to the university or college.

References

Anderson, E. L. (2003). Changing US Demographics and American Higher Education. *New Directions in Higher Education*, no. 121, Spring 2003. Wiley Periodicals, Inc. http://dx.doi.org/10.1002/he.97

Barksdale, C. L., & Molock, S. D. (2009). Perceived norms and mental health help seeking among African American college students. *Journal of Behavioral Health Services and Research*, 36, 285–299. http://dx.doi.org/10.1007/s11414-008-9138-y

Barr, V., Rando, R., Krylowicz, B., & Winfield, E. (2010). The Association for University and College Counseling Center Directors annual survey. http://files.cmcglobal.com/aucccd_directors_survey_monograph_2010_public.pdf.

Boone, M. S., Edwards, G. R., Haltom, M., Hill, J. S., Liang, Y. S., Mier, S. R., Shropshire, S. Y., Belizaire, L. S., Kamp, L. C., Murthi, M., Wong, W. K., & Yau, T. Y. (2011). Let's talk: Getting out of the counseling center to serve hard-to-reach students. *Journal of Multicultural Counseling and Development*, 39, 194–205. http://dx.doi.org/10.1002/j.2161-1912.2011.tb00634.x

Brownson, C., Drum, D. J., Swanbrow Becker, M. A., Saathoff, A., & Hentschel, E. (2016). Distress and suicidality in higher education: Implications for population-oriented prevention paradigms. *Journal of College Student Psychotherapy*, 30, 98–113. https://doi.org/10.1080/87568225.2016.1140978

Brunner, J. L., Wallace, D. L., Reymann, L. S., Sellers, J., & McCabe, A. G. (2014). College counseling today: Contemporary students and how counseling centers meet their needs. *Journal of College Student Psychotherapy*, 28(4), 257–324, http://dx.doi.org/10.1080/87568225.2014.948770

Cabral, R. R., & Smith, T. B. (2011). Racial/ethnic matching of clients and therapists in mental health services: A meta-analytic review of preferences, perceptions, and outcomes. *Journal of Counseling Psychology, 58,* 537–554. http://dx.doi.org/10.1037/a0025266

Cheng, H. L., Kwan, K. L. K., Sevig, T. (2013). Racial and ethnic minority college student stigma associated with seeking help: Examining psychocultural correlates. *Journal of Counseling Psychology, 60,* 98–111. http://dx.doi.org/10.1037/a0031169

Choi, K.-H. (2010). Evaluation of counseling outcomes at a university counseling center: The impact of clinically significant change on problem resolution and academic functioning. *Journal of Counseling Psychology, 57,* 297–303. http://dx.doi.org/10.1037/a0020029

Comas-Díaz, L. (2014). Multicultural psychotherapy. In F. T. L. Leong, L. Comas-Díaz, G. C. Nagayama Hall, V. C. McLoyd, & J. E. Trimble (Eds.), *APA handbook of multicultural psychology,* Vol. 2: *Applications and training* (pp. 419–441). New York, NY: American Psychological Association.

Constantine, M. G. (2002). Predictors of satisfaction with counseling: Racial and ethnic minority clients' attitudes towards counseling and ratings of their counselors' general and multicultural counseling competence. *Journal of Counseling Psychology, 49,* 255–263. http://dx.doi.org/10.1037/0022-0167.49.2.255

Constantine, M. G. (2007). Racial microaggressions against African American clients in cross-racial counseling relationships. *Journal of Counseling Psychology, 54*(1), 1–16. http://dx.doi.org/10.1037/0022-0167.54.1.1

Daughters, S. B., Lejuez, C. W., Bornovalova, M. A., Kahler, C. W., Strong, D. R., & Brown, R. A. (2005). Distress tolderance as a predictor of early treatment dropout in a residential substance abuse treatment facility. *Journal of Abnormal Psychology, 114,* 729–734. http://dx.doi.org/10.1037/0021-843X.114.4.729

Erdur, O., Rude, S. S., & Baron, A. (2003). Symptom improvement and length of treatment in ethnically similar and dissimilar client-therapist pairings. *Journal of Counseling Psychology, 50,* 52–58. http://dx.doi.org/10.1037/0022-0167.50.1.52

Flores, S. M., Park, T. J., & Baker, D. (2017). The racial college completion gap. *Journal of Higher Education.* http://dx.doi.org/10.1080/00221546.2017.1291259.

Forrest, L. (1989). Guiding, supporting, and advising students: The counselor role. In U. Delworth & G. R. Hanson (Eds.), *Student services: A handbook for the helping professions* (pp. 265–283). San Francisco: Jossey-Bass.

Fuertes, J. N., Stracuzzi, T. I., Bennett, J., Scheinholtz, J., Mislowack, A., Hersh, M., & Cheng, D. (2006). Therapist multicultural competence: A study of therapy dyads. *Psychotherapy: Theory, Research, Practice, Training, 43,* 480–490. http://dx.doi.org/10.1037/0033-3204.43.4.480

Garrett, M. L., Portman, T. A. A., Williams, C., Lisa Grayshield, L., Rivera, E. T., & Parrish, M. (2012). Native American adult lifespan perspectives: Where power moves. In E. C. Chang & C. A. Downery (Eds.) *Handbook of race and development in mental health.* New York, NY: Springer. http://dx.doi.org/10.1007/978-1-4614-0424-8

Garroutte, E. M., Kunovich, R. M., Jacobsen, C, & Goldberg, J. (2004). Patient satisfaction and ethnic identity among American Indian older adults. *Social Science and Medicine, 59,* 2233–2244. http://dx.doi.org/10.1016/j.socscimed.2004.03.032

Goldston, D. B., Walrath, C. M., McKeon, R., Puddy, R. W., Lubell, K. M., Potter, L. B., & Rodi, M. S. (2010). The Garrett Lee Smith memorial suicide prevention programs. *Suicide and Life-Threatening Behavior, 40,* 245–256. http://dx.doi.org/10.1521/suli.2010.40.3.245

Gummadam, P., Pittman, L. D., & Ioffe, M. (2015). School belonging, ethnic identity, and psychological adjustment among ethnic minority college students. *Journal of Experimental Education, 84,* 289–306. https://doi.org/10.1080/00220973.2015.1048844

Gushue, G. V. (2004). Race, color-blind racial attitudes, and judgments about mental health: A shifting standards perspective. *Journal of Counseling Psychology, 51,* 398–407. http://dx.doi.org/10.1037/0022-0167.51.4.398

Haviland, M. G., Horswill, R. K., O'Connell, J. J., & Dynneson, V. V. (1983). Native American college students' preference for counselor race and sex and the likelihood of their use of a counseling center. *Journal of Counseling Psychology, 30,* 267–270. http://dx.doi.org/10.1037/0022-0167.30 .2.267

Hayes, J. A., Chun-Kennedy, C., Edens, A., & Locke, B. D. (2011). Do double minority students face double jeopardy? Testing minority stress theory. *Journal of College Counseling, 14,* 117–126. http:// dx.doi.org//10.1002/j.2161-1882.2011.tb00267.x

Hayes, J. A., McAleavey, A. A., Castonguay, L. G., Locke, B. D. (2016). Psychotherapists' outcomes with White and racial/ethnic minority clients: First, the good news. *Journal of Counseling Psychology, 63,* 261–268. http://dx.doi.org/10.1037/cou0000098

Hayes, J. A., Owen, J., & Bieschke, K. J. (2015). Therapist differences in symptom change with racial/ ethnic minority clients. *Psychotherapy, 52,* 308–314. http://ds.doi.org/10.1037/a0037957

Hayes, J. A., Youn, S. J., Castonguay, L. G., Locke, B. D., McAleavey, A. A., & Nordberg, S. (2011). Rates and predictors of counseling center use among college students of color. *Journal of College Counseling, 14,* 105–116. http://dx.doi.org/10.1002/j.2161-1882.2011.tb00266.x

Hook, J. N, Davis, D. E., Owen, J., Worthington, E. L., & Utsey, S. O. (2013). Cultural humility: Measuring openness to culturally diverse clients. *Journal of Counseling Psychology, 60,* 353–366. http://dx.doi.org/10.1037/a0032595

Kearney, L. K., Draper, M., & Baron, A. (2005). Counseling utilization by ethnic minority college students. *Cultural Diversity and Ethnic Minority Psychology, 11,* 272–285. http://dx.doi.org/10.1037 /1099-9809.11.3.272

Kim, P. Y., & Lee, D. (2014). Internalized model minority myth, Asian values, and help-seeking attitudes among Asian American students. *Cultural Diversity and Ethnic Minority Psychology, 20,* 98–105. http://dx.doi.org/10.1037/a0033351

Kim, J. E., & Zane, N. (2016). Help-seeking intentions among Asian American and White American students in psychological distress: Application of the health belief model. *Cultural Diversity and Ethnic Minority Psychology, 22,* 311–321. http://dx.doi.org/10.1037/t08324-000

King, C. A., Eisenberg, D., Zheng, K., Czyz, E., Kramer, A., Horwitz, A., & Chermack, S. (2015). Online suicide risk screening and intervention with college students: A pilot randomized controlled trial. *Journal of Consulting and Clinical Psychology, 83,* 630–636. http://dx.doi.org/10 .1037/a0038805.

Kraft, D. P. (2011). One hundred years of college mental health. *Journal of American College Health, 59,* 477–481. http://dx.doi.org/10.1080/07448481.2011.569964

Lambert, M. J., Smart, D. W., Campbell, M. P., Hawkins, E. J., Harmon, C., & Slade, K. L. (2006). Psychotherapy outcome as measured by the OQ-45, in African American, Asian/Pacific Islander, Latino/a, and Native American clients compared with matched Caucasian clients. *Journal of College Student Psychotherapy, 20,* 17–29. http://dx.doi.org/10.1300/J035v20n04_3

Larrison, C. R., Schoppelrey, S. L., Hack-Ritzo, S., & Korr, W. S. (2011). Clinician factors related to outcome differences between black and white patients at CMHCs. *Psychiatric Services, 62,* 525– 531. http://dx.doi.org/10.1176/ps.62.5.pss6205_0525

Lee, D., Olson, E. A., Locke, B., Michelson, S. T., & Odes, E. (2009). The effects of college counseling services on academic performance and retention. *Journal of College Student Development, 50,* 305– 319. http://dx.doi.org/10.1353/csd.0.0071

Lipson, S. K., Speer, N., Brunwasser, S., Hahn, E., & Eisenberg, D. (2014). Gatekeeper training and access to mental health care at universities and colleges. *Journal of Adolescent Health, 55,* 612–619. http://dx.doi.org/10.1016/j.jadohealth.2014.05.009

López, S. R., Barrio, C., Kopelowicz, A., & Vega, W. A. (2012). From documenting to eliminating disparities in mental health care for Latinos. *American Psychologist, 67,* 511–523. http://dx.doi.org /10.1037/a0029737

Maramba, G., & Hall, G. (2002). Meta-analysis of ethnic match as a predictor of dropout, utilization, and level of functioning. *Cultural Diversity and Ethnic Minority Psychology, 8*, 290–297. http:// dx.doi.org/10.1037/1099-9809.8.3.290.

Masson, P. C., Perlman, C. M., Ross, S. A., & Gates, A. L. (2007). Premature termination of treatment in an inpatient eating disorder programme. *European Eating Disorder Review, 15*, 275–282. http:// dx.doi.org/10.1002/erv.762

McLeod, J., & McLeod, J. (2015). Research on embedded counselling: An emerging topic of potential importance for the future of counselling psychology. *Counselling Psychology Quarterly, 28*, 27–43. http://dx.doi.org/10.1080/09515070.2014.942774

Moffitt, L. B., Garcia-Williams, A., Berg, J. P., Calderon, M. E., Haas, A. P., & Kaslow, N. J. (2014). Reaching graduate students at risk for suicidal behavior through the interactive screening program. *Journal of College Student Psychotherapy, 28*, 23–34. http://dx.doi.org/10.1080/87568225 .2014.854675

Mokkarala, S., O'Brien, E. K., & Siegel, J. T. (2015). The relationship between shame and perceived biological origins of mental illness among South Asian and white American young adults. *Psychology, Health & Medicine, 21*, 448–459. http://dx.doi.org/10.1080/13548506.2015.1090615

Mokrue, K., & Acri, M. (2013). Feasibility and effectiveness of a brief cognitive behavioral skills group on an ethnically diverse campus. *Journal of College Student Psychotherapy, 27*, 254–269. https://doi .org/10.1080/87568225.2013.766114

Mosher, D. K., Hook, J. N., Captari, L. E., Davis, D. E., DeBlaere, C., & Owen, J. (2017). Cultural humility: A therapeutic framework for engaging diverse clients. *Practice Innovations, 2*, 221–233. http://dx.doi.org/10.1037/pri0000055

National Center for Education Statistics. (2010). Retrieved from https://nces.ed.gov/pubs2010/2010015 /indicator6_24.asp.

National Commission on Asian American and Pacific Islander Research Education (2011). Retrieved from http://care.gseis.ucla.edu/wp-content/uploads/2015/08/2011_CARE_Report.pdf.

Neimeyer, G. J., & Gonzales, M. (1983). Duration, satisfaction and perceived effectiveness of cross-cultural counseling. *Journal of Counseling Psychology, 30*, 91–95. http://dx.doi.org/10.1037/0022 -0167.30.1.91.

Owen, J., Imel, Z., Adelson, J., & Rodolfa, E. (2012). "No-Show": Therapist racial-ethnic disparities in client unilateral termination. *Journal of Counseling Psychology, 59*, 314–320. http://dx.doi.org/10 .1037/a0027091

Owen, J., Leach, M. M., Wampold, B., & Rodolfa, E. (2011). Client and therapist variability in clients' perceptions of their therapists' multicultural competencies. *Journal of Counseling Psychology, 58*, 1–9. http://dx.doi.org/10.1037/a0021496

Owen, J., Smith, A. A., & Rodolfa, E. (2009). Clients' expected number of sessions, treatment effectiveness, and termination status: Using empirical evidence to inform session limit policies. *Journal of College Student Psychotherapy, 23*, 118–134. http://dx.doi.org/10.1080/87568220902743660

Presnell, A., Harris, G., & Scogin, F. (2012). Therapist and client race/ethnicity match: An examination of treatment of treatment outcome and process with rural older adults in the deep south. *Psychotherapy Research, 22*, 458–463. http://dx.doi.org/10.1080/10503307.2012.6773022

Quintana, S. M., Kilmartin, C., Yesenosky, J., & Macias, D. (1991). Factors affecting referral decisions in a university counseling center. *Professional Psychology: Research and Practice, 22*, 90–97. http:// dx.doi.org/10.1037/0735-7028.22.1.90

Reetz, D. R., Bershad, C., LeViness, P., & Whitlock, M. (2016). *The Association for University and College Counseling Center Directors Annual Survey*. Indianapolis, IN: Association for University and College Counseling Center Directors, Inc. Retrieved from https://www.aucccd.org/assets /documents/aucccd%202016%20monograph%20-%20public.pdf

Rogers, C. R. (1951). *Client-centered therapy: Its current practice, implications, and theory.* Boston: Houghton-Mifflin.

Shimokawa, K., Lambert, M. J., & Smart, D. W. (2010). Enhancing treatment outcome of patients at risk of treatment failure: Meta-analytic and mega-analytic review of a psychotherapy quality assurance system. *Journal and Consulting and Clinical Psychology, 78*, 298–311. http://dx.doi.org/10.1037/a0019247

Smith, T. B., Rodriguez, M. M. D., & Bernal, G. (2011). Culture. In J. C. Norcross (Ed.), *Psychotherapy relationships that work* (2nd ed.) (pp. 316–335). New York, NY: Oxford University Press. http://dx.doi.org/10.1093/acprof:oso/9780199737208.003.0016.

Smith, T. B., & Trimble, J. E. (2016). *Foundations of multicultural psychology: Research to inform effective practice.* Washington, DC: American Psychological Association. http://dx.doi.org/10.1037/14733-000

Sue, D. W. (1981). *Counseling the culturally diverse: Theory and practice.* New York, NY: Wiley.

Tate, E. (2017). Graduation rates and race. *Inside Higher Ed*, April 26, 2017. Retrieved from https://www.insidehighered.com/news/2017/04/26/college-completion-rates-vary-race-and-ethnicity-report-finds

Terrell, F., & Terrell, S. (1984). Race of counselor, client sex, cultural mistrust level, and premature termination from counseling among Black students. *Journal of Counseling Psychology, 31*, 371–375. http://dx.doi.org/10.1037/0022-0167.31.3.371

Thompson, R. A., & Cimbolic, P. (1978). Black students' counselor preference and attitudes toward counseling center use. *Journal of Counseling Psychology, 25*, 570–575. http://dx.doi.org/10.1037/0022-0167.25.6.570

Ting, J. Y., & Hwang, W. C. (2009). Cultural influences on help-seeking attitudes in Asian American students. *American Journal of Orthopsychiatry, 79*, 125–132. http://dx.doi.org/10.1037/a0015394

Townes, D. L., Chavez-Korell, S., & Cunningham, N. J. (2009). Reexamining the relationships between racial identity, cultural mistrust, help-seeking attitudes, and preference for a Black counselor. *Journal of Counseling Psychology, 56*, 330–336. http://dx.doi.org./10.1037/a0015449

Vermeersch, D., Whipple, J. L., Lambert, M. J., Hawkins, E. J., Burchfield, C. M., Okiishi, J. C. (2004). Outcome questionnaire: Is it sensitive to changes in counseling center clients? *Journal of Counseling Psychology, 51*, 38–49. http://dx.doi.org/10.1037/0022-0167.51.1.38

Wade, P., & Bernstein, B. L. (1991). Culture sensitivity training and counselor's race: Effects on Black clients' perceptions and attrition. *Journal of Counseling Psychology, 38*, 9–15. http://dx.doi.org/10.1037/0022-0167.38.1.9

Watson, N. N., & Hunter, C. D. (2015). Anxiety and depression among African American women: The costs of strength and negative attitudes toward psychological help-seeking. *Cultural Diversity and Ethnic Minority Psychology, 21*, 604–612. http://dx.doi.org./10.1037/cdp0000015

Williamson, E. G., (1939). *How to counsel students.* New York, NY: McGraw Hill.

CHAPTER 16

Mental Health Treatment Disparities in Racial and Ethnic Minority Military Service Members and Veterans

Elizabeth M. Goetter,
Massachusetts General Hospital

Allyson M. Blackburn,
Harvard Medical School

Introduction

Racial and ethnic minorities comprise nearly 30 percent of the 2.5 million active duty and reserve personnel serving in US military (Department of Defense, 2015) and 22 percent of the total veteran population (US Census Bureau, 2014). The military population is growing more diverse, and racial and ethnic minorities are expected to make up over a third of the veteran population by 2040 (National Center for Veterans Analysis and Statistics [NCVAS], 2017). Minority veterans are more likely to be women and younger, underscoring the implications of race-based mental health disparities (NCVAS, 2017).

In 2015, 9.6 million veterans (44 percent) were using at least one Department of Veterans Affairs (VA). VA health care and disability comprised 75 percent of all service use (NCVAS, 2016). In the same year, more than 1.6 million veterans were receiving specialized mental health treatment from the VA, which represents a nearly two-fold increase since 2006 (NCVAS, 2009). Veterans from all eras disproportionately experience higher rates of mental illness than civilians (Jordan et al., 1991; Tanielian et al., 2008), and minority veterans have higher rates of post-traumatic stress disorder (PTSD) than nonminority veterans (NCVAS, 2017).

The number of minority veterans who use at least one VA service or benefit has grown from 35 percent in 2005 to 44 percent in 2014 (National Center for Veterans Analysis, 2017). In 2015, African American and Hispanic veterans were more likely to utilize VA service benefits than any other racial group, while American Indians and

Native Alaskans were least likely to utilize VA benefits (NCVAS, 2016). While health disparities within the VA have been documented (Luncheon & Zack, 2012; Nayback, 2008; Saha et al., 2008; Sheehan, Hummer, Moore, Husyer & Butler, 2015), literature on mental health disparities within the VA and veteran populations remains unorganized and without systematic review.

As the population of veterans and service members grows more diverse, and mental health service use increases among VA users, our understanding of the unique mental health needs of racial and ethnic minority veterans becomes increasingly important. Veterans who identify as racial and ethnic minorities experience a lack of cultural sensitivity (Castro et al., 2015), less favorable feelings toward disability examiners (Rosen et al., 2013), dissatisfaction with treatment access, and dissatisfaction with the communication and helpfulness of providers (Jones et al., 2016). Service members of color also experience discrimination in the military, and discrimination is a predictor of future physical and mental health problems (Foynes, Shipherd, & Harrington, 2013; Foynes, Smith, & Shipherd, 2015; Loo et al., 2001; Loo, Singh, Scurfield, & Kilauano, 1998; Sohn & Harada, 2008). Understanding the unique mental health needs of minority veterans is crucial.

Treatment Access

Studies of civilian populations have found that racial and ethnic minorities access treatment at lower rates than nonminorities (De Luca, Blosnich, Hentschel, King & Amen, 2016) and perceive more barriers to mental health treatment (Goetter et al., under review; Williams et al., 2012). Within veteran populations, mental health treatment utilization disparities among racial and ethnic minorities initially appear smaller than in civilian populations. In a large cross-sectional telephone survey of veterans and civilians with varied mental health problems, there were no race-based differences among veterans in current or past mental health treatment utilization, and racial minority veterans were significantly more likely to utilize mental health resources than minority civilians (De Luca et al., 2016). Another study found that among male veterans with a probable need for mental health treatment, non-White race was positively associated with VA mental health treatment use (Di Leone et al., 2013). Similarly, results from the 1992 National Survey of Veterans revealed that African American and Hispanic veterans were more likely to use VA outpatient care than similar cohorts of White veterans, even after controlling for enabling, need, and predisposing factors (Harada et al., 2002).

These findings have been replicated in samples of veterans with more specific mental health problems. For example, among sexual assault victims in the military, Black race was positively associated with treatment-seeking behavior (Zinzow et al., 2015). An electronic medical review of over 1,500 depressed Operation Enduring Freedom and Operation Iraqi Freedom veterans treated in the VA found no ethnic or gender differences in specialty mental health service utilization (Davis, Deen, Fortney, Sullivan, &

Hudson, 2014). A smaller study comparing African American and White combat veterans with PTSD at a VA outpatient clinic found no differences in VA service use by race (Frueh, Elhai, Monnier, Hamner, & Knapp, 2004). A retrospective cohort study comparing 84,000 American Indian, Alaska Native, Native Hawaiian, Pacific Islanders to a non-Native reference group (which included White and minority veterans) found that native veterans were more likely to utilize the VA for PTSD, traumatic brain injury, depression, anxiety, and substance use concerns (Brooks et al., 2015). More compelling still are results from a prospective, longitudinal study of National Guard soldiers who had returned from deployment, which found that being female, Black, and Hispanic predicted mental health treatment use in the subsequent year (Goodwin et al., 2014).

The majority of the aforementioned research occurred in VA settings and thus raises the question that these smaller disparities may reflect equalization of access afforded by the VA. For example, African American veterans may be less likely to access non-VA mental health services than White veterans (Tsai, Desai, Cheng, & Chang, 2014). In fact, the most common reason endorsed for not utilizing VA health services is that veterans have other resources to access health care, and White veterans are more likely to be covered by Medicare or private insurance (Tsai et al., 2014). Thus, these findings raise the possibility that the "overrepresentation" of minorities within the VA health care system could actually be caused by the underrepresentation of White veterans or the mitigation of disparities resulting from fewer financial and insurance related barriers (Tsai et al., 2014).

BARRIERS TO TREATMENT

Additionally, there is mixed evidence to suggest that racial and ethnic minority veterans may differentially perceive barriers to care relative to nonminority populations. For example, in a study of 490 veterans with PTSD, non-White males reported more logistical barriers (e.g., ease of use) than White veterans, though the effects were small (Ouimette et al., 2011). These findings were in contrast to those of a smaller study that found that perceived logistical barriers did not differ significantly by race and ethnicity (Pierre-Louis, Moore, & Hamilton, 2015). Another large survey of veterans, controlling for demographic and health factors, found no differences in perceived barriers to care, including stigma, between Asian American and Pacific Islander veterans and White, Hispanic, Black, or Native American and Native Alaskan veterans (Tsai, Whealin, & Pietrzak, 2014). Another study of post-9/11 veterans with PTSD, depression, and alcohol use disorder found that non-White veterans were more likely to seek help from pastoral counselors, and that pastoral counselor use was associated with more negative views about the mental health care system (Nieuwsma et al., 2014). Although incidental, these findings speak to the importance of gaining a more thorough understanding of the perceived barriers (both logistical and non-logistical) among racial and ethnic minority veterans, even though veteran status appears to mitigate treatment access disparities for racial and ethnic minorities.

Treatment Engagement

SELECTION AND UTILIZATION

Several studies have documented racial and ethnic disparities with respect to types of mental health service use. For instance, in a study examining electro-convulsive shock therapy (ECT), an efficacious treatment for severe or treatment-resistant depression, Black patients were significantly less likely than Whites to receive ECT (Pfeiffer et al., 2011). Similarly, disparities have been found in the utilization of adequate psychopharmacological treatments. Racial and ethnic minority patients are less likely than White veterans to receive adequate antidepressant treatment for chronic depression (Quiñones et al., 2014) and are less likely to be prescribed atypical antipsychotics for schizophrenia (Copeland, Zeber, Velenstein, & Blow, 2003). Native American veterans are also less likely than White veterans to receive psychiatric medication treatment (Spoont, Hodges, Murdoch, & Nugent, 2009). Some suggest that disparities in psychiatric medication use is a function of negative treatment beliefs about medication rather than minority status (Spoont et al., 2015), speaking to the importance of understanding differences in treatment preferences and increasing trust and credibility of the mental health system in minority veterans with PTSD.

Research has also revealed that White and non-White veterans engage in different treatments for substance abuse problems. For example, in a large study of veterans with opioid use disorder, Black race was negatively associated with the odds of receiving buprenorphine compared to methadone (Manhapra, Quiñones, & Rosenheck, 2016). These findings persisted even after controlling for income, age, and rural location, leading the authors to conclude that these disparities were shaped by race and ethnicity characteristics rather than individual medical, psychiatric, or other access factors. Another study found that Black veterans were significantly less likely than White veterans to receive medication-assisted treatments for alcohol use disorder (Williams et al., 2017). This is alarming, as Black veterans were shown to have the highest prevalence of documented alcohol-related care when compared to White and Hispanic veterans (Williams et al. 2012). Taken together, more research is needed to determine if these race-based disparities in treatment selection reflect differences in treatment preferences or system-wide biases in treatment practices as some (e.g., Kales, Blow, Bingham, Copeland, & Mellow, 2000) have suggested.

SUSTAINED INVOLVEMENT IN TREATMENT

Research on disparities in treatment engagement in racial and ethnic minority veteran populations is mixed. In a prospective national cohort study of nearly seven thousand VA patients with PTSD, African American and Latinx veterans were less likely to receive a minimally adequate trial of psychiatric medication, and African American veterans were less likely to receive a minimal trial of any type of mental health treatment in the first six months after receiving a PTSD diagnosis (Spoont et al., 2015).

In a study of 152 African American and White veterans seeking psychopharmacology for various mental health conditions, race was significantly associated with working alliance, medication adherence, and patient activation (one's ability and willingness to manage their health care), such that African Americans reported lower alliance, adherence, and activation in their care (Eliacin et al., 2016).

Similar patterns have been found in various studies of outpatient psychotherapy. In a large, naturalistic, longitudinal study of several VA PTSD Clinical Team programs, Black veterans had significantly lower program participation and were seen, on average, for shorter periods of time and fewer sessions than White veterans (Rosenheck, Fontana, & Cottrol, 1995). Another study found that African American patients with psychotic disorders had significantly fewer outpatient psychiatric visits even though there were no differences by race in inpatient treatment utilization (Kales, Blow, Bingham, Roberts, Copeland, & Mellow, 2000).

However, results from another study found that African Americans, Native Hawaiians, and Pacific Islanders were more likely than Whites were to engage in psychotherapy for PTSD, and African Americans were more likely than Whites to receive at least eight psychotherapy sessions for PTSD (Spoont et al., 2009). Additionally, in a study of Black and White veterans who screened positive for PTSD but who had not yet initiated trauma-focused treatment, participants were randomly assigned to a waitlist or a cognitive behavioral engagement intervention (Stecker et al., 2016). Black veterans were significantly more likely than White veterans to engage in treatment following the intervention. Additionally, although they completed fewer sessions of PTSD treatment compared to White veterans overall, they had greater PTSD symptom reduction than White veterans, which led the authors to conclude that dropout was related to feeling better (Stecker et al., 2016).

DROPOUT

Within veteran samples, research examining the association between race and ethnicity and early dropout from treatment is mixed. One study of 117 Iraq and Afghanistan veterans (69 percent racial and ethnic minorities) receiving treatment in a PTSD clinic in the southern United States found no effect of race or ethnicity on rates of dropout (Garcia, Kelley, Rentz, & Lee, 2011). However, in one of the largest studies of its kind—a study of over two hundred thousand mixed-era veterans who had a diagnosis of primary PTSD seen in the VA between 2004 and 2007 (approximately 9 percent of the sample identified as a racial or ethnic minority)—African American veterans faced a higher risk of dropping out of treatment within the first year after initial diagnosis (Harpaz-Rotem & Rosenheck, 2011).

These discrepant findings may speak to regional differences in cultural sensitivity among providers or a generally small effect of race and ethnicity on dropout. Reasons for early termination are various and may actually be related to symptom improvement (Lester, Artz, Resick, & Young-Xu, 2010). However, inadequate treatment engagement and early dropout may be mediated by low therapeutic alliance (Meier, Donmall, McElduff, Barrowclough, & Heller, 2006), lack of provider cultural sensitivity (Damashek, Bard, & Hecht, 2011), low outcome expectancy (e.g., Diala et al., 2000), or differential treatment preferences between provider and patient (Kwan, Dimidijian, & Rizvi, 2010; Steidtmann et al., 2012). Taken together, results on dropout are less conclusive than results suggesting that racial and ethnic minorities, and African Americans in particular, are at higher risk of receiving minimally adequate psychotherapy and medication treatment. The results of these studies underscore the importance of identifying potential mediators of low treatment engagement among racial and ethnic minorities and facilitating patient involvement in mental health care in culturally sensitive ways.

Diagnostic Disparities

Consistent with research on civilian populations (Breslau et al., 2005; US Department of Health and Human Services, 2001), veterans of color are diagnosed with mental health-related problems at a different rate than White veterans. Koo, Hebenstreit, Madden, Seal, and Maguen (2015) found that veterans from racial minority backgrounds were less likely to be diagnosed with a mental health disorder by providers at the VA than their White counterparts. In a sample of elderly veterans in a VA inpatient psychiatric program, African American patients were less than half as likely as their White counterparts to receive a diagnosis for a mood disorder (Kales, Blow, Bingham, Copeland, & Mellow, 2000). The reverse pattern has emerged in psychotic disorders. For example, in a study of veterans with serious mental illness, Black and Hispanic patients were significantly more likely to have a diagnosis of schizophrenia than White veterans (Blow et al., 2004). Another study found that psychotic symptoms in combat-related PTSD were more commonly diagnosed among Black and Hispanic veterans than in White veterans (David, Kutcher, Jackson, & Mellman, 1999). Finally, in a study of Iraq and Afghanistan veterans, Black and Hispanic veterans had higher incidence of PTSD, depression, and alcohol use–related diagnoses for older veterans (forty-five to sixty-four years old), but lower incidence for younger veterans (age eighteen to twenty-nine), relative to White veterans (Ramsey et al., 2017).

Despite these diagnostic disparities, several studies have revealed that African American veterans receive service-connected disability at a significantly lower rate than White veterans, even after controlling for PTSD severity and functional limitations (Marx et al., 2017; Murdoch, Hodges, Cowper, Fortier & van Ryn, 2003). Black veterans also rate the quality of their examinations and the interpersonal quality of their examiners lower than their White counterparts (Rosen et al., 2013). This raises concern not only about the financial implications of diagnostic disparities (Marx et al., 2017) but also about the potential issues of access to mental health treatment, as there is a well-documented correlation between service-connected disability status and treatment use (Gorman et al., 2016).

Disparities in Symptom Severity and Suicidality

A significant body of research suggests that ethnic and racial minority veterans are at increased risk of PTSD symptom severity following a traumatic incident, though the reasons for this are not clear (Davis et al., 2012; Koenen, Stellman, Stellman & Sommer, 2003; Ortega & Rosenheck, 2002). Research on disparities in symptom severity for minority veterans, however, is not unequivocal. In a small study of veterans seeking PTSD treatment at a VA medical center, there were no racial differences in self-reported anxiety, depression, PTSD symptom severity, dissociation, paranoia, or schizophrenia (Monnier, Elhai, Frueh, Sauvageot, & Magruder, 2002). Finally, another study found that, among a sample of medically ill veterans, Black veterans were least likely to report feelings of depression compared to other racial groups. Black patients were also more likely to report being satisfied with life than other racial groups (Karel & Moye, 2002). Additional research is needed to determine if these potential differences in symptom severity reflect differences in assessment or psychometric properties, cultural attitudes regarding psychological symptoms, or differences in the greater ecological context for particular minority groups (e.g., differences in social support or culturally sanctioned beliefs about mental illness) and whether these differences vary with respect to specific mental health conditions (e.g., PTSD).

Finally, there have been differential rates of suicidality among veterans and active-duty service members of differing racial backgrounds. In a sample of nearly ninety thousand VA patients who underwent surgery from 2005 to 2006, African Americans were at an increased risk for suicidal behavior and ideation compared to their White and Hispanic counterparts (Copeland et al., 2014). In a study of over five thousand Iraq and Afghanistan veteran suicides, there were substantially higher suicide rates for Native Americans (30.6 per 100,000) than for non-Hispanic White (20.17), Asian American and Pacific Islander (12.82), Hispanic (12.12), or non-Hispanic Black (10.53) veterans (Reger et al., 2015), corroborating findings from another study demonstrating increased suicide mortality risk among Native American soldiers (Schoenbaum et al., 2014). Finally, in a large study of veterans from the Army Study to Assess Risk and Resilience in Service Members (ARMY STARSS), soldiers who identified their race as "other" had significantly higher odds for pre-enlistment suicidal ideation than non-Hispanic Whites (Ursano et al,. 2015).

Special Considerations for At-risk Populations

WOMEN

There is a dearth of empirical study of the mental health needs of women of color in the Veterans Health Administration (Carter et al., 2016). Previous research has suggested that, generally, female veterans are more likely than their male counterparts to utilize the VA (Tsai, Mota, & Pietrzak, 2015), though this may not be the case for veterans of the more recent conflicts (Hoff & Rosenheck, 1998) or for women veterans of color. A study of 3,611 veteran women found that those of racial and ethnic minority backgrounds were 1.3 times more likely than their White counterparts to delay accessing health care from the VA (Washington, Bean-Mayberry, Riopelle, & Yano, 2001). This study also found that minority women veterans were more likely to have an unmet health need in the past twelve months.

Minority military service members are more likely to be women (NCVAS, 2017), and women of color are at risk for intersecting or "double-jeopardy" discrimination (race-based discrimination and sex-based discrimination). This places minority women service members at increased risk for mental illness (Foynes et al., 2013). One study found that Native American and Native Hawaiian women were more likely endorse having experienced military sexual trauma (MST) than non-Native controls (Brooks et al., 2015). Another small study found that Black female veterans who experienced MST endorsed more sexual dysfunction and sexual health concerns than White controls (Gobin & Allard, 2016). However, research has shown that female veterans of color respond to and engage in trauma-focused therapy just as well as their White counterparts (Holliday, Holder, Williamson, & Surís, 2017).

GENDER AND SEXUAL MINORITIES

Research on the health needs of gender and sexual minority veterans is in its early stages (e.g., Mattocks et al., 2013; Ray-Sannerud, Bryan, Perry, & Bryan, 2015), and research on the experience of racial and ethnic minority veterans who also identify as gender or sexual minorities is lacking. One study found that racial and ethnic minorities (and women) were disproportionately impacted by the military's Don't Ask, Don't Tell policy, which prohibits disclosure of lesbian, gay, or bisexual identity among those serving in the US military (Gates, 2010). Another study of 5,135 transgender veterans found that Black transgender veterans were 1.33 times more likely to experience MST than White transgender veterans (Brown & Jones, 2014). Black transgender veterans also faced increased odds for alcohol abuse, tobacco use, HIV, infection, and serious mental illness. These findings point to the increased mental health risks for sexual and gender minority veterans, and the intersection of these identities should be carefully considered.

HOMELESS VETERANS

Roughly 23 percent of homeless individuals are veterans (Jones et al., 2017), and rates of mental illness are significant among this subset of veterans (Pending Health Legislation, Including the Heather French Henry Homeless Veteran's Assistance Act, 2001). Relative to non-homeless veterans, homeless veterans are more likely to be racial and ethnic minorities (Jones et al., 2017; Murphy, 2000). Homeless veterans face unique challenges with respect to accessing mental health care and have negative experiences with primary care services (Jones et al., 2017). Some researchers have suggested that homeless veterans, relative to homeless nonveterans, may have more personal resources, perhaps due to access to various benefits and a large health care system (Tessler, Rosenheck, & Gamache, 2002). Nonetheless, racial and ethnic minority homeless veterans face additional challenges relative to their non-homeless counterparts. This may be particularly true for homeless minority veterans who reside in nonmetropolitan areas, where access to VA services may be more difficult relative to nonminority veterans (Gordon, Haas, Luther, Hilton, & Goldstein, 2010). Yet, somewhat discordant findings from another study found that of nearly 36,000 veterans who screened positive for homelessness over a one-year period between 2012 and 2013, unsheltered status was associated with being White (Byrne, Montgomery, & Fargo, 2016). Encouraging findings from a study of 381 homeless veterans with various mental health conditions revealed no differences in psychiatric treatment outcomes and alcohol use disorder symptoms between Black and White homeless veterans following participation in a residential program (Rosenheck, Leda, Frisman, & Gallup, 1997).

INCARCERATED VETERANS

Between 2011 and 2012, veterans made up approximately 8 percent of the US incarcerated population, representing a historically declining rate (Bronson, Carson, Noonan, & Berzofsky, 2015). Veterans may be at risk for incarceration due to mental health conditions like PTSD and substance use disorders (McGuire, Rosenheck, & Kasprow, 2003). In fact, nearly half of all incarcerated veterans have been diagnosed with a mental health disorder (Bronson et al., 2015). Disparities exist between veterans based on racial and ethnic identity, just as they do in civilian populations (Pettit & Western, 2004), such that African American veterans and Hispanic veterans have higher rates of incarceration than White veterans (Tsai, Rosenheck, Kasprow, & McGuire, 2013). However, veteran status may be both protective against and associated with risk for incarceration, depending on race and ethnicity. For instance, White veterans have a higher risk of incarceration than nonveteran Whites (Greenberg & Rosenheck, 2012), whereas the risk for incarceration for Black and Hispanic veterans is lower than their nonveteran peers (Greenberg & Rosenheck, 2012). The authors propose that military membership may provide individuals with access to more benefits and opportunities (e.g., financial benefits, work opportunities, housing vouchers) than would be otherwise inaccessible to civilians. Access to these resources may reduce the risk for incarceration for some veterans.

Conclusion

In summary, racial and ethnic minorities comprise 30 percent to 35 percent of the active-duty and veteran military population (Department of Defense, 2015). The universal health care coverage afforded by the federally-funded VA health care system appears to mitigate racial and ethnic disparities that exist regarding mental health treatment access. Nonetheless, evidence suggests that race-based disparities exist for certain mental health treatments (e.g., ECT, pharmacotherapy), diagnosis rates, access to compensation and pension benefits, and suicide (i.e., rates are highest among Native American veterans). Veterans of color who have intersecting identities such as women, sexual minorities, and gender identity minorities face additional challenges, but research on unique mental health needs is lacking. Minority veterans are overrepresented in other vulnerable populations (i.e., incarcerated and homeless veterans); however, mental health disparities are smaller than in the civilian nonveteran population.

Solutions and Future Directions

CLINICAL PRACTICE CONSIDERATIONS

Broadly, research suggests that ethnic minority veterans have more negative views about mental health treatment and more distrust of the mental health system (Nieuwsma et al., 2014). Lack of cultural sensitivity by providers might further deter mental health service use (Castro et al., 2015). Racial and ethnic minority veterans would benefit from targeted efforts to improve their active engagement in mental health care. Additional research is needed to determine which engagement campaigns may be most effective and for which minority groups. Engagement interventions that use CBT strategies to target treatment beliefs (e.g., Stecker et al., 2016) have the potential to facilitate racial and ethnic minority veterans' access to evidence-based treatments. See chapter 4 for more information about engaging people of color in mental health care.

As discussed in chapter 9, providers are encouraged to actively assess for cultural, social, and ecological factors as part of their routine clinical assessment. Providers could ask questions like "What is your cultural background?" and "What cultural traditions or values were you raised with, and how do these interact with your military experiences?" and "How do your cultural values and experiences in the military influence your current experience with your mental health symptoms?" Providers should avoid making assumptions; assessing for level of assimilation and the patient's own identity with respect to their cultural background is important (Asnaani & Hofmann, 2012). Providers could also collaboratively and openly discuss patient beliefs about treatment and outcome expectancy. When considering risk assessment, clinicians should consider research suggesting that ethnic minority status may generally be associated with reduced risk for suicidal behavior (Ursano et al. 2015), except among those who identify as Native American or "other," for whom the risk is higher and special attention is warranted (O'Keefe & Reger, 2017). Of course, well-intentioned clinicians should avoid making assumptions about any one individual based on their racial or ethnic identity. As some have suggested, veterans' experience and expectations of VA health care may be better informed by their veteran and military identity than their racial identity (Damron-Rodriguez et al., 2004).

Additionally, it is worth noting that there are race-based disparities suggesting racial and ethnic minority veterans may have less access to VA primary care services (Davis et al., 2014) and lower satisfaction with primary care (Jones et al., 2016). Given the larger movement within the VA to integrate mental health services with primary care (Zeiss & Karlin, 2008), it will be increasingly important to attend to potential disparities in access and to address unmet needs for racial and ethnic minorities in all VA health settings. Providers are encouraged to facilitate minority veterans' access to primary medical care, which could increase mental health access.

Finally, evidence-based treatments (EBTs) have the potential to mitigate race-based disparities. Evidence suggests that treatment outcomes for a variety of mental health conditions do not differ by race or ethnicity (e.g., Horrell, 2008; Huey & Polo, 2008; Huey, Tilley, Jones, & Smith, 2014; Lesser et al., 2011; Pan, Huey, & Hernandez, 2011). A small focus-group study of White and African American veterans found that there were no racial differences with respect to unfavorable or favorable views of manualized treatments (Castro et al., 2015). EBTs are an effective way to mitigate health disparities, as they've been shown to be acceptable by many different populations. While some cultural adaptations of existing evidence-based protocols have been both warranted and effective at increasing treatment engagement in military and veteran populations (Kaufmann, Buck Richardson, Floyd & Shore, 2014; Onoye et al., 2017; Rosenheck et al., 1995), adapting every single evidence-based treatment for the myriad and diverse cultures represented by the veteran population would not be feasible, and focusing on reducing health care disparities through clinician-based cultural competence may be most effective (Harris, 2011). See chapters 7 and 8 for more about building cultural competence.

FUTURE RESEARCH DIRECTIONS

Future research should attend to limitations evident in the literature on race-based mental health disparities among veterans. First, many studies collapse racial and ethnic minority groups when making comparisons to White veterans (e.g., Davis et al., 2014; Tsai, Desai, Cheng, & Chang, 2014), which ignores the heterogeneity of minority groups. Asian American, Pacific Islanders, and Native American veterans are underrepresented in the literature examining race-based disparities in mental health. Asian American and Pacific Islander veterans are the fastest growing racial and ethnic group within the larger veteran population (Tsai, Whealin, & Pietrzak, 2014), and more research is needed to understand the unique experiences faced by this subpopulation of veterans (Tsai & Kong, 2012). Additionally, most studies do not include measures of acculturation, racial and ethnic identification, or mental health treatment beliefs informed by cultural background. Including such measures has the potential to provide a richer and more informative view on the nature of racial and ethnic minorities' experience with mental health care and existing disparities. Most research on veteran mental health disparities occurs among VA samples. Researchers are encouraged to recruit diverse groups of racial and ethnic minorities across treatment settings when conducting research with veterans. Attending to these limitations will provide better understanding of race-based disparities among veteran and military populations. Lastly, the VA has served as a model in the dissemination of evidence-based treatments for PTSD (Karlin et al., 2010). Future dissemination and implementation studies should guide the development and dissemination of effective trainings in other evidence-based practices that produce culturally competent mental healthcare providers.

KEY POINTS FOR CLINICIANS

- Racial and ethnic minorities comprise approximately a quarter to a third of the US military and veteran population, and the military is growing more diverse.

- Within military and veteran populations, mental health treatment utilization disparities among racial and ethnic minorities may be smaller than in civilian populations due to the likely equalization of access to health care afforded by the Veterans Administration Healthcare System.

- As a group, racial and ethnic minority veterans may face other barriers to mental health treatment, including more negative views about mental health treatment and unequitable access to particular types of mental health treatments.

- Among vulnerable populations (incarceration and homelessness), veteran status may offer a protective benefit for racial and ethnic minorities relative to their civilian counterparts.

- Ethnic and racial minority veterans are at increased risk of PTSD symptom severity, but African American veterans receive service-connected disability at a significantly lower rate than White veterans. Suicide rates appear to be especially high for Native American veterans.

- Using open-ended questions, clinicians should assess for the ways in which their client's military background might interact with their cultural background. Clinicians should, however, be careful to not make assumptions as to whether their veteran status or racial and ethnic identity is more important to them.

References

Asnaani, A., & Hofmann, S. G. (2012). Collaboration in multicultural therapy: Establishing a strong therapeutic alliance across cultural lines. *Journal of Clinical Psychology*, 68(2), 187–197.

Blow, F. C., Zeber, J. E., McCarthy, J. F., Valenstein, M., Gillon, L., & Bingham, C. R. (2004). Ethnicity and diagnostic patterns in veterans with psychoses. *Social Psychiatry and Psychiatric Epidemiology*, 39(10), 841–851.

Breslau, J., Aguilar-Gaxiola, S., Kendler, K. S., Su, M., Williams, D., & Kessler, R. C. (2005). Specifying race-ethnic differences in risk for psychiatric disorder in a USA national sample. *Psychological Medicine*, 36(1), 57. doi:10.1017/s0033291705006161

Bronson, J., Carson, A., Noonan, M., & Berzofsky, M. (2015). Veterans in prison and jail, 2011–12. *US Department of Justice, Bureau of Justice Statistics*.

Brooks, E., Kaufman, C., Nagamoto, H. T., Dailey, N. K., Bair, B. D., & Shore, J. (2015). The impact of demographic differences on native veterans' outpatient service utilization. *Psychological Services*, 12(2), 134–140. https://doi.org/10.1037/a0038687

Brown, G. R., & Jones, K. T. (2014). Racial health disparities in a cohort of 5,135 transgender veterans. *Journal of Racial and Ethnic Health Disparities, 1*(4), 257–266.

Byrne, T., Montgomery, A. E., & Fargo, J. D. (2016). Unsheltered homelessness among veterans: Correlates and profiles. *Community Mental Health Journal, 52*(2), 148–157. https://doi.org/10.1007/s10597-015-9922-0

Carter, A., Borrero, S., Wessel, C., Washington, D. L., Bean-Mayberry, B., Corbelli, J. (2016). Racial and ethnic health care disparities among women in the Veterans Affairs Healthcare System: A systematic review. *Womens Health Issues, 26*(4), 401–409.

Castro, F., AhnAllen, C. G., Wiltsey-Stirman, S., Lester-Williams, K., Klunk-Gillis, J., Dick, A. M., & Resick, P. A. (2015). African American and European American veterans' perspectives on receiving mental health treatment. *Psychological Services, 12*(3), 330–338. https://doi.org/10.1037/a0038702

Copeland, L. A., McIntyre, R. T., Stock, E. M., Zeber, J. E., MacCarthy, D. J., & Pugh, M. J. (2014). Prevalence of suicidality among Hispanic and African American veterans following surgery. *American Journal of Public Health, 104 Suppl 4*, S603–608. https://doi.org/10.2105/AJPH.2014.301938

Copeland, L. A., Zeber, J. E., Valenstein, M., & Blow, F. C. (2003). Racial disparity in the use of atypical antipsychotic medications among veterans. *The American Journal of Psychiatry, 160*(10), 1817–1822. https://doi.org/10.1176/appi.ajp.160.10.181

Damashek, A., Bard, D., & Hecht, D. (2011). Provider cultural competency, client satisfaction, and engagement in home-based programs to treat child abuse and neglect. *Child Maltreatment, 17*(1), 56–66. doi:10.1177/1077559511423570

Damron-Rodriguez, J., White-Kazemipour, W., Washington, D., Villa, V. M., Dhanani, S., & Harada, N. D. (2004). Accessibility and acceptability of the Department of Veteran Affairs health care: diverse veterans' perspectives. *Military Medicine, 169*(3), 243–250.

David, D., Kutcher, G. S., Jackson, E. I., & Mellman, T. A. (1999). Psychotic symptoms in combat-related posttraumatic stress disorder. *The Journal of Clinical Psychiatry, 60*(1), 29–32.

Davis, T. D., Deen, T. L., Fortney, J. C., Sullivan, G., & Hudson, T. J. (2014). Utilization of VA mental health and primary care services among Iraq and Afghanistan veterans with depression: the influence of gender and ethnicity status. *Military Medicine, 179*(5), 515–520. https://doi.org/10.7205/MILMED-D-13-00179

Davis, T. D., Sullivan, G., Vasterling, J. J., Tharp, A. L. T., Han, X., Deitch, E. A., & Constans, J. I. (2012). Racial variations in postdisaster PTSD among veteran survivors of Hurricane Katrina. *Psychological Trauma: Theory, Research, Practice, and Policy, 4*(5), 447–456. https://doi.org/10.1037/a0025501

De Luca, S. M., Blosnich, J. R., Hentschel, E. A. W., King, E., & Amen, S. (2016). Mental health care utilization: How race, ethnicity and veteran status are associated with seeking help. *Community Mental Health Journal, 52*(2), 174–179. https://doi.org/10.1007/s10597-015-9964

Department of Defense. (2015). *Military Demographics Report.*

Di Leone, B. A. L., Vogt, D., Gradus, J. L., Street, A. E., Giasson, H. L., & Resick, P. A. (2013). Predictors of mental health care use among male and female veterans deployed in support of the wars in Afghanistan and Iraq. *Psychological Services, 10*(2), 145–151. https://doi.org/10.1037/a0032088

Diala, C., Muntaner, C., Walrath, C., Nickerson, K. J., LaVeist, T. A., & Leaf, P. J. (2000). Racial differences in attitudes toward professional mental health care and in the use of services. *American Journal of Orthopsychiatry, 70*(4), 455–464.

Eliacin, J., Coffing, J. M., Matthias, M. S., Burgess, D. J., Bair, M. J., & Rollins, A. L. (2016). The relationship between race, patient activation, and working alliance: Implications for patient engagement in mental health care. *Administration and Policy in Mental Health.* https://doi.org/10.1007/s10488-016-0779-5

Foynes, M. M., Shipherd, J. C., & Harrington, E. F. (2013). Race and gender discrimination in the Marines. *Cultural Diversity & Ethnic Minority Psychology*, 19(1), 111–119. https://doi.org/10.1037/a0030567

Foynes, M. M., Smith, B. N., & Shipherd, J. C. (2015). Associations between race-based and sex-based discrimination, health, and functioning: A longitudinal study of Marines. *Medical Care, 53* (4 Suppl 1), S128–135. https://doi.org/10.1097/MLR.0000000000000300

Frueh, B. C., Elhai, J. D., Monnier, J., Hamner, M. B., & Knapp, R. G. (2004). Symptom patterns and service use among African American and Caucasian veterans with combat-related PTSD. *Psychological Services*, 1(1), 22–30. https://doi.org/10.1037/1541-1559.1.1.22

Garcia, H. A., Kelley, L. P., Rentz, T. O., & Lee, S. (2011). Pretreatment predictors of dropout from cognitive behavioral therapy for PTSD in Iraq and Afghanistan war veterans. *Psychological Services*, 8(1), 1–11.

Gates G. J. (2010). Discharges under the Don't Ask, Don't Tell policy: Women and racial/ethnic minorities. The Williams Institute. http://williamsinstitute.law.ucla.edu/category/research/military-related/#sthash.ikBT7Fr9. dpuf

Gobin, R. L., & Allard, C. B. (2016). Associations between sexual health concerns and mental health symptoms among African American and European American women veterans who have experienced interpersonal trauma. *Dr. Sybil Eysenck Young Researcher Award, 100* (Supplement C), 37–42. https://doi.org/10.1016/j.paid.2016.02.007

Goetter, E. M., Frumkin, M., Swee, M. B., Palitz, S., Baker, A. W., Bui, E., & Simon, N. M. (under review). Barriers to treatment among individuals with social anxiety disorder and generalized anxiety disorder. *Psychological Services.*

Goodwin, R. D., Cohen, G. H., Tamburrino, M., Calabrese, J. R., Liberzon, I., & Galea, S. (2014). Mental health service use in a representative sample of National Guard soldiers. *Psychiatric Services (Washington, DC)*, 65(11), 1347–1353. https://doi.org/10.1176/appi.ps.201300282.

Gordon, A. J., Haas, G. L., Luther, J. F., Hilton, M. T., & Goldstein, G. (2010). Personal, medical, and healthcare utilization among homeless veterans served by metropolitan and nonmetropolitan veteran facilities. *Psychological Services*, 7(2), 65–74. https://doi.org/10.1037/a0018479

Gorman, L. A., Sripada, R. K., Ganoczy, D., Walters, H. M., Bohnert, K. M., Dalack, G. W., & Valenstein, M. (2016). Determinants of National Guard mental health service utilization in VA versus non-VA settings. *Health Services Research*, 51(5), 1814–1837. doi:10.1111/1475-6773.12446

Greenberg, G. A., & Rosenheck, R. A. (2012). Incarceration among male veterans: Relative risk of imprisonment and differences between veteran and nonveteran inmates. *International Journal of Offender Therapy and Comparative Criminology*, 56(4), 646–667. https://doi.org/10.1177/0306624X11406091

Harada, N. D., Villa, V. M., Damron-Rodriguez, J., Washington, D., Makinodan, T., Dhanani, S., … & Andersen, R. (2002). The influence of military service on outpatient care use among racial/ethnic groups in Department of Veterans Affairs medical centers. *Military Medicine*, 167(7), 525–531.

Harpaz-Rotem, I., & Rosenheck, R. A. (2011). Serving those who served: Retention of newly returning veterans from Iraq and Afghanistan in mental health treatment. *Psychiatric Services*, 62(1), 22–27. doi:10.1176/ps.62.1.pss6201_0022

Harris, G. L. A. (2011). Reducing healthcare disparities in the military through cultural competence. *Journal of Health and Human Services Administration*, 34(2), 145–181.

Hoff, R. A., & Rosenheck, R. A. (1998). The use of VA and non-VA mental health services by female veterans. *Medical Care, 7*(11), 1524–1533.

Holliday, R. P., Holder, N. D., Williamson, M. L. C., & Surís, A. (2017). Therapeutic response to cognitive processing therapy in White and Black female veterans with military sexual trauma-related PTSD. *Cognitive Behaviour Therapy*, 46(5), 432–446. https://doi.org/10.1080/16506073.2017.1312511

Horrell, S. C. V. (2008). Effectiveness of cognitive-behavioral therapy with adult ethnic minority clients: A review. *Professional Psychology: Research and Practice, 39*(2), 160–168. https://doi.org/10.1037/0735-7028.39.2.160

Huey, S. J., & Polo, A. J. (2008). Evidence-based psychosocial treatments for ethnic minority youth. *Journal of Clinical Child and Adolescent Psychology: The Official Journal for the Society of Clinical Child and Adolescent Psychology, American Psychological Association, Division 53, 37*(1), 262–301. https://doi.org/10.1080/15374410701820174.

Huey, S. J., Tilley, J. L., Jones, E. O., & Smith, C. A. (2014). The contribution of cultural competence to evidence-based care for ethnically diverse populations. *Annual Review of Clinical Psychology, 10*, 305–338. https://doi.org/10.1146/annurev-clinpsy-032813-153729

Jones, A. L., Hausmann, L. R. M., Haas, G. L., Mor, M. K., Cashy, J. P., Schaefer, J. H., & Gordon, A. J. (2017). A national evaluation of homeless and nonhomeless veterans' experiences with primary care. *Psychological Services, 14*(2), 174–183. https://doi.org/10.1037/ser0000116

Jones, A. L., Mor, M. K., Cashy, J. P., Gordon, A. J., Haas, G. L., Schaefer, J. H., & Hausmann, L. R. M. (2016). Racial/ethnic differences in primary care experiences in patient-centered medical homes among veterans with mental health and substance use disorders. *Journal of General Internal Medicine, 31*(12), 1435–1443. https://doi.org/10.1007/s11606-016-3776-1

Jordan, B. K., Schlenger, W. E., Hough, R., Kulka, R. A., Weiss, D. Fairbank, J. A., & Marmar, C. R. (1991). Lifetime and current prevalence of specific psychiatric disorders among Vietnam veterans and controls. *Archives of General Psychiatry, 48*(3), 207. doi:10.1001/archpsyc.1991.01810270019002

Kales, H. C., Blow, F. C., Bingham, C. R., Copeland, L. A., & Mellow, A. M. (2000). Race and inpatient psychiatric diagnoses among elderly veterans. *Psychiatric Services (Washington, DC), 51*(6), 795–800. https://doi.org/10.1176/appi.ps.51.6.795

Kales, H. C., Blow, F. C., Bingham, C. R., Roberts, J. S., Copeland, L. A., & Mellow, A. M. (2000). Race, psychiatric diagnosis, and mental health care utilization in older patients. *The American Journal of Geriatric Psychiatry: Official Journal of the American Association for Geriatric Psychiatry, 8*(4), 301–309.

Karel, M., & Moye, J. (2002). Assessing depression in medically ill elderly male veterans: Item-scale properties across and within racial groups. *Journal of Mental Health and Aging, 8*(2), 121–138.

Karlin, B. E., Ruzek, J. I., Chard, K. M., Eftekhari, A., Monson, C. M., Hembree, E. A., … & Foa, E. B. (2010). Dissemination of evidence-based psychological treatments for posttraumatic stress disorder in the Veterans Health Administration. *Journal of Traumatic Stress, 23*(6), 663–673.

Kaufmann, L. J., Buck Richardson, W. J., Floyd, J., & Shore, J. (2014). Tribal Veterans Representative (TVR) training program: The effect of community outreach workers on American Indian and Alaska Native Veterans access to and utilization of the Veterans Health Administration. *Journal of Community Health, 39*(5), 990–996. https://doi.org/10.1007/s10900-014-9846-6

Koenen, K. C., Stellman, J. M., Stellman, S. D., & Sommer, J. F. (2003). Risk factors for course of posttraumatic stress disorder among Vietnam veterans: A 14-year follow-up of American Legionnaires. *Journal of Consulting and Clinical Psychology, 71*(6), 980–986. https://doi.org/10.1037/0022-006X.71.6.980

Koo, K. H., Hebenstreit, C. L., Madden, E., Seal, K. H., & Maguen, S. (2015). Race/ethnicity and gender differences in mental health diagnoses among Iraq and Afghanistan veterans. *Psychiatry Research, 229*(3), 724–731. https://doi.org/10.1016/j.psychres.2015.08.013

Kwan, B. M., Dimidjian, S., & Rizvi, S. L. (2010). Treatment preference, engagement, and clinical improvement in pharmacotherapy versus psychotherapy for depression. *Behaviour Research and Therapy, 48*(8), 799–804. doi:10.1016/j.brat.2010.04.003

Lesser, I. M., Zisook, S., Gaynes, B. N., Wisniewski, S. R., Luther, J. F., Fava, M., … Trivedi, M. (2011). Effects of race and ethnicity on depression treatment outcomes: The CO-MED trial. *Psychiatric Services, 62*(10), 1167–1179. https://doi.org/10.1176/ps.62.10.pss6210_1167

Lester, K., Artz, C., Resick, P. A., & Young-Xu, Y. (2010). Impact of race on early treatment termination and outcomes in posttraumatic stress disorder treatment. *Journal of Consulting and Clinical Psychology, 78*(4), 480–489.

Loo, C. M., Fairbank, J. A., Scurfield, R. M., Ruch, L. O., King, D. W., Adams, L. J., & Chemtob, C. M. (2001). Measuring exposure to racism: Development and validation of a Race-Related Stressor Scale (RRSS) for Asian American Vietnam veterans. *Psychological Assessment, 13*(4), 503–520.

Loo, C. M., Singh, K., Scurfield, R., & Kilauano, B. (1998). Race-related stress among Asian American veterans: A model to enhance diagnosis and treatment. *Cultural Diversity and Mental Health, 4*(2), 75–90.

Luncheon, C., & Zack, M. (2012). Health-related quality of life among US veterans and civilians by race and ethnicity. *Preventing Chronic Disease, 9*, E108.

Manhapra, A., Quiñones, L., & Rosenheck, R. (2016). Characteristics of veterans receiving buprenorphine vs. methadone for opioid use disorder nationally in the Veterans Health Administration. *Drug and Alcohol Dependence, 160*, 82–89. https://doi.org/10.1016/j.drugalcdep.2015.12.035

Marx, B. P., Engel-Rebitzer, E., Bovin, M. J., Parker-Guilbert, K. S., Moshier, S., Barretto, K., … & Keane, T. M. (2017). The influence of veteran race and psychometric testing on veterans affairs posttraumatic stress disorder (PTSD) disability exam outcomes. *Psychological Assessment, 29*(6), 710–719. https://doi.org/10.1037/pas0000378

Mattocks, K. M., Sadler, A., Yano, E. M., Krebs, E. E., Zephyrin, L., Brandt, C., … & Allison, J. (2013). Sexual victimization, health status, and VA healthcare utilization among lesbian and bisexual OEF/OIF veterans. *Journal of General Internal Medicine, 28*(2), 604–608.

McGuire, J., Rosenheck, R. A., & Kasprow, W. J. (2003). Health status, service use, and costs among veterans receiving outreach services in jail or community settings. *Psychiatric Services, 54*(2), 201–207.

Meier, P. S., Donmall, M. C., McElduff, P., Barrowclough, C., & Heller, R. F. (2006). The role of the early therapeutic alliance in predicting drug treatment dropout. *Drug and Alcohol Dependence, 83*(1), 57–64. doi:10.1016/j.drugalcdep.2005.10.010

Monnier, J., Elhai, J. D., Frueh, B. C., Sauvageot, J. A., & Magruder, K. M. (2002). Replication and expansion of findings related to racial differences in veterans with combat-related PTSD. *Depression and Anxiety, 16*(2), 64–70. https://doi.org/10.1002/da.10060

Murdoch, M., Hodges, J., Cowper, D., Fortier, L., & van Ryn, M. (2003). Racial disparities in VA service connection for posttraumatic stress disorder disability. *Medical Care, 41*(4), 536–549. https://doi.org/10.1097/01.MLR.0000053232.67079.A5

Murphy, F. M. Statement of Frances M. Murphy, MD, MPH, Acting Deputy Under Secretary for Policy and Management. 3–9–2000; Committee on Veterans' Affairs, Subcommittee on Health and Subcommittee on Benefits, US House of Representatives, 2000.

National Center for Veterans Analysis and Statistics. (2009). *Analysis of unique veterans utilization of VA benefits and services.* Office of Policy and Planning at the United States Department of Veterans Affairs.

National Center for Veterans Analysis and Statistics. (2016). *Unique veteran users provile, fiscal year, 2015.* United States Department of Veteran Affairs.

National Center for Veterans Analysis and Statistics. (2017). *Minority veterans report: Military service history and VA benefit utilization statistics.* United States Department of Veteran Affairs.

Nayback, A. M. (2008). Health disparities in military veterans with PTSD: influential sociocultural factors. *Journal of Psychosocial Nursing and Mental Health Services, 46*(6), 41–51.

Nieuwsma, J. A., Fortune-Greeley, A. K., Jackson, G. L., Meador, K. G., Beckham, J. C., & Elbogen, E. B. (2014). Pastoral care use among post-9/11 veterans who screen positive for mental health problems. *Psychological Services, 11*(3), 300–308. https://doi.org/10.1037/a0037065

O'Keefe, V. M., & Reger, G. M. (2017). Suicide among American Indian/Alaska Native military service members and veterans. *Psychological Services, 14*(3), 289–294. https://doi.org/10.1037/ser0000117

Onoye, J. M., Spoont, M., Whealin, J. M., Pole, N., Mackintosh, M.-A., Spira, J. L., & Morland, L. A. (2017). Improving assessment of race, ethnicity, and culture to further veteran PTSD research. *Psychological Trauma: Theory, Research, Practice and Policy, 9*(2), 222–229. https://doi.org/10.1037/tra0000181

Ortega, A. N., & Rosenheck, R. (2000). Posttraumatic stress disorder among Hispanic Vietnam veterans. *The American Journal of Psychiatry, 157*(4), 615–619. https://doi.org/10.1176/appi.ajp.157.4.615

Ouimette, P., Vogt, D., Wade, M., Tirone, V., Greenbaum, M. A., Kimerling, R., ... & Rosen, C. S. (2011). Perceived barriers to care among veterans health administration patients with posttraumatic stress disorder. *Psychological Services, 8*(3), 212–223. https://doi.org/10.1037/a0024360

Pan, D., Huey, S. J., & Hernandez, D. (2011). Culturally adapted versus standard exposure treatment for phobic Asian Americans: Treatment efficacy, moderators, and predictors. *Cultural Diversity & Ethnic Minority Psychology, 17*(1), 11–22. https://doi.org/10.1037/a0022534

Pending Health Legislation, Including the Heather French Henry Homeless Veteran's Assistance Act, Senate, S. Hrg. 107–653, (2001).

Pettit, B., & Western, B. (2004). Mass imprisonment and the life course: Race and class inequality in US incarceration. *American Sociological Review, 69*(2), 151–169.

Pfeiffer, P. N., Valenstein, M., Hoggatt, K. J., Ganoczy, D., Maixner, D., Miller, E. M., & Zivin, K. (2011). Electroconvulsive therapy for major depression within the Veterans Health Administration. *Journal of Affective Disorders, 130*(1–2), 21–25. https://doi.org/10.1016/j.jad.2010.09.023

Pierre-Louis, B. J., Moore, A. D., & Hamilton, J. B. (2015). The military health care system may have the potential to prevent health care disparities. *Journal of Racial and Ethnic Health Disparities, 2*(3), 280–289. https://doi.org/10.1007/s40615-014-0067-6

Quiñones, A. R., Thielke, S. M., Beaver, K. A., Trivedi, R. B., Williams, E. C., & Fan, V. S. (2014). Racial and ethnic differences in receipt of antidepressants and psychotherapy by veterans with chronic depression. *Psychiatric Services (Washington, DC), 65*(2), 193–200. https://doi.org/10.1176/appi.ps.201300057

Ramsey, C., Dziura, J., Justice, A. C., Altalib, H. H., Bathulapalli, H., Burg, M., ... & Brandt, C. (2017). Incidence of mental health diagnoses in veterans of Operations Iraqi Freedom, Enduring Freedom, and New Dawn, 2001–2014. *American Journal of Public Health, 107*(2), 329–335. https://doi.org/10.2105/AJPH.2016.303574

Ray-Sannerud, B. N., Bryan, C. J., Perry, N. S., & Bryan, A. O. (2015). High levels of emotional distress, trauma exposure, and self-injurious thoughts and behaviors among military personnel and veterans with a history of same sex behavior. *Psychology of Sexual Orientation and Gender Diversity, 2*(2), 130–137. https://doi.org/10.1037/sgd0000096

Reger, M. A., Smolenski, D. J., Skopp, N. A., Metzger-Abamukang, M. J., Kang, H. K., Bullman, T. A., ... & Gahm, G. A. (2015). Risk of suicide among US military service members following Operation Enduring Freedom or Operation Iraqi Freedom deployment and separation from the US military. *JAMA Psychiatry, 72*(6), 561–569. https://doi.org/10.1001/jamapsychiatry.2014.3195

Rosen, M. I., Afshartous, D. R., Nwosu, S., Scott, M. C., Jackson, J. C., Marx, B. P., ... & Speroff, T. (2013). Racial differences in veterans' satisfaction with examination of disability from posttraumatic stress disorder. *Psychiatric Services (Washington, DC), 64*(4), 354–359. https://doi.org/10.1176/appi.ps.201100526

Rosenheck, R., Fontana, A., & Cottrol, C. (1995). Effect of clinician-veteran racial pairing in the treatment of posttraumatic stress disorder. *The American Journal of Psychiatry, 152*(4), 555–563. https://doi.org/10.1176/ajp.152.4.555

Rosenheck, R., Leda, C., Frisman, L., & Gallup, P. (1997). Homeless mentally ill veterans: Race, service use, and treatment outcomes. *The American Journal of Orthopsychiatry, 67*(4), 632–638.

Saha, S., Freeman, M., Toure, J., Tippens, K. M., Weeks, C., & Ibrahim, S. (2008). Racial and ethnic disparities in the VA health care system: a systematic review. *Journal of General Internal Medicine, 23*(5), 654–671. https://doi.org/10.1007/s11606-008-0521-4

Schoenbaum, M., Kessler, R. C., Gilman, S. E., Colpe, L. J., Heeringa, S. G., Stein, M. B., … & Army STARRS Collaborators. (2014). Predictors of suicide and accident death in the Army Study to Assess Risk and Resilience in Servicemembers (Army STARRS): Results from the Army Study to Assess Risk and Resilience in Servicemembers (Army STARRS). *JAMA Psychiatry, 71*(5), 493–503. https://doi.org/10.1001/jamapsychiatry.2013.4417

Sheehan, C. M., Hummer, R. A., Moore, B. L., Huyser, K. R., & Butler, J. S. (2015). Duty, honor, country, disparity: Race/ethnic differences in health and disability among male veterans. *Population Research and Policy Review, 34*(6), 785–804. https://doi.org/10.1007/s11113-015-9358-9

Sohn, L., & Harada, N. D. (2008). Effects of racial/ethnic discrimination on the health status of minority veterans. *Military Medicine, 173*(4), 331–338.

Spoont, M. R., Hodges, J., Murdoch, M., & Nugent, S. (2009). Race and ethnicity as factors in mental health service use among veterans with PTSD. *Journal of Traumatic Stress, 22*(6), 648–653. https://doi.org/10.1002/jts.20470

Spoont, M. R., Nelson, D. B., Murdoch, M., Sayer, N. A., Nugent, S., Rector, T., & Westermeyer, J. (2015). Are there racial/ethnic disparities in VA PTSD treatment retention? *Depression and Anxiety, 32*(6), 415–425. https://doi.org/10.1002/da.22295

Stecker, T., Adams, L., Carpenter-Song, E., Nicholson, J., Streltzov, N., & Xie, H. (2016). Intervention efficacy in engaging Black and White veterans with post-traumatic stress disorder into treatment. *Social Work in Public Health, 31*(6), 481–489. https://doi.org/10.1080/19371918.2016.1160340

Steidtmann, D., Manber, R., Arnow, B. A., Klein, D. N., Markowitz, J. C., Rothbaum, B. O., … & Kocsis, J. H. (2012). Patient treatment preference as a predictor of response and attrition in treatment for chronic depression. *Depression and Anxiety, 29*(10), 896–905. doi:10.1002/da.21977

Tanielian, T., Jaycox, J. H., Schell, T., Marshall, G. N., Burnam, M. A., Eibner, C., Karney, B., Meredith, L. S., Ringel, J., & Vaiana, M. E. (2008). *Invisible wounds: Mental health and cognitive care needs of America's returning veterans.* RAND Corporation.

Tessler, R., Rosenheck, R., & Gamache, G. (2002). Comparison of homeless veterans with other homeless men in a large clinical outreach program. *The Psychiatric Quarterly, 73*(2), 109–119.

Tsai, J., Desai, M. U., Cheng, A. W., & Chang, J. (2014). The effects of race and other socioeconomic factors on health service use among American military veterans. *The Psychiatric Quarterly, 85*(1), 35–47. https://doi.org/10.1007/s11126-013-9268-0

Tsai, J., & Kong, G. (2012). Mental health of Asian American and Pacific Islander military veterans: brief review of an understudied group. *Military Medicine, 177*(11), 1438–1444.

Tsai, J., Rosenheck, R. A., Kasprow, W. J., & McGuire, J. F. (2013). Risk of incarceration and clinical characteristics of incarcerated veterans by race/ethnicity. *Social Psychiatry and Psychiatric Epidemiology, 48*(11), 1777–1786. https://doi.org/10.1007/s00127-013-0677-z

Tsai, J., Whealin, J. M., & Pietrzak, R. H. (2014). Asian American and Pacific Islander military veterans in the United States: health service use and perceived barriers to mental health services. *American Journal of Public Health, 104* Suppl 4, S538–547. https://doi.org/10.2105/AJPH.2014.302124

Ursano, R. J., Heeringa, S. G., Stein, M. B., Jain, S., Raman, R., Sun, X., … & Kessler, R. C. (2015). Prevalence and correlates of suicidal behavior among new soldiers in the US Army: Results from the Army Study to Assess Risk and Resilience in Servicemembers (Army STARRS). *Depression and Anxiety, 32*(1), 3–12. https://doi.org/10.1002/da.22317

US Census Bureau. (2014). Evaluation of the Revised Veteran Status Question in the 2013 American Community Survey.

US Department of Health and Human Services. (2001). *Mental health: Culture, race, and ethnicity: A supplement to mental health: A report of the surgeon general.* Substance Abuse and Mental Health Services Administration, National institute of Mental Health.

Washington, D. L., Bean-Mayberry, B., Riopelle, D., & Yano, E. M. (2011). Access to care for women veterans: Delayed healthcare and unmet need. *Journal of General Internal Medicine, 26*(2), 655.

Williams, E. C., Gupta, S., Rubinsky, A. D., Glass, J. E., Jones-Webb, R., Bensley, K. M., & Harris, A. H. S. (2017). Variation in receipt of pharmacotherapy for alcohol use disorders across racial/ethnic groups: A national study in the US Veterans Health Administration. *Drug and Alcohol Dependence, 178*, 527–533. https://doi.org/10.1016/j.drugalcdep.2017.06.011

Williams, E. C., Lapham, G. T., Hawkins, E. J., Rubinsky, A. D., Morales, L. S., Young, B. A., & Bradley, K. A. (2012). Variation in documented care for unhealthy alcohol consumption across race/ethnicity in the Department of Veterans Affairs Healthcare System. *Alcoholism, Clinical and Experimental Research, 36*(9), 1614–1622. https://doi.org/10.1111/j.1530-0277.2012.01761.x

Zeiss, A., & Karlin, B. (2008). Integrating mental health and primary care services in the department of Veterans Affairs Health Care System. *Journal of Clinical Psychology in Medical Settings, 15*(1), 73–78.

Zinzow, H. M., Britt, T. W., Pury, C. L. S., Jennings, K., Cheung, J. H., & Raymond, M. A. (2015). Barriers and facilitators of mental health treatment-seeking in US active duty soldiers with sexual assault histories. *Journal of Traumatic Stress, 28*(4), 289–297. https://doi.org/10.1002/jts.22026

CHAPTER 17

Refugee Communities

Victoria A. Schlaudt,
Nova Southeastern University and University of Michigan

Alisa B. Miller,
Boston Children's Hospital and Harvard Medical School

Purpose of This Chapter

In this chapter, we provide the definition of a refugee, detail the historical context of refugees in the United States, and present a brief overview of their unique experiences. We then offer a critique of the mental health services currently available for refugees, including analyzing their access to and quality of care, describing their treatment, discussing strategies that have been shown to combat the inequality of care, and proposing approaches for care moving forward. Implications for clinical work and researchers will be outlined. Readers will walk away with an understanding of the unique experiences of refugees before, during, and after migration, barriers to care in resettlement, and what they can do to eliminate disparities in care.

Overview of Refugee Populations and the US Context

In order to understand refugees and their mental health, it is vital to comprehend the context of this unique population. Refugees, as defined by the 1951 Refugee Convention, are those who "owing to well-founded fear of being persecuted for reasons of race, religion, nationality, membership of a particular social group or political opinion, [are] out of the country of [their] nationality and [are] unable to or, owing to such fear, [are] unwilling to avail [themselves] of the protection of that country" (United Nations General Assembly, 1951). As of 2017, the United Nations High Commissioner for Refugees (UNHCR) reported that there were 22.5 million refugees worldwide (UNHCR, 2017). Over half of refugees are under the age of eighteen (UNHCR, 2017). The United States has resettled over 3.25 million refugees since 1975, making it, historically, one of the most refugee-welcoming countries. The number of refugees accepted in the United

States can change over time, based on world events, the need that the UNHCR identifies, and presidential decisions. The United States has admitted less than 30,000 refugees in some years, and over 200,000 in others (Epatko, 2017). For example, according to the UNHCR (2017), in 2015 the United States accepted 70,000 refugees with most coming from the Middle East and South Asia (e.g., Iraq, Afghanistan), Africa (e.g., Somalia, Democratic Republic of Congo), and East Asia (e.g., Burma).

Prior to Arrival in the United States

Individuals achieve the legal status of refugee by applying prior to arrival in the United States. This process includes requesting refugee status when arriving in a new country (neither the home country nor the country of resettlement), explaining the reasons that refugee status is necessary, and providing evidence related to the claim of eligibility (UNHCR, 2011a). Once a person has established his or her status as a refugee, there are many steps to take before he or she can be resettled in the United States. Before recommending resettlement, the UNHCR verifies the individual's refugee status and registration and conducts an assessment regarding his or her need to resettle (UNHCR, 2011b). This information is reviewed by a supervisor, and any additional information needed is requested, which may include a medical assessment. If a refugee passes these steps, he or she then completes a resettlement interview with the UNHCR (UNHCR, 2011b). The UNHCR then identifies the most vulnerable refugees (e.g., women, children, and disabled individuals) and communicates this information to countries who have agreed to resettle refugees (UNHCR, 2013).

Once the United States decides to accept refugees, it begins a vetting process. First, workers from Resettlement Support Centers travel to the refugee in the host country to conduct an interview, check facts, and provide this information to the US Department of State (DOS). Next, a background check is run by several US organizations. Then the Department of Homeland Security (DHS) completes an interview to verify information provided and to collect fingerprints. DHS checks the refugee's fingerprints through several databases to ensure that the refugee has not been involved in crime or terror (DOS, n.d.). After interviews and finger printing is completed, a refugee has a cultural orientation (i.e., refugees learn about "American culture, customs, and practices") and is screened for diseases that present public health concerns (DOS, n.d.). Next, travel is booked for the refugee by the International Organization for Migration (IOM) (DOS, n.d.). Refugees are expected to pay back their travel expenses to the IOM within forty-six months (IOM, 2010). Upon arrival in the United States, refugee resettlement agencies help refugees to find employment and secure housing (DOS, n.d.). The process for resettlement to United States, takes between one and a half and two years, but it can often take longer (Epatko, 2017). Many, many refugees are never resettled; over 99 percent are not given this opportunity (UNHCR, 2007; Murray, Davidson, & Schweitzer, 2010).

REFUGEES AND TRAUMA EXPOSURE

Refugees experience a variety of traumas and stressors from the time they decide to flee their home country, throughout migration, and during and after resettlement. In their countries of origin, refugees may experience torture, grief, and "threats to life, traumatic loss, dispossession, and eviction" (Davidson, Murray, & Schweitzer, 2008, p. 161; Lustig et al., 2004). Once refugees leave their country of origin, new and different challenges await them; they may face long waits in a refugee camp, arduous travel, and separation from family (Fazel, Reed, Panter-Brick, & Stein, 2012; Lustig et al., 2004). Upon resettlement in a new nation, refugees may be victims of racism, often experience acculturative stress, feel isolated, encounter resettlement stressors (e.g., adequate housing, navigating transportation), and struggle to develop and maintain economic stability (Kim, 2016; Fazel et al., 2012).

Refugees and Psychological Distress

Worldwide, refugees often experience multiple, ongoing traumatic experiences and prolonged stress due to the political, racial, or religious persecution they face, which makes them at high risk for the development of mental health problems (Porter & Haslam, 2005).

ADULTS

Overall, the rates of mental health difficulties in refugees are extremely high, though the rates vary by country of origin and across studies. In a review of the literature, Hollifield and colleagues (2002) reported depression prevalence rates between 5 percent and 31 percent. For post-traumatic stress disorder (PTSD), these numbers are even more wide-ranging, with estimates between 4 percent and 86 percent (Hollifield et al., 2002). Reasons for these disparities include methodological issues such as varying measures, difficulties regarding language of assessments, lack of resources to properly complete studies, and cultural differences and biases (Hollifield et al., 2002). In a study of Bhutanese refugees, Ao and colleagues (2016) found that 21 percent were experiencing depression, 19 percent anxiety, and 4.5 percent PTSD, and 3 percent endorsed suicidal ideation. In Cambodian refugees who had been resettled twenty years prior, 62 percent met the criteria for PTSD, 51 percent for major depression, and 4 percent for alcohol use disorders (Marshall, Schell, Elliott, Berthold, & Chun, 2005). A more recent study placed the co-morbidity rate of PTSD and depression in a group of Cambodian refugees at 64 percent (Berthold et al., 2014). A study of Iraqi refugees found that 50 percent of the sample screened positive for anxiety, depression, and emotional distress, and 31 percent screened positive for PTSD (Taylor, et al., 2014). In a study of Vietnamese refugees, 20.3 percent scored in the clinical range for anxiety and 20.8 percent for depression (Birman & Tran, 2008).

A meta-analysis of studies of over 64,000 refugees from many countries (and who resettled to many Western countries) by Steel and colleagues (2009) reported an overall weighted PTSD rate of 30.6 percent and a depression rate of 30.8 percent. Although this review incorporated information about refugees resettled inside and outside the United States, it provides an estimate of the mental health difficulties present in this population. Of note, the Center for Behavioral Health Statistics and Quality (2016) reports that 17.9 percent of US adults will experience a mental health condition in any given year. Therefore, refugees generally endorse a higher rate of mental health difficulties than the average American adult.

CHILDREN

Betancourt and colleagues (2012) reported that in a sample of children refugees (mean age = 13.1 years) from several regions of the world, 30.3 percent presented with PTSD, 21.4 percent with traumatic grief, 26.8 percent each with generalized anxiety and somatization, 21.4 percent with externalizing problems, and 12.5 percent each with depression and dissociation. Further, co-morbid conditions, such as displaying symptoms of both PTSD and anxiety or depression, was very common. Berthold (2000) reported that in a sample of Cambodian adolescents, 30 percent had behavioral problems in school, 33 percent experienced symptoms of PTSD, and 63 percent endorsed symptoms of depression. Unaccompanied Sudanese refugees reported a 20 percent PTSD rate (Geltman et al., 2005). Importantly, mental health symptoms may be expressed somatically in refugee populations (Lustig et al., 2004), such as respiratory or gastrointestinal issues without physical or organic cause (Van Ommeren et al., 2002). A sample of Cuban adolescents who had been detained in refugee camps at Guantanamo experienced somatic symptoms at a rate of 52 percent, while 57 percent experienced PTSD (Rothe et al., 2002).

In a review of refugee children's mental health symptoms, Lustig and colleagues (2004) reported that in studies of Cubans, Cambodians, and Bosnians resettled in the United States, child refugees endorsed rates of PTSD ranging between 30 percent and 57 percent. The study of Cambodian children placed the depression rate at 53 percent, while the others did not report on these symptoms (Lustig et al., 2004). Reasons for these disparities in rates of mental health issues may include problems with measurement, individual resilience factors, disparities in trauma exposure, differences in difficulties upon resettlement, and expectations about resettlement (Lustig et al., 2004). A nationally representative sample of US children demonstrated that the rate of any mental health disorder in the past year was 13.1 percent (Merikangas et al., 2010), which reveals the heightened rate of mental health difficulties among refugee children.

BEYOND TRAUMA AND PSYCHOLOGICAL DISTRESS

Miller and Rasmussen (2010) asserted that in therapy, professionals may focus excessively on the major life events of refugee patients without realizing that everyday stressors are more impactful on their mental health functioning. Thus, although refugees have unique war- and trauma-related experiences, evidence suggests that in order to help them heal, it is important to focus on the difficulties they experience upon resettlement (Kim, 2016). Similarly, Ellis, Miller, Baldwin, and Abdi (2011) described that refugees often prioritize resettlement stressors over mental health needs. Although services for both mental health and resettlement difficulties may be offered, they are usually not provided collaboratively (Ellis et al., 2011). In addition, mental health clinicians may not see it as their role to help with fundamental needs. Taken together, this may decrease the likelihood that refugee families will seek mental health care (Ellis et al., 2011).

CULTURAL TRAUMA

Scholars have argued that the psychological and psychiatric community's understanding of trauma and mental health often does not apply to the intense, diverse, and prolonged traumatic experiences that refugees encounter (Hollifield et al., 2002; Kira, 2010; Porter & Haslam, 2005). For example, when discussing the diagnostic criteria of PTSD, Herman (1992) argued that complex traumas are not taken into account in our diagnosis of PTSD, and, thus, we may not have a label that accurately describes the mental health issues of those who have experienced ongoing traumas. Alexander, Everman, Giesen, Smelser, and Sztompka (2004) stated that the multiple, complex traumas that some groups face can create "cultural trauma." This term describes what hapapens when "members of a collectivity feel they have been subjected to a horrendous event that leaves indelible marks upon their group consciousness, marking their memories forever and changing their future identity in fundamental and irrevocable ways" (Alexander et al., 2004, p. 1). It is vital to foster an understanding in the psychological community of the best ways to ameliorate mental health difficulties, and it should be considered that cultural trauma may present in this vulnerable population.

Risk Factors for Psychological Distress in Adult and Child Refugees

Demographic and situational factors affect the psychological outcomes of refugees; understanding an individual's risk factors is critical in order to create research and therapy protocols that allow for best mental health outcomes.

ADULTS

Difficulty finding work or financial stress is an important risk factor for suicidal ideation, depression, and PTSD among Bhutanese refugees, whereas family conflict or not having resources to resolve conflict were risk factors for depression and suicidal ideation (Ao et al., 2016; Blair, 2000; Marshall et al., 2005; Vonnahme et al., 2015). Trauma was predictive of PTSD and depression in Cambodian refugees (Blair, 2000) and anxiety in

Vietnamese refugees (Birman & Tran, 2008). Cambodian individuals were more at risk for PTSD and depression due to difficulties such as transportation troubles, limited English proficiency (Blair, 2000), older age, having a disability, or living in poverty (Marshall et al., 2005). Bhutanese refugees were at higher risk for suicidal ideation when they did not have access to therapy or government financial support and perceived an inability to control their futures (Ao et al., 2016). Depression in Bhutanese refugees was associated with poor health, a perceived loss of cultural traditions, and worrying about family members back home (Vonnahme et al., 2015). Birman and Tran (2008) found that Vietnamese refugees were at higher risk for anxiety if they were female and were more behaviorally acculturated to Vietnamese culture (e.g., preferring Vietnamese food to American food) or participating in traditional Vietnamese activities (e.g., watching Vietnamese television programs). Overall, trauma, gender, financial and cultural stressors, family difficulties, language difficulties, and perceived lack of control seem to be risk factors for mental health concerns in adult refugees in the United States.

CHILDREN AND ADOLESCENTS

An important risk factor for refugee youth (ages eleven to twenty) seems to be exposure to violence for symptomology such as PTSD (Berthold, 2000; Ellis et al., 2010), depression (Ellis et al., 2010), and withdrawn behavior (Rothe et al., 2002). Lack of social support or feeling lonely or isolated predicted PTSD in Sudanese teenage refugees (Geltman et al., 2005) and predicted PTSD and depression in Cambodian teens (Berthold, 2000). Separation from one's family and being in foster care without others from a similar ethnic background predicted PTSD in Sudanese teenage refugees (Geltman et al., 2005). Perceived discrimination has been associated with both PTSD and depression in adolescent Somali refugees (Ellis et al., 2010).

Interestingly, a longer stay in the United States was associated with more PTSD in Cambodian adolescents (Berthold, 2000) and less depression in Somali adolescents (Ellis et al., 2010). Other risk factors for child refugees include older age (Rothe et al., 2002), female sex (Berthold, 2000), and personal injury premigration (Geltman et al., 2005). In sum, issues such as exposure to violence, lack of social support, and injury, along with demographic characteristics such as age and sex all appear to be significant risk factors for child refugees.

Disparities in Mental Health Treatment

ACCESS TO CARE

Ovitt, Larrison, and Nackerud (2003) reported that refugees struggle to engage with the mental health care system due to cultural differences, difficulty finding care, language barriers, and priorities upon resettlement. Wong, Marshall, Schell, Berthold, and Hambarsoomians (2015) reported that only 52 percent of Cambodian refugees who met criteria for PTSD sought any type of care for their mental health concerns, which they speculated may be due to language barriers. This number is similar to the percentage of Americans (56 percent) who do not receive treatment for mental illness (Nguyen & Davis, 2016). Agrawal and Venkatesh (2016) stated that 40 percent of refugees are resettled in states that did not expand Medicaid with the Affordable Care Act (ACA), which was intended to increase the capacity for vulnerable individuals such as refugees to obtain affordable health care. Therefore, refugees in these states are less likely to be able to obtain coverage and may not be able to afford care (Agrawal & Venkatesh, 2016). With the uncertainty of the ACA, the expansions of Medicaid may be eliminated by 2020 (Williams, 2017); other effects of this uncertainty for refugees and their access to mental health care are hard to predict.

QUALITY OF CARE

When considering the care received by refugees, it is important to note the quality of mental health screening provided upon arrival in the United States as well as the overall care. State refugee health coordinators in the United States were asked to discuss the mental health screening provided to incoming refugees (Shannon et al., 2012), and almost half of the sample (43.2 percent) stated that they did not offer any screening for mental health. Of those who did, 70.8 percent used an informal conversation to assess mental health (Shannon et al., 2012). This type of informal conversation in place of a formalized assessment may present a significant challenge in terms of the accuracy and effectiveness of screening procedures. Refugees are also likely to receive poor quality of clinical intervention due to a lack of training and support provided to mental health care providers (de Anstiss, Ziaian, Procter, Warland & Baghurst, 2009).

In a study with Cambodian refugees, Wong and colleagues (2015) reported that over half sought some type of clinical care for their mental health difficulties from multiple different types of providers. Of this group, 45 percent received "minimally adequate care," which was defined as (1) at least two months of medication and at least four visits to the care provider; or (2) at least eight psychotherapy visits with a mean length of at least thirty minutes (Wong et al., 2015).

Reasons for Mental Health Disparity

LANGUAGE

Upon arrival in the United States, refugees often are expected to learn the English language. Capps and colleagues (2015) reported that only 33 percent of refugees resettled between 2008 and 2013 described that they spoke "some" English upon arrival. Therefore, a main barrier to accessing mental health care for refugees is finding a clinician who can properly communicate with them. When bilingual clinicians are not available, an interpreter is necessary, though properly trained interpreters are not always available. The use of an interpreter can complicate a thorough understanding of the mental health difficulties of the client if training and communication between interpreter and therapist is not efficient and effective (Guregård & Seikkula, 2014). Additionally, issues can arise when informal interpreters such as friends and family are used, due to the refugee's discomfort sharing private information with community members, lack of training in interpretation of family and friends, and true meanings being lost.

CULTURAL ISSUES

In a recent study measuring barriers to mental health treatment for Somali and Congolese refugee adults, several cultural issues were cited, including use of non-Western services such as traditional healing, friends and family, or religious figures for healing, and the confusing nature of Western mental health services (Piwowarczyk, Bishop, Yusuf, Mudymba, & Raj, 2014). Stigma was also a significant barrier to mental health treatment, as refugees felt they would be ostracized by their communities for their choice to seek mental health services and because disclosing personal information to a stranger is undesirable (Piwowarczyk et al., 2014).

An important cultural consideration in understanding access to mental health care is specific expectations refugees may have regarding care. The type of care received for physical and mental health may vary widely between cultures, and, thus, refugees may be confused and even disappointed by Western medical and mental health practices (Morris, Popper, Rodwell, Brodine, & Brouwer, 2009). These issues may decrease trust in mental health care providers and decrease the ability to provide quality care for refugee individuals (McKeary & Newbold, 2010). Further, the individual nature of Western therapy (e.g., one-on-one counseling) may seem strange to people from collectivistic cultures in which the focus is on the well-being of the group instead of the individual (Leong & Kalibatseva, 2011).

Service providers' lack of patience with refugee clients' cultural differences or simply a lack of cultural understanding is another significant challenge (Mirza & Heinemann, 2012). In order to provide proper care, clinicians must understand the impact of culture on the conceptualization of mental health, symptom manifestation, and attitudes toward mental health difficulties, as well as the etiology for the illness from the cultural perspective and corresponding mechanisms for healing based on culture (Kleinman, 1977). When not taken into account, these factors can lead to the selection of improper interventions, over- and under-pathologizing, and a gap in the clients' ability to understand how to access and utilize their care (Lowman, 2013).

ECONOMIC ISSUES

As with the non-refugee population in the United States, issues of insurance coverage and expensive co-pays and prescriptions constitute significant issues within access to care for refugees' mental health and physical health (Morris et al., 2009). For the first eight months after resettlement, refugees are covered by a temporary Refugee Medical Assistance that allows them access to Medicaid (Office of Refugee Resettlement, 2015). After eight months, some refugees are eligible for Medicaid; if not, they must find their own insurance through the marketplace (Office of Refugee Resettlement, 2015). Relatedly, transportation, scheduling, and childcare are important considerations for refugees (and non-refugees) attempting to access mental health care (Morris et al., 2009).

STRUCTURAL ISSUES

One significant structural issue regarding refugee mental health is awareness of how to access services and what services are provided. According to Mirza and Heinemann (2012), while discussing refugee physical and mental health, there was a lack of understanding among refugees of the health care system, the resources available, and how to access them. Additionally, they reported that due to the high caseload and pressure for time, many service providers were unable to provide appropriate, full-ranging services and also to connect refugees to other necessary intervention services (Mirza & Heinemann, 2012).

Eliminating Disparities among Refugees

COORDINATION OF CARE AND COMMUNITY INTERVENTION

Of paramount importance in refugee health care is increasing access to and engagement with mental health care. Bosson and colleagues (2017) outlined an integrative, holistic approach used at their global health clinic at the University of Louisville that aimed to solve issues related to refugees' acceptance of mental health services by integrating physical and mental health in the primary care setting. Their strategy was to provide both family and individual therapy, facilitate support groups, provide referrals to agencies that help create a social support network, and offer clinical care from a multidisciplinary team (e.g., nurse practitioners, physicians, social workers, psychologists, cultural health care experts). This integrative, multidisciplinary approach may diminish some of the issues regarding stigma and social acceptableness of involvement in psychotherapy and can facilitate a more holistic, person-centered method.

Another promising approach is community-based interventions. One example of a community-based intervention comes from Goodkind and colleagues' (2013) "learning circles." This intervention allowed refugees to discuss important cultural, political, and resettlement-related topics (Goodkind et al., 2013) along with one-on-one learning with undergraduate mentors. It also consisted of advocacy, in which students helped to increase the refugees' ability to self-advocate in the future (Goodkind et al., 2013). After the intervention, the authors noted high acceptability of the intervention, less psychopathology, and increases in language capacity and quality of life.

Another community-based effort, Project SHIFA (Supporting the Health of Immigrant Families and Adolescents), is an intervention originally designed for Somali middle school children in Boston that also provides a broad range of services (Ellis et al., 2011). Project SHIFA is a refugee adaptation of trauma systems therapy (TST-R) and includes four tiers of services: community outreach, school-based acculturation groups, individual outpatient therapy, and home-based therapy. Clinicians are paired with a cultural broker who has knowledge of the Somali culture, language, and resettlement community. The school's teachers and staff received school-wide trainings and individual consultation, as needed, in relation to topics relevant to the experience of the Somali refugee community (e.g., trauma, culture, refugee process, acculturation). Project SHIFA addressed issues contributing to disparities in care, such as mistrust of authorities, by basing services in a trusted location (e.g., school) and stigma by providing preventative and psychosocial groups (e.g., children who are struggling are not singled out for services), which also allowed families to get to know and begin to trust providers. Preliminary findings support high acceptability of Project SHIFA to a refugee group that is often difficult to engage in services (Ellis et al., 2011). Further outcome data demonstrated a 100 percent acceptance rate of referrals and reduced PTSD and depression symptoms (Ellis et al., 2013).

Relatedly, Shannon, Vinson, Cook, and Lennon (2015) described strategies that contribute to refugees accepting referrals to mental health care. They reported that an alliance with the refugee, cultural competence in care, and helping to coordinate the care (e.g., location, transportation, interpreters) were all factors that made it more likely that a refugee would accept a mental health referral (Shannon et al., 2015). Thus, offering services that are community-based, multidisciplinary, and coordinated may be among the most helpful ways to increase the likelihood that refugees will access effective care.

THERAPY TECHNIQUES AND OUTCOMES

While results are mixed as to the efficacy of mental health treatment for adult and child refugees, researchers have noted that although a small number of studies have reported significant changes in mental health outcomes due to treatment, many studies find no change in mental health symptoms over time (Carlsson, Mortensen, & Kastrup, 2005; Sullivan & Simonson, 2016). A main issue in tracking treatment outcomes for refugees is that most studies lack scientific rigor, including lack of blindness to condition, insufficient sample sizes, and lack of effect size reporting (Nickerson, Bryant, Silove, & Steele, 2011).

Importantly, a review of the literature by Murray and colleagues (2010) demonstrated that some types of treatment have shown efficacy in addressing the mental health difficulties of refugees resettled in Western countries. Cognitive behavioral therapy (CBT) has been demonstrated as a highly effective form of care to help with symptoms of PTSD, depression, and anxiety in adults and depression in children (Fox, Rossetti, Burns, & Popovich, 2005; Hinton et al. 2005; Murray et al., 2010). Somewhat to highly effective (based on moderate to large effect sizes) treatments include family therapy (Weine et al., 2003) and community-based interventions (Goodkind, 2005; Murray et al., 2010).

One feature that has been cited as an important aspect of treatment is cultural adaptation based on cultural needs (Murray et al., 2010). Bernal, Jiménez-Chafey, and Domenech Rodríguez (2009) define "cultural adaptation" as "the systematic modification of an evidence-based treatment (EBT) or intervention protocol to consider language, culture, and context in such a way that it is compatible with the client's cultural patterns, meanings, and values" (p. 362). Griner and Smith (2006) found that clinical programs that adapted for one culture were more effective than those that encompassed many cultures, which were more effective than non-adapted treatments; clinical work is most effective when using culture-specific adaptations. Additionally, language matching of clients and clinicians evidenced twice the effectiveness rates as in studies that did not match by language (Griner & Smith, 2006). Hall, Ibaraki, Huang, Marti, and Stice (2016) found that culturally adapted interventions were more effective than non-adapted interventions and that "culturally adapted interventions had 4.68 times greater odds than other conditions to produce remission from psychopathology" (p. 999).

However, there are issues present when adapting a treatment, including understanding the amount of adaptation necessary, how adaptation is useful in different clinical disorders, and the resources needed for adaptation (Bernal et al., 2009). Therefore, although cultural adaptation is an important venture to improving mental health services and outcomes for refugee populations, there are many challenges to face to understand the most effective way to carry it out.

To date, scholars have theorized and provided exploratory research regarding treatment outcomes with several modes of therapy. For example, Hinton, Ojserkis, Jalal, Peou, and Hofmann (2013) theorize that mindfulness techniques, such as loving-kindness meditations, would be extremely useful to refugee adults due to the ability of these techniques to enhance emotional and psychological flexibility, aid in emotion regulation, and decrease rumination (Hinton et al., 2013). Additionally, self-efficacy, or the belief that one can achieve what they would like to despite existing challenges, has been linked to lower psychological distress and greater well-being among Afghan adult refugees (Sulaiman-Hill & Thompson, 2013). Currently, no studies have been aimed at attempting to increase self-efficacy. Sulaiman-Hill and Thompson (2013) suggest that using positive refugee role models who have successfully acculturated could be a fruitful way to increase self-efficacy in this group and potentially decrease symptomology.

Other suggested types of interventions that are in need of empirical support for refugee groups are psycho-education, psychosocial counseling, suicide prevention and intervention, classroom-based intervention, women's empowerment groups, capacity development (Reiffers et al., 2013), group-based family interventions, testimonial therapy, stress inoculation training programs, and community-based comprehensive services programs (Murray et al., 2010).

COLLABORATION WITH SPIRITUAL HEALERS

Another important aspect of culturally responsive mental health care is collaboration with spiritual or traditional healers, when indicated. This may allow for a non-stigmatized and culturally acceptable form of alleviation of mental health difficulties. Therapists willing to work with spiritual healers may find that their clients are more willing to engage in psychotherapy and that the therapeutic alliance may be strengthened (Pouchly, 2012).

Conclusion

Refugees represent a group of individuals who have experienced a disproportionate amount of difficult experiences, trauma, and anguish and, therefore, are at a heightened risk for experiencing symptoms of psychological disorders. Refugees often lack access to appropriate care, experience a low quality of care, and have poor mental health outcomes due to a whole host of clinician-related, cultural, economic, and structural factors. The scant literature available demonstrates that there are certain strategies that can at least partially improve refugee mental health outcomes, such as collaboration with spiritual leaders, coordination of care, and community intervention. In sum, future studies are vital in order to determine the best type of care for refugees, who experience mental health difficulties at a high rate due to traumatic experiences and significant stressors. Research must determine the cultural factors that affect treatment and the best methods to combat them in order to facilitate better mental health outcomes in this population. Ensuring that refugees are able to readily access and engage with culturally and linguistically responsive effective mental health care is critical for the mental health community and for the larger US society. By doing so, the conditions are created under which vulnerable individuals will be able to overcome psychological distress and acculturative and resettlement stressors. At the same time, they will have the capacity to achieve their potentials as vital assets to the US society. Enabling refugees to thrive will not only enhance the lives of these individuals but also contribute to our success as a nation and our capacity to respect human dignity.

Table 1. Disparities in care, reasons for disparity, and strategies for achieving health equality.

Disparity in Care	Reasons for Disparity	Strategies for Achieving Health Equality
Access to care	• Lack of knowledge of services • Stigma of mental illness • Lack of or insufficient health insurance • Lack of finances • Transportation difficulties	• Provision of psychoeducation and preventative care for refugees • Collaboration of care • Provision of referrals (with personal handoffs when possible) • Provision of care in one location • Involvement of family and community in care (e.g., support groups) • Alliance building with refugees
Quality of care	• Lack of professionally trained interpreters • Lack of provider training in working with interpreters • Low levels of cultural competence and humility in service provision	• Cultural humility training for providers • Education for providers in cultural and linguistic responsiveness • Availability of bilingual therapists and interpreters, cultural brokers • Discourage use of community or family members as interpreters, especially children
Outcomes	• Increased prevalence rates of mental illness • Limited knowledge of outcomes due to methodology issues (e.g., language barriers, lack of streamlined assessment, etc.) in research studies with refugee groups	• Availability of culturally adapted treatments • Availability of culturally and linguistically responsive providers • Attend to scientific rigor in treatment outcome studies

KEY POINTS FOR CLINICIANS

- Refugees are those who are forced to leave their country of origin due to persecution based on race, religion, nationality, political views, or other group membership and who legally remain outside their home country as they are unable to be protected from the persecution feared.

- Refugees are often exposed to multiple potentially traumatic events prior to migration, in transit, and during the acculturation process to the host nation.

- Refugees, both children and adults, experience high rates of psychopathology, including depression, anxiety, and PTSD.

- Despite high rates of psychopathology, refugees underutilize mental health services for a multitude of reasons, including issues related to access, cultural barriers, structural challenges, and an overall paucity of linguistically and culturally responsive interventions.

- Several proposed solutions to enable refugees in receiving proper care are (1) coordination of care, (2) community-based interventions, (3) collaboration with spiritual healers, and (4) knowledge of therapeutic techniques that have been shown to be useful for refugees.

- Providing affordable, accessible, and effective linguistically and culturally responsive mental health care for refugees will aid them on their journey to achieve their potentials as new, contributing members of the US society.

References

Agrawal, P., & Venkatesh, A. K. (2016). Refugee resettlement patterns and state-level health care insurance access in the US. *American Journal of Public Health*, 106(4), 662–663.

Alexander, J. C., Everman, R., Giesen, B., Smelser, N. J., & Sztompka, P. (2004). *Collective trauma and collective identity*. Berkeley: University of California Press.

Ao, T., Shetty, S., Sivilli, T., Blanton, C., Ellis, H., Geltman, P. L., … & Cardozo, B. L. (2016). Suicidal ideation and mental health of Bhutanese refugees in the United States. *Journal of Immigrant and Minority Health*, 18(4), 828–835.

Bernal, G., Jiménez-Chafey, M. I., & Domenech Rodríguez, M. M. (2009). Cultural adaptation of treatments: A resource for considering culture in evidence-based practice. *Professional Psychology: Research and Practice*, 40(4), 361.

Berthold, S. M., Kong, S., Mollica, R. F., Kuoch, T., Scully, M., & Franke, T. (2014). Comorbid mental and physical health and health access in Cambodian refugees in the US *Journal of Community Health*, 39(6), 1045–1052.

Berthold, S. M. (2000). War traumas and community violence. *Journal of Multicultural Social Work*, 8:1–2, 15–46, doi:10.1300/J285v08n01_02

Betancourt, T. S., Newnham, E. A., Layne, C. M., Kim, S., Steinberg, A. M., Ellis, H., & Birman, D. (2012). Trauma history and psychopathology in war-affected refugee children referred for trauma-related mental health services in the United States. *Journal of Traumatic Stress*, *25*(6), 682–690.

Birman, D., & Tran, N. (2008). Psychological distress and adjustment of Vietnamese refugees in the United States: Association with pre- and postmigration factors. *American Journal of Orthopsychiatry*, *78*(1), 109.

Blair, R. G. (2000). Risk factors associated with PTSD and major depression among Cambodian refugees in Utah. *Health & Social Work*, *25*(1), 23–30.

Bosson, R., Williams, M. T., Lippman, S., Carrico, R., Kanter, J., …& Ramirez, J. (2017). Addressing refugee mental health needs: From concept to implementation. *The Behavior Therapist*, *40*(3), 110–112.

Capps, R., Newland, K., Fratzke, S., Groves, S., Fix, M. McHugh, M., & Auclair, G. (2015). The integration outcomes of US refugee: Successes and challenges. *Migration Policy Institute*. Retrieved from https://www.migrationpolicy.org/research/integration-outcomes-us-refugees-successes-and-challenges

Carlsson, J. M., Mortensen, E. L., & Kastrup, M. (2005). A follow-up study of mental health and health-related quality of life in tortured refugees in multidisciplinary treatment. *The Journal of Nervous and Mental Disease*, *193*(10), 651–657.

Center for Behavioral Health Statistics and Quality. (2016). *Key substance use and mental health indicators in the United States: Results from the 2015 National Survey on Drug Use and Health* (HHS Publication No. SMA 16-4984, NSDUH Series H-51). Retrieved from http://www.samhsa.gov/data/

Davidson, G. R., Murray, K. E., & Schweitzer, R. (2008). Review of refugee mental health and well-being: Australian perspectives. *Australian Psychologist*, *43*(3), 160–174.

de Anstiss, H., Ziaian, T., Procter, N., Warland, J., & Baghurst, P. (2009). Help-seeking for mental health problems in young refugees: A review of the literature with implications for policy, practice, and research. *Transcultural psychiatry*, *46*(4), 584–607.

Ellis, B. H., MacDonald, H. Z., Klunk-Gillis, J., Lincoln, A., Strunin, L., & Cabral, H. J. (2010). Discrimination and mental health among Somali refugee adolescents: The role of acculturation and gender. *American Journal of Orthopsychiatry*, *80*(4), 564.

Ellis, B. H., Miller, A. B., Abdi, S., Barrett, C., Blood, E. A., & Betancourt, T. S. (2013). Multi-tier mental health program for refugee youth. *Journal of Consulting and Clinical Psychology*, *81*(1), 129–140.

Ellis, B. H., Miller, A. B., Baldwin, H., & Abdi, S. (2011). New directions in refugee youth mental health services: Overcoming barriers to engagement. *Journal of Child & Adolescent Trauma*, *4*(1), 69–85.

Epatko, L. (2017). You asked: How are refugees vetted? *PBS News Hour*. Retrieved from https://www.pbs.org/newshour/world/asked-refugees-vetted-today

Fazel, M., Reed, R. V., Panter-Brick, C., & Stein, A. (2012). Mental health of displaced and refugee children resettled in high-income countries: Risk and protective factors. *The Lancet*, *379*(9812), 266–282.

Fox, P. G., Rossetti, J., Burns, K. R., & Popovich, J. (2005). Southeast Asian refugee children: A school-based mental health intervention. *The International Journal of Psychiatric Nursing Research*, *11*(1), 1227–1236.

Geltman, P. L., Grant-Knight, W., Mehta, S. D., Lloyd-Travaglini, C., Lustig, S., Landgraf, J. M., & Wise, P. H. (2005). The "lost boys of Sudan": Functional and behavioral health of unaccompanied refugee minors resettled in the United States. *Archives of Pediatrics & Adolescent Medicine*, *159*(6), 585–591.

Goodkind, J. R. (2005). Effectiveness of a community-based advocacy and learning program for Hmong refugees. *American Journal of Community Psychology*, *36*(3–4), 387–408.

Goodkind, J. R., Hess, J. M., Isakson, B., LaNoue, M., Githinji, A., Roche, N., ... & Parker, D. P. (2013). Reducing refugee mental health disparities: A community-based intervention to address postmigration stressors with African adults. *Psychological Services*, *11*(3), 333.

Griner, D., & Smith, T. B. (2006). Culturally adapted mental health intervention: A meta-analytic review. *Psychotherapy*, *43*(4), 531–548.

Guregård, S., & Seikkula, J. (2014). Establishing therapeutic dialogue with refugee families. *Contemporary Family Therapy*, *36*(1), 41–57.

Hall, G. C. N., Ibaraki, A. Y., Huang, E. R., Marti, C. N., & Stice, E. (2016). A meta-analysis of cultural adaptations of psychological interventions. *Behavior Therapy*, *47*(6), 993–1014.

Herman, J. L. (1992). *Trauma and recovery*. New York, NY: BasicBooks.

Hinton, D. E., Chhean, D., Pich, V., Safren, S. A., Hofmann, S. G., & Pollack, M. H. (2005). A randomized controlled trial of cognitive-behavior therapy for Cambodian refugees with treatment-resistant PTSD and panic attacks: A cross-over design. *Journal of Traumatic Stress*, *18*(6), 617–629.

Hinton, D. E., Ojserkis, R. A., Jalal, B., Peou, S., & Hofmann, S. G. (2013). Loving-kindness in the treatment of traumatized refugees and minority groups: A typology of mindfulness and the nodal network model of affect and affect regulation. *Journal of Clinical Psychology*, *69*(8), 817–828.

Hollifield, M., Warner, T. D., Lian, N., Krakow, B., Jenkins, J. H., Kesler, J., ... & Westermeyer, J. (2002). Measuring trauma and health status in refugees: a critical review. *JAMA*, *288*(5), 611–621.

International Organization of Migration (2010). *Migration Activities*. Retrieved from https://www.iom .int/countries/united-states-america#rtl

Kim, I. (2016). Beyond trauma: Post-resettlement factors and mental health outcomes among Latino and Asian refugees in the US. *Journal of Immigrant and Minority Health*, *18*(4), 740–748.

Kira, I. A. (2010). Etiology and treatment of post-cumulative traumatic stress disorders in different cultures. *Traumatology*, *16*(4), 128.

Kleinman, A. M. (1977). Depression, somatization and the "new cross-cultural psychiatry." *Social Science and Medicine*, *11*(1), 3–10.

Leong, F. T., & Kalibatseva, Z. (2011). Cross-cultural barriers to mental health services in the US. In *Cerebrum: The Dana Forum on Brain Science* (Vol. 2011). New York: Dana Foundation.

Lowman, M. E. (2013). Mental health screening and barriers to care of refugees in the Triangle Area of North Carolina: A community survey & program intervention approach. University of North Carolina at Chapel Hill. Retrieved from http://globalmigration.web.unc.edu/files/2013/09 /Refugee-Mental-Health-Screenings-and-Intervention.pdf

Lustig, S. L., Kia-Keating, M., Knight, W. G., Geltman, P., Ellis, H., Kinzie, J. D., ... & Saxe, G. N. (2004). Review of child and adolescent refugee mental health. *Journal of the American Academy of Child & Adolescent Psychiatry*, *43*(1), 24–36.

Marshall, G. N., Schell, T. L., Elliott, M. N., Berthold, S. M., & Chun, C. A. (2005). Mental health of Cambodian refugees 2 decades after resettlement in the United States. *JAMA*, *294*(5), 571–579.

McKeary, M., & Newbold, B. (2010). Barriers to care: The challenges for Canadian refugees and their health care providers. *Journal of Refugee Studies*, *23*(4), 523–545.

Merikangas, K. R., He, J., Burstein, M., Swanson, S. A., Avenevoli, S., Cui, L. ... & Swendsen, J. (2010). Lifetime prevalence of mental disorders in US adolescents: Results from the National Comorbidity Survey Replication–Adolescent Supplement (NCS-A). *Journal of the American Academy of Child & Adolescent Psychiatry*, *49*(10), 980–989. http://doi.org/10.1016/j.jaac.2010.05.017

Miller, K. E., & Rasmussen, A. (2010). War exposure, daily stressors, and mental health in conflict and post-conflict settings: Bridging the divide between trauma-focused and psychosocial frameworks. *Social Science & Medicine*, *70*(1), 7–16.

Mirza, M., & Heinemann, A. W. (2012). Service needs and service gaps among refugees with disabilities resettled in the US. *Disability and Rehabilitation*, *34*(7), 542–552.

Morris, M. D., Popper, S. T., Rodwell, T. C., Brodine, S. K., & Brouwer, K. C. (2009). Healthcare barriers of refugees post-resettlement. *Journal of Community Health, 34*(6), 529.

Murray, K. E., Davidson, G. R., & Schweitzer, R. D. (2010). Review of refugee mental health interventions following resettlement: Best practices and recommendations. *American Journal of Orthopsychiatry, 80*(4), 576–585.

Nguyen, T., & Davis, K. (2016). *The State of Mental Health in America 2017.* Retrieved from http://www .mentalhealthamerica.net/issues/state-mental-health-america

Nickerson, A., Bryant, R. A., Silove, D., & Steel, Z. (2011). A critical review of psychological treatments of posttraumatic stress disorder in refugees. *Clinical Psychology Review, 31*(3), 399–417.

Office of Refugee Resettlement. (2015). *Health Insurance.* Retrieved from https://www.acf.hhs.gov/orr /health

Ovitt, N., Larrison, C. R., & Nackerud, L. (2003). Refugees' responses to mental health screening: A resettlement initiative. *International Social Work, 46*(2), 235–250.

Piwowarczyk, L., Bishop, H., Yusuf, A., Mudymba, F., & Raj, A. (2014). Congolese and Somali beliefs about mental health services. *The Journal of Nervous and Mental Disease, 202*(3), 209–216.

Porter, M., & Haslam, N. (2005). Predisplacement and postdisplacement factors associated with mental health of refugees and internally displaced persons: A meta-analysis. *Journal of the American Medical Association, 294*(5), 602–612.

Pouchly, C. A. (2012). A narrative review: Arguments for a collaborative approach in mental health between traditional healers and clinicians regarding spiritual beliefs. *Mental Health, Religion & Culture, 15*(1), 65–85.

Reiffers, R., Dahal, R. P., Koirala, S., Gerritzen, R., Upadhaya, N., Luitel, N. P., … & Jordans, M. J. (2013). Psychosocial support for Bhutanese refugees in Nepal. *Intervention, 11*(2), 169–179.

Rothe, E. M., Lewis, J., Castillo-Matos, H., Martinez, O., Busquets, R., & Martinez, I. (2002). Posttraumatic stress disorder among Cuban children and adolescents after release from a refugee camp. *Psychiatric Services, 53*(8), 970–976.

Shannon, P., Im, H., Becher, E., Simmelink, J., Wieling, E., & O'Fallon, A. (2012). Screening for war trauma, torture, and mental health symptoms among newly arrived refugees: A national survey of US refugee health coordinators. *Journal of Immigrant & Refugee Studies, 10*(4), 380–394. doi:10.10 80/15562948.2012.674324.

Shannon, P. J., Vinson, G. A., Cook, T. L., & Lennon, E. (2015). Characteristics of successful and unsuccessful mental health referrals of refugees. *Administration and Policy in Mental Health and Mental Health Services Research, 43*(4), 555–568.

Steel, Z., Chey, T., Silove, D., Marnane, C., Bryant, R. A., & Van Ommeren, M. (2009). Association of torture and other potentially traumatic events with mental health outcomes among populations exposed to mass conflict and displacement: A systematic review and meta-analysis. *JAMA, 302*(5), 537–549.

Sulaiman-Hill, C. M., & Thompson, S. C. (2013). Learning to fit in: An exploratory study of general perceived self-efficacy in selected refugee groups. *Journal of Immigrant and Minority Health, 15*(1), 125–131.

Sullivan, A. L., & Simonson, G. R. (2016). A systematic review of school-based social-emotional interventions for refugee and war-traumatized youth. *Review of Educational Research, 86*(2), 503–530.

Taylor, E. M., Yanni, E. A., Pezzi, C., Guterbock, M., Rothney, E., Harton, E., … & Burke, H. (2014). Physical and mental health status of Iraqi refugees resettled in the US. *Journal of Immigrant and Minority Health, 16*(6), 1130–1137.

United Nations General Assembly. (1951). *Convention relating to the status of refugees.* United Nations Treaty Series, 189.

United Nations High Commissioner for Refugees. (2017). *Figures at a glance.* Retrieved from http:// www.unhcr.org/en-us/figures-at-a-glance.html

United Nations High Commissioner for Refugees. (2013). *Frequently asked questions about resettlement.* Retrieved from https://www.unhcr.org/en-us/protection/resettlement/524c31666/frequently-asked -questions-resettlement.html?query=resettlement%20process

United Nations High Commissioner for Refugees (2011a). *Handbook and guidelines on procedures and criteria for determining refugee status under the 1951 convention and the 1967 protocol relating to the status of refugees.* Retrieved from http://www.unhcr.org/en-us/publications/legal/3d58e13b4/hand book-procedures-criteria-determining-refugee-status-under-1951-convention.html.

United Nations High Commissioner for Refugees (2011b). *UNHCR resettlement handbook.* Retrieved from http://www.unhcr.org/46f7c0ee2.pdf

United Nations High Commissioner for Refugees. (2007). *2006 global trends: Refugees, asylum-seekers, returnees, internally displaced and stateless persons.* Retrieved from http://www.unhcr.org/4676a71d4 .html

United States Department of State. *US refugee admissions program.* Retrieved October 28, 2017, https:// www.state.gov/j/prm/ra/admissions/

Van Ommeren, M., Sharma, B., Sharma, G. K., Komproe, I., Cardeña, E., & de Jong, J. T. (2002). The relationship between somatic and PTSD symptoms among Bhutanese refugee torture survivors: examination of comorbidity with anxiety and depression. *Journal of Traumatic Stress, 15*(5), 415–421.

Vonnahme, L. A., Lankau, E. W., Ao, T., Shetty, S., & Cardozo, B. L. (2015). Factors associated with symptoms of depression among Bhutanese refugees in the United States. *Journal of Immigrant and Minority Health, 17*(6), 1705–1714.

Weine, S. M., Raina, D., Zhubi, M., Delesi, M., Huseni, D., Feetham, S., ... & Pavkovic, I. (2003). The TAFES multi-family group intervention for Kosovar refugees: A feasibility study. *The Journal of Nervous and Mental Disease, 191*(2), 100–107.

Williams, K. (2017). The uncertainty of health-care reform and the Affordable Care Act. *Government Finance Review,* 51–54.

Wong, E. C., Marshall, G. N., Schell, T. L., Berthold, S. M., & Hambarsoomians, K. (2015). Characterizing the mental health care of US Cambodian refugees. *Psychiatric Services, 66*(9), 980–984.

About Authors

Editor **Monnica T. Williams, PhD, ABPP**, is a board-certified clinical psychologist and associate professor at the University of Ottawa in the school of psychology, where she holds the Canadian Research Chair for Mental Health Disparities. She received her master's and doctoral degrees from the University of Virginia, where she conducted research in the areas of major mental illness, tests and measurement, and ethnic differences. She has started clinics in Virginia, Pennsylvania, and Connecticut, and a refugee mental health clinic in Kentucky. Her clinical work and research focus on African American mental health, culture, trauma, and obsessive-compulsive disorder (OCD).

Williams serves on the scientific advisory board of the International OCD Foundation, where she cofounded their diversity council. She is on the editorial board of several scientific journals, and is currently associate editor of *the Behavior Therapist* and *New Ideas in Psychology*. Williams has published over one hundred peer-reviewed articles and book chapters focused on psychopathology and cultural differences. She gives diversity trainings nationally. Her work has been featured in several major media outlets, including NPR, CNN, and *The New York Times*.

Editor **Daniel C. Rosen, PhD**, is chair and professor in the department of counseling and health psychology at Bastyr University, and director of the Daniel K. Church Center for Social Justice and Diversity. He earned a PhD in counseling psychology from Arizona State University after completing his predoctoral internship at the Center for Multicultural Training in Psychology at Boston Medical Center/Boston University School of Medicine. He completed his postdoctoral fellowship in the behavioral medicine program at Cambridge Health Alliance/Harvard Medical School. Rosen's scholarship is focused in multicultural psychology, and has explored issues of social justice in mental health, addressing disparities in access to and quality of mental health services; and anti-Semitism-related stress. He has a private practice in Seattle, WA.

Editor **Jonathan W. Kanter, PhD**, received his doctorate in clinical psychology from the University of Washington in 2002, and then moved to the University of Wisconsin-Milwaukee where he spent several years collaborating closely with members of the Black, Latinx, and Muslim communities on issues of social and political activism (including police brutality and voter rights), racism and discrimination, and culturally appropriate treatments of depression. In 2013, Kanter came to the University of Washington to direct the Center for the Science of Social Connection (CSSC), where he approaches projects with a contextual behavioral science (CBS) model that integrates disciplines—including evolution science, neuroscience, anthropology, and psychology—within a behavioral science foundation. Kanter is regularly invited to give talks and workshops nationally and internationally on topics of interest to the Center, including anti-racism workshops, workshops for therapists on how to improve psychotherapy relationships and help clients with relational problems, and culturally tailored behavioral treatments for depression.

Foreword writer **Patricia Arredondo, EdD, NCC,** has published extensively on cultural competency models and guidelines, Latinx mental health, women's leadership, and organizational change through diversity. She is a scholar-practitioner and a multicultural competency and social justice advocate. Arredondo is a licensed psychologist and has been a full professor and senior administrator at research universities and president of a professional school of psychology. She is a fellow of the American Counseling Association (ACA) and the American Psychological Association (APA). She was named a Living Legend by the ACA, and Changemaker: Top 25 Women of Color Psychologists by the APA.

Index

A

about this book, ix–xii, 2–4
academic advisors, 251–252
acceptability of treatment, 31, 32
acceptance, practice of, 154
acceptance and commitment therapy (ACT), 148; defusion and acceptance in, 153; model of psychological flexibility, 102, 119; prejudice targeted through, 163; present moment awareness in, 150
access to care, 10–11, 31, 32; for military veterans, 308–309; outpatient psychotherapy, 278–279; for people of color, 27, 61, 279; for refugees, 332–333, 339; strategies for increasing, 297–299; university counseling center, 293–294
accountable care organizations (ACOs), 19
activation of patients. See patient activation
ADDRESSING framework, 171–172, 189
adopted children: family of origin considerations for, 207–208; transracial families and, 203, 207–208
Affordable Care Act (ACA), 12, 279, 333
African Americans: assessment and evaluation of, 35–36; cultural competence with, 34–38; distinction between Blacks and, 28; kinship in the culture of, 206; mental health of, 28–31, 138, 139; mistrust of mental health treatment among, 29–31, 50; Model of Treatment Initiation for, 31–34; outreach to communities of, 36–37; pathological stereotypes of, 134–135; patient activation with, 66; racism experienced by, 79, 135–136; raised by White parents, 203–220; VA services used by, 307, 308, 312. See also Blacks
alcohol use disorders, 87
Alegría, Margarita, 9, 61
Ali, Naomi, 61
Alvarez, Kiara, 9
American Indians and Alaska Natives (AI/ANs): mental health disparities for, 294; motivational interviewing with, 70–71; percentage below poverty level, 232; prevalence of mental health disorders in, 10; VA services used by, 307–308
American Muslims, 85
American Psychological Association (APA), 35, 227
Americans with Disabilities Act (1990), 292
anxiety, intergroup, 51, 100, 104, 115
appropriateness of treatment, 31, 32, 34
Arney, Erin N., 227
Arredondo, Patricia, ix
Asian Americans: microaggressions toward, 177; racism experienced by, 79, 85; reluctance to seek psychological help, 294; stigma interventions for, 298
assessment: ADDRESSING framework for, 171–172; African American evaluation and, 35–36; awareness and knowledge related to, 171–177; culturally responsive diagnosis and, 181–182; of impact of race-based discrimination, 178; measures of race-based discrimination, 178–179; multicultural counseling competencies for, 171; neuropsychological, 45–46; psychodiagnostic, 44–45; racial and ethnic disparities in, 44–46; RESPECTFUL interview model for, 172–173; role in therapy retention, 180–181; stereotype threat and, 179–180
attitudes, cultural, 131
availability of treatment, 31, 32
aversive racism, 101, 245
avoidance of internal experiences: clinical challenge of, 151–152; proposed CBS interventions for, 153–155. See also experiential avoidance
awareness: of attitudes and beliefs, 171–176; of power and privilege issues, 189–191; of the present moment, 150

B

barriers: to language understanding, 12, 14, 283; to outpatient psychotherapy treatment, 277–286; to receiving mental health treatment, 31–34; to treating military veterans, 309

Behavioral Model of Health Service Use, 31

behaviors, cultural, 131

biases: clinician, 15–16, 47–53, 54; explicit, 47–48; implicit, 48–53, 89, 103–104; key points and conclusions about, 54–55; microaggressions as form of, 245–246; in psychological assessment, 44–46; in treatment planning and service delivery, 46–47

Big White Wall website, 68

Biopsychosocial Model of Racism, 82

biracial couples, 203

Black Lives Matter, 215, 219

Blackburn, Allyson M., 307

Blacks: campus-life experiences of, 255; clinician biases with, 45, 47, 48, 49; college faculty percentage of, 249; distinction between African Americans and, 28; mental health access disparities for, 61, 294; percentage below poverty level, 232; police interactions with, 218–219; raised by White parents, 203–220; school dropout rates for, 212. See also African Americans

Branstetter, Heather M. L., 99

Breland-Noble, Alfiee M., 277

C

campus climate: departmental assessments of, 262–263; experienced by students of color, 229–231; psychologist's role in addressing, 265–267; suggestions for improving, 248–265

care-manager interventions, 67

Casados, Ava T., 43

CBS. See contextual behavioral science

chief diversity officers, 255

children: Black, raised by White parents, 203–220; family of origin for adopted, 207–208; psychological distress of refugee, 330; risk factors for refugee, 332

Ching, Terence H. W., 187

Chronic Care Model, 67

chronic-contextual stress, 81

Civil Rights Act (1964), ix

Clark, Kenneth and Mamie, 255

Clark, Rodney, 82

CLAS standards, 283, 284

clients: activation of, 64–67; engagement of, 67–71; patient-level factors for, 11–13; racism from, 193–194

clinical challenges: avoidance of internal experiences, 151–152; fusion with self-as-content, 155–156; objectification, 149–150; rigid and unexamined self-identity, 155–156; social distance and disconnection, 158–159

clinicians: awareness and knowledge of, 171–177; communication disparities among, 62; racial/ethnic biases of, 44, 45, 47–53, 54. See also mental health providers; psychologists

coaching, individualized, 66

cognitive behavioral therapy (CBT), 70, 284–285, 336

cognitive/affective assaults, 86

collective experiences, 81

collectivist societies, 108

colleges and universities: academic advisors at, 251–252; admission structures/criteria of, 232–233; campus climate issues of, 229–231, 248–265; counseling center disparities at, 291–301; disciplining racist acts at, 264–265; diversity training for faculty at, 256–258; environmental microaggressions at, 258–261; faculty diversity needed at, 249–250; financial constraints on attending, 232–233; forums for racial dialogue at, 255–256; graduation rates from, 292–293; mentorship options offered by, 235–237; minority outreach and communications by, 231–233; providing diversity courses at, 252–254; racism and discrimination at, 243–248; retaining racial minorities at, 233–237; role of psychologist in serving, 265–267; student course evaluations used at, 262; underrepresentation of SOC in, 227–228

color-blind racial ideology (CBRI), 230

color-blindness, 104–105; CBS view of, 105–106, 114; college campuses and, 230; conceptualized self and, 114; discussing in trainings, 132–133; problem with strategy of, 51–52, 177; supervisory relationship and, 192; White privilege related to, 107 communication: minority patients and differences in, 62; patient activation related to, 67; psychology program outreach and, 231–233

communities of support, 208–209

community outreach, 36–37

community-based interventions, 335–336

compassion, culturally responsive, 182

Comprehensive Addiction and Recovery Act, 19

conceptualized self, 108, 113–114, 155–156

Confederate monument story, 260–261

conflict theory, 216

connectedness, 163

contact techniques, 150

contact theory, 159

contextual behavioral science (CBS), 2, 111–117; color-blindness and, 105–106, 114; experiential avoidance and, 116–117; implicit bias and, 103–104; intergroup anxiety and, 115; microaggressions and, 110, 117; perceptual processes and, 114; racism interventions based on, 102, 111–112, 149–163; White privilege and, 108–109, 114

Corey, Mariah D., 99

Counseling the Culturally Diverse (Sue), 292

covert and subtle racism, 80

criminal justice system, 88

critical thinking skills, 182

cultural adaptation, 337

cultural attitudes and behaviors, 131

cultural competence: evidence-based strategies to enhance, 34–38; lack of training and tools for, 14–15; psychotherapy based on, 37–38; reducing provider bias through, 283; responsiveness and, 169–171; training approach for, 129–143

Cultural Formulation Interview (CFI), 36, 179

cultural genograms, 234

cultural humility, 143, 182, 297

cultural immersion activities, 234

cultural mistrust, 29–31

cultural racism: definition of, 80–81; mental health and, 89–90

cultural sensitivity, 34, 297

cultural stigma, 282–283

cultural symbols, 131

cultural taxation, 250

culture: defining elements of, 131; kinship in African American, 206; refugee issues related to, 334

D

daily racism microstressors, 81

defusing from difficult thoughts, 153

depression, 46, 62, 64, 87, 310

diagnosis: culturally responsive, 181–182; military veteran disparities in, 312; role in therapy retention, 180–181. See also assessment

Diagnostic and Statistical Manual of Mental Disorders (DSM-5), 36

disconnection. See social distance and disconnection

discrimination: assessing the impact of, 178; college climate marred by, 243–248; definition of, 80; implicit bias and unconscious, 89; measures of race-based, 178–179; psychological disorders and, 86

distress, psychological, 83, 84–85, 329–330

diversity: acknowledging many forms of, 187; college faculty training on, 256–258; of counseling center staff, 297; forums to discuss issues of, 255–256; hiring college faculty based on, 249–250; increasing student body, 267; integrating into course curriculums, 254–255; military service member, 307; providing college courses on, 252–254

diversity training, 101, 256–258

Douglas, Courtland, 27

Dovidio, John F., 43

drop-in consultations, 298

dropouts: school, 211–212; veteran treatment, 311–312

Du Bois, W. E. B., 106

E

eating disorders, 87

economic or socioeconomic status, 11–12. See also financial issues education: Black students in special, 211; clinician process of multicultural, 176–177; culturally competent training and, 14–15, 129–143. *See also* colleges and universities; school issues

eHealth technologies, 68

electroconvulsive shock therapy (ECT), 310

emic approach to counseling, 170

emotions, exploring, 154

engagement of patients. *See* patient engagement

environmental microaggressions, 258–261

Epidemiologic Catchment Area (ECA) Survey, 83

ethnicity: definition of, 131; discussing in therapy, 37, 52; identity based on, 133–134; matching for therapy, 33–34, 140, 294, 296. *See also* race

ethnoracial, use of term, 132

etic approach to counseling, 170

eugenics movement, 28–29

evaluation: of African Americans, 35–36; supervisor's power of, 189

evidence-based treatments (EBTs), 19, 181, 297, 317, 337

expectations of therapy, 32–33

experiential avoidance (EA), 100, 116–117, 152, 164. *See also* avoidance of internal experiences

experiential exercises, 141

explanatory models, 35–36

explicit bias, 47–48

eye contact, 114

F

faculty: hiring ethnically and racially diverse, 249–250; listening to racial complaints by, 263–264; mentoring students of color by, 235–236; providing diversity training for, 256–258; student course evaluations of, 262

Faith Based Mental Health Promotion (FBMHP), 283–284

families, transracial. *See* transracial families

female veterans, 313–314

financial issues: for refugee populations, 334–335; for students of color, 232–233

flexibility, 150

forums for racial dialogue, 255–256

foster families, 208

Fuentes, Larimar, 61

functional analytic psychotherapy (FAP), 129–130, 160

fusion with self-as-content: clinical challenge of, 155–156; proposed CBS intervention for, 156–158

G

gatekeeper training programs, 298–299

gender and sexual minorities, 314

General Ethnic Discrimination Scale (GEDS), 178

generalized anxiety disorder, 86

Goetter, Elizabeth M., 307

Golden Rule, new version of, 133

graduate psychology programs: admission structures/criteria for, 232–233; faculty of color in, 250; financial issues related to, 232; mentoring of students in, 235–237; outreach and communication by, 231–233; recruiting racial minorities into, 229–231; retaining racial minorities in, 233–237; underrepresentation of SOC in, 227–228

Graduate Record Exam (GRE) scores, 233

graduation rates from college, 292–293

Graham-LoPresti, Jessica R., 169

Grawemeyer, H. Charles, 258

group identity, 133, 170

H

Harb, Camelia, 277

Harrell, Camara Jules P., 79

Harrell, Shelly, 81

Hays, Pamela, 189

health, social determinants of, 18

health care systems, 17

Hispanics: census categorization of, 132; VA services used by, 307, 308, 312. *See also* Latinx

homeless veterans, 314–315

Housing First programs, 18

humility, cultural, 143, 182

I

identity: development of, 108, 113–114, 216–218; racial and ethnic, 35, 133–134; rigid and unexamined self-, 155–156; three levels of, 133; transracial families and, 216–218; tripartite model of, 170
impactful interactions, 234–235
Implicit Association Test (IAT), 48, 103, 136
implicit bias: Black students and, 210–211; CBS view of, 103–104; descriptions of, 48–50, 103; implications of, 50–53; negative stereotypes and, 89; quality of care related to, 280
incarceration: mental health impacts of, 88–89; military veterans subjected to, 315
individual identity, 133, 170
individual racism, 80, 82, 85
individualistic societies, 108
individualized coaching, 66
Individualized Education Program (IEP), 211
in-group favoritism, 108–109, 112–113
Institute of Medicine, 278
institutional and systemic factors, 16–17; health care systems, 17; insurance plans, 16
institutional racism: definition of, 80; higher education and, 244–245, 252; mental health and, 87–89; trainees of color and, 196–197
insurance coverage, 12, 16, 18–19
intake sessions, 63
interactions: of Blacks with police, 218–219; college faculty and peer, 234–235
intergroup anxiety (IGA), 51, 100, 104, 115
internalized racism, 81, 89, 90
International Organization for Migration (IOM), 328
Interpersonal Process Model (IPM), 159
interracial therapeutic dyad, 141
invalidation, 138, 195, 196

J

Jackson, Jessica, 277
Jim Crow laws, 135
Jones, Shawn C. T., 79

K

Kanter, Jonathan W., 1, 2, 99, 147, 243
King, Martin Luther, Jr., 104
kinship, African American, 206
knowledge, clinician, 176–177
Kuczynski, Adam M., 99
Kune, M. R. Natacha Foo, 291
Kwong, Agnes, 291

L

language barriers: CLAS standards addressing, 283; mental health disparities and, 12, 14; refugees and, 333–334, 337
Latinx: college faculty percentage of, 249; mental health access disparities for, 27, 61, 294; mistrust of mental health community by, 50; motivational interviewing with, 71; patient activation with, 66; racism experienced by, 79; VA services used by, 307, 308, 312
Lee, Sharon Y., 227
Let's Talk program, 298
life-events, racism-related, 81
linked lives hypothesis, 85
Loudon, Mary Plummer, 147

M

major depressive disorder, 87
Malone, Celeste M., 27
Manbeck, Katherine E., 99
Manichean Psychology: Racism and the Minds of People of African Descent (Harrell), 79
manualized treatments, 280
marginalized populations, 177
matching by race/ethnicity. *See* racial/ethnic matching
McIntosh, Peggy, 106
medical care for multicultural families, 209
meditation on discomfort with racism and privilege, 154–155
Menafee, Corey, 259
mental health: cultural racism and, 89–90; individual racism and, 80, 82, 85; institutional racism and, 87–89; social-historical racism and, 28–31; stigma related to, 13, 181, 282–283, 334

mental health disorders. *See* psychological disorders

mental health disparities: approaches to addressing, 17–19; definition of, 278; institutional and system factors in, 16–17; military service members and, 307; patient-level factors in, 11–13; provider-level factors in, 13–16; psychological assessment and, 44–46; refugees and, 332–333; statistics on, 9–11, 61; teaching students about, 138–140; in treatment planning and service delivery, 46–47; in university counseling centers, 291–301

mental health literacy, 284

mental health providers: bias and discrimination of, 15–16; lack of racial and ethnic, 14; training and tools lacking for, 14–15. *See also* clinicians

mental health services: access to and utilization of, 10–11; disparities and bias in delivery of, 46–47; quality issues related to, 11

mental health treatment: barriers to receiving, 31–34; disparities and bias in, 46–47; mistrust of, 13, 29–31, 50

mental illness: stigma related to, 13, 181, 282–283, 334. *See also* psychological disorders

mentorship: faculty, 235–236; peer, 236–237

microaggressions, 30–31, 109–110; bias engaged through, 245–246; CBS view of, 110, 117; clinician education about, 177; covert or subtle racism and, 80; descriptions of, 47, 101, 109; environmental, 258–261; student of color experience of, 255–256; teaching students about, 137–138; trainee of color experience of, 187

microstressors, daily racism, 81

military service members and veterans, 307–318; barriers to treatment for, 309; clinical practice considerations for, 316–317; current and future diversity of, 307; diagnostic disparities among, 312; engagement in treatment for, 310–312; future research directions on, 317; key points for clinicians about, 318; overview of

mental health disparities among, 307–308; special considerations for at-risk populations, 313–315; suicidality disparities among, 313; symptom severity disparities among, 313; treatment access for, 308–309

military sexual trauma (MST), 314

Miller, Alisa B., 327

mindfulness techniques, 150, 151, 337

minority development models, 174–175

mistrust of mental health treatment, 13, 29–31, 50

Model of Treatment Initiation (MTI), 31–34

motivational enhancement therapies (METs), 69

motivational interviewing (MI), 69–71

multicultural counseling competencies, 171. *See also* cultural competence

multicultural counseling competency (MCC) model, ix

Multicultural Guidelines of the APA, 35

multiculturalism, 133, 266

multiracial families. *See* transracial families

N

National Comorbidity Survey (NCS), 33, 83

National Health Service (NHS), 68

National Institutes of Health (NIH), 14

National Survey of American Life (NSAL), 34

nationalism, resurgence of, 100

nationality, definition of, 131

Native Americans. *See* American Indians and Alaska Natives

Neblett, Enrique W., Jr., 79

NeMoyer, Amanda, 9

neuropsychological assessment, 45–46

O

Obama, Barack, 85

objectification: clinical challenge of, 149–150; proposed CBS intervention for, 150–151

obsessive compulsive disorder, 87

Oshin, Linda A., 187

outcomes. *See* treatment outcomes

out-group rejection, 112–113

outpatient psychotherapy, 277–286; access to care with, 278–279; cultural stigma related to, 282–283; mental health disparities and, 278; quality of care with, 279–280; strategies for improving access to, 283–285; treatment outcomes with, 280–281; youth of color and, 281–282

outreach: college, 231–233, 298; community, 36–37

overt and blatant racism, 80

P

parents in transracial families, 203–220

pathological stereotypes, 134–135, 245

patient activation, 64–67; definition of, 64; models for improving, 65–67; racial/ethnic disparities in, 65; role of, 64–65

Patient Activation Measure (PAM), 65

patient adherence, 69

patient engagement, 67–71; approaches to improving, 67–71; military veterans and, 310–312; patient activation distinguished from, 64

Patient Health Engagement (PHE) model, 68

patient-centered medical homes, 67

patient-level factors, 11–13; insurance status, 12; language proficiency, 12; patient preferences, 13; socioeconomic status, 11–12; stigma or mistrust, 13

Patient-Provider Encounter Study, 63

peers: college student interactions with, 234–235; increasing activation through support of, 66; mentoring in colleges by, 236–237; racism experienced from, 194–195

people of color (POC): academic advisors as, 251–252; access to care for, 279; college faculty hirings of, 249–250; diagnostic disparities among, 312; impact of racism on mental health of, 79–91; listening to racial complaints by, 263–264; mental health disparities of, 278; outpatient treatment and, 281–282; quality of care for, 279–280; stigma of mental illness among, 13, 181, 282–283; students in college as, 227–237; supervising as trainees, 187–199. *See also specific ethnic and racial groups*

perceptual processes, 114

Personalized Patient Activation and Empowerment (P-PAE) model, 65–66

perspective taking, 157

police interactions, 218–219

Positive Behavior Intervention System (PBIS), 213

post-traumatic stress disorder (PTSD): military veterans with, 307, 309, 311, 312, 313; motivation enhancement for treating, 70; refugees with, 329–330, 331–332; studies of racism and, 86

power: awareness of supervisory, 189–191; description of privilege and, 175

prejudice: ACT interventions for, 163; clinician awareness of, 176; color-blindness and, 105; definition of, 80

present moment awareness, 150–151

primary care behavioral health (PCBH), 284

primary care mental health integration (PC-MHI), 284

Printz, Destiny M. B., 227

privilege: description of power and, 175; meditation on discomfort with, 154–155. *See also* White privilege

privilege walk, 106

progressive dyads, 199

Project SHIFA, 336

provider-level factors, 13–16; bias and discrimination, 15–16; lack of minority providers, 14; lack of training and tools, 14–15

psychiatric medications: disparities in prescribing of, 46; military veteran treatment with, 310–311

psychodiagnostic assessment, 44–45

psychological disorders: ethnic/racial prevalence of, 10; racism and, 85–87; stigma related to, 181, 282–283

psychological distress, 83, 84–85, 329–330

psychological well-being, 83–85

psychologists: ethnic/racial biases of, 44, 45, 47–53, 54; misuse of science by early, 28–29; racism on campuses addressed by, 265–267. *See also* clinicians

psychology programs. *See* graduate psychology programs

psychotherapy: barriers to outpatient, 277–286; culturally competent, 37–38
psychotic disorders, 87
PTSD. *See* post-traumatic stress disorder

Q

quality of care: approaches to improving, 19–20; outpatient psychotherapy and, 279–280; racial/ethnic disparities in, 11, 279–280, 294; refugee populations and, 333, 339

R

race: definition of, 132; discussing in therapy, 37, 52; explicitly teaching about, 209; identity based on, 133–134; matching for therapy, 33–34, 140, 294. *See also* ethnicity
race-based traumatic stress, 86, 138
Race-Based Traumatic Stress Symptom Scale (RBTSSS), 178
Racial and Ethnic Microaggressions Scale (REMS), 179
racial frame paradigm, 216
Racial Harmony Workshop, 130–143; color-blindness discussed in, 132–133; considerations on racism in, 135–137, 140–141; defining key concepts in, 131–132; experiential exercises used in, 141; introducing participants to, 130–131; mental health disparities discussed in, 138–140; microaggressions discussed in, 137–138; multiculturalism introduced in, 133; pathological stereotypes reviewed in, 134–135; practical implications of, 142; racial/ethnic identity discussed in, 133–134
Racial Microaggressions Scale (RMS), 179
racial socialization, 133
racial/ethnic concordance, 63
racial/ethnic matching: for supervising TOCs, 188; for therapy, 33–34, 140, 294, 296
racialized habits, 220
racism: assessing the impact of, 178; chart of historical, 247; college climate marred by, 243–248; color-blindness and, 105, 132–133; cultural, 80–81, 89–90; definitions of, 80, 137; disciplining acts of,

264–265; environmental, 258–261; experiential avoidance and, 116–117; forms and types of, 80–81; identity development and, 113–114; individual, 80, 82, 85; institutional, 80, 87–89, 196–197; intergroup anxiety and, 115; meditation on discomfort with, 154–155; mental health and, 28–31, 82–90, 138; microaggressions and, 109–110, 117, 137–138, 245–246; perceptual processes and, 114; pervasive context of, 112–113; psychological disorders and, 85–87; psychological distress/well-being and, 84–85; resurgence of explicit acts of, 100; sensitivity training to reduce, 257; social-historical context of, 28–31; stress related to, 81, 85, 86; supervision and, 192–197; teaching students about, 135–137, 140–141; vicarious, 81
racist-incident trauma, 86
reciprocity process, 159
refugees, 327–340; access to care for, 332–333, 339; collaboration with spiritual healers for, 338; community-based interventions for, 335–336; cultural issues for, 334; definition of, 327; economic issues for, 334–335; eliminating disparities among, 335–338, 339; key points for clinicians about, 340; language issues for, 333–334; psychological distress of, 329–330; quality of care for, 333, 339; resettlement process for, 328; risk factors for, 331–332; structural issues for, 335; therapy techniques and outcomes for, 336–337; trauma experienced by, 329, 331; U.S. acceptance of, 327–328
regressive dyads, 199
religious affiliation, 131
religious/spiritual beliefs, 34
residential segregation, 87–88
RESPECTFUL interview model, 172–173
responsiveness: cultural competency and, 169–171; diagnosis and cultural, 181–182
rigid and unexamined self-identity: clinical challenge of, 155; proposed CBS intervention for, 156–158
role expectations, 32–33
Rosen, Daniel C., 1, 99, 147, 169

S

same-race providers, 33–34

Schedule of Racist Event (SRE), 178

Schlaudt, Victoria A., 327

school issues: therapeutic suggestions for, 212–214; transracial families and, 209–212. *See also* colleges and universities; education

school-based mental health (SBMH), 284

segregation, residential, 87–88

self-as-content, 108, 113–114, 155–156

self-as-context, 156–158

self-efficacy, 337

self-focused orientation, 51

self-identity: rigid and unexamined, 155–156. *See also* identity

self-reflection, 174, 176

sensitivity training, 257

sexual and gender minorities, 314

Shuttleworth, Sylvie P., 227

Skinta, Matthew D., 147

social connection, 160–161

social determinants of health, 18

social distance and disconnection: clinical challenge of, 158–159; proposed CBS interventions for, 160–163

social effectiveness therapy (SET), 170

social-historical context of racism, 28–31

social identity theory, 100

social justice framework, 37–38

social psychopathology, 134

socioeconomic status (SES), 11–12

special education issues, 211

spiritual healers, 338

Steketee, Anne Blakely, 203

stereotypes: clinician awareness of, 176; internalized racism based on, 89, 90; neuropsychological assessment and, 46; pathological, 134–135, 245; threat related to, 90, 179–180

Stewart, Catherine E., 227

stigma considerations, 13, 181, 282–283, 298, 334

stress, racism-related, 81, 85, 86

structural racism, 81, 244–245

structured interviews, 35, 36

students of color (SOC): academic advisors for, 251–252; campus climate and recruitment of, 229–231; faculty mentoring of, 235–236; financial limitations of, 232–233; forums for racial dialogue with, 255–256; impactful interactions for, 234–235; increasing the number of, 267, 291–292; listening to racial complaints by, 263–264; outreach to and communication with, 231–233; peer mentorships for, 236–237; retaining in graduate psychology programs, 233–237; underrepresentation in graduate programs, 227–228

Substance Abuse and Mental Health Services Administration (SAMHSA), 27

substance use disorders, 87, 310

Sue, Derald Wing, 292

suicidal ideation and behavior, 87, 313

supervising trainees of color, 187–199; avoiding color-blind supervision in, 192; awareness of power and privilege in, 189–191; ethnoracial matching for, 188; increasing comfort and skills in, 191–192; overview of considerations for, 188; racism related to, 192–197

supervisors: evaluation power of, 189; racism from, 195–196

symbols, cultural, 131

systemic factors. *See* institutional and systemic factors

T

Taylor, Ellen B., 291

technological mechanisms, 68

termination of therapy, 295

textbooks, racial bias in, 254

therapeutic alliance: cultural competence and, 37; importance of creating, 163–164; patient engagement and, 69; positive outcomes and, 52

therapy retention, 180–181

thoughts: defusing from difficult, 153; tactic of suppressing, 152

trainees of color (TOC): microaggressions experienced by, 187; racism experienced by, 187, 192–197; supervision of, 187–199

training: culturally competent, 14–15, 129–143. *See also* education

transgender veterans, 314

transgenerational stress, 81

transracial families, 203–220; adulthood transition in, 218–219; community of support for, 208–209; explicit racial teaching for, 209; family of origin considerations for, 207–208; identity development in, 216–218; importance of communication in, 215–216; medical care issues and, 209; police interactions considered in, 218–219; school issues and, 209–214; social issues and, 214, 215

trauma: cultural, 331; racist-incident, 86, 138; refugee experience of, 329, 331

Trauma Symptoms and Discrimination Scale (TSDS), 179

trauma systems therapy (TST-R), 336

treatment outcomes: disparities in, 280–281, 295; expectations of, 32–33; refugee populations and, 339

tripartite model of identity, 170

Turner, Erlanger A., 27

Tuskegee Syphilis Study, 29, 180

U

underrepresented racial minority (URM) students: faculty and peer mentoring of, 235–237; outreach to and communication with, 231–232. See also students of color

unilateral termination, 295

United Nations High Commissioner for Refugees (UNHCR), 327, 328

universal identity, 133, 170

university counseling centers, 291–301; access to care disparities in, 293–294; causes of disparities in, 295–296; future directions for research on, 299–300; key points for clinicians about, 301; overview of care delivery in, 291–293; quality of care disparities in, 294; strategies for increasing access to care and engagement in, 297–299; treatment outcome disparities in, 295. See also colleges and universities

UnRESTS instrument, 179

V

validation, 162

veterans. See military service members and veterans

Veterans Affairs (VA) services, 307, 308, 312, 316–317

vicarious racism, 81

Villatte, Matthieu, 147

vulnerability, participating with, 163

W

well-being, psychological, 83–85

West, Lindsey M., 187

White fragility, 117, 152

White privilege, 106–109; CBS view of, 108–109, 114; description of, 106–108; racial identity and, 133

Williams, Monnica T., 1, 129, 169, 243

willingness, stance of, 154

women veterans, 313–314

workshop on cultural competence. See Racial Harmony Workshop

Y

Yale Child Center Study, 149

youth of color: outpatient treatment and, 281–282; raised by White parents, 203–220

MORE BOOKS *from*
NEW HARBINGER PUBLICATIONS

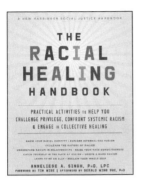
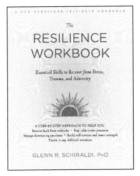
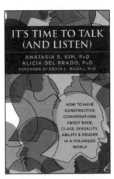
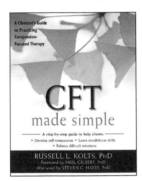
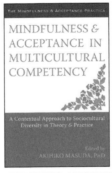
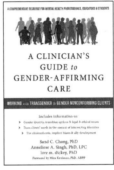

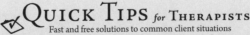

Register your **new harbinger** titles for additional benefits!

When you register your **new harbinger** title—purchased in any format, from any source—you get access to benefits like the following:

- Downloadable accessories like printable worksheets and extra content
- Instructional videos and audio files
- Information about updates, corrections, and new editions

Not every title has accessories, but we're adding new material all the time.

Access free accessories in 3 easy steps:

1. Sign in at NewHarbinger.com (or **register** to create an account).

2. Click on **register a book**. Search for your title and click the **register** button when it appears.

3. Click on the **book cover or title** to go to its details page. Click on **accessories** to view and access files.

That's all there is to it!

If you need help, visit:

NewHarbinger.com/accessories

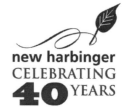

new harbinger
CELEBRATING
40 YEARS